Alterations of Excitation-Contraction Coupling in the Failing Human Heart

G. Hasenfuss · H. Just
Editors

Alterations of Excitation-Contraction Coupling in the Failing Human Heart

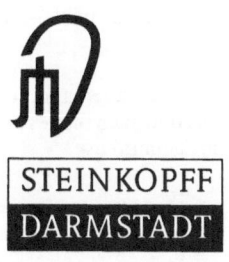

STEINKOPFF
DARMSTADT

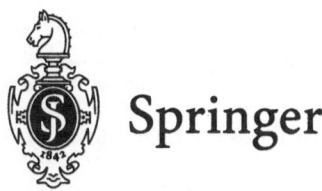

Editors' addresses:

Prof. Dr. G. Hasenfuss · Prof. Dr. H. Just
Universität Freiburg – Med. Klinik III
Abt. Kardiologie und Angiologie
Hugstetter Straße 55
79106 Freiburg

Die Deutsche Bibliothek – CIP-Einheitsaufnahme

Alterations of excitation contraction coupling in the failing human heart / G. Hasenfuss ; H. Just, ed. – Darmstadt : Steinkopff ; New York : Springer, 1998
ISBN-13: 978-3-642-48672-2   e-ISBN-13: 978-3-642-48670-8
DOI: 10.1007/978-3-642-48670-8

© 1998 by Dr. Dietrich Steinkopff Verlag GmbH & Co. KG, Darmstadt
Softcover reprint of the hardcover 1st edition 1998

Medical Editor: Beate Rühlemann – English Editor: James C. Willis – Production: Heinz J. Schäfer
Cover Design: Erich Kirchner, Heidelberg

Typesetting: Typoservice, Griesheim

Printed on acid-free paper

Preface and Introduction

Alteration of excitation-contraction coupling in the failing human heart was deemed an interesting subject for a dialogue between basic scientists and clinical researchers in continuation of previous Gargellen Conferences concerned with the function of the normal and failing human myocardium.

In 1987 basic mechanisms and clinical implications of then new insights into cardiac energetics was followed by a comprehensive review of inotropic stimulation and myocardial energetics in 1989. Here, we undertook a re-evaluation of the principles of inotropic stimulation and of its potential therapeutic value, based on new observations from experiments with human myocardium. In 1992 the risk due to myocardial phenotype change as a consequence of adaptation in heart failure was published. Here, alterations of subcellular structures and functions as a consequence of chronic heart failure, summarized as phenotype change, could be described as an essential characteristic of the failing human myocardium. This topic was discussed in greater depth in the volume "Cellular and Molecular Alterations in the Failing Human Heart", considering both the sarcolemma and the phosphodiesterases, as well as excitation-contraction coupling and contractile proteins, extracellular matrix, and mitochondrial function. Since it soon became apparent that myocardial ischemia represents a special case of chronic alteration to the human myocardium and that an intimate connection exists between excitation-contraction coupling and contractile performance within the framework of myocardial phenotype change on the one hand and the propensity to develop arrhythmias on the other hand, yet another conference was conducted and published on the topic of "Myocardial Ischemia and Arrhythmia" in 1994.

The rapid development of new observations and concepts has prompted us to again deal with the alteration of excitation-contraction coupling in the failing human heart and the proceedings are presented here.

This series of supplements to Basic Research in Cardiology has been the result of a larger series of conferences dedicated to the dialogue between basic scientists and clinicians and is named, according to the little village where the conferences take place, the "Gargellen" conferences. These conferences have been concerned with a rather wide spectrum of topics and is always characterized by an open dialogue between experts from all parts of the world, organized by the Society for Cooperation in Medical Sciences. This Society and its numerous conferences is based on the personal initiative of Prof. H. Just, the late Prof. Dr. med. Felix Burkart, Basel, Prof. Dr. jur. Albin Eser, Freiburg, Prof. Dr. med. Detlef Ganten, Berlin, Prof. Dr. med. H. R. Kirchheim, Heidelberg, Prof. Dr. med. Thomas Meinertz, Hamburg, Prof. Dr. med. Wilhelm Rutishauser, Genf, Prof. Dr. med. Hasso Scholz, Hamburg, and Prof. Dr. med. Stanley H. Taylor, Leeds. The broader, more general interest of the Society in the interdisciplinary exchange of thought in various fields of medicine and natural science is focused on specific topics with the collaboration of experts in the field to be dealt with.

My Co-worker Prof. Dr. med. Gerd Hasenfuss, Freiburg, organized the conference in 1995. It represents a field of research which has been subject of intense efforts of our group in Freiburg. Both conference and extended publication of its proceedings would not have been possible without the generous support of the Boehringer

Ingelheim Pharmaceutical Company through its affiliate Dr. Carl Thomae GmbH, Biberach/Riss, Germany, as well as the Bayer AG, Leverkusen, Germany. In particular we thank Dr. Manfred Haehl from Boehringer Ingelheim Zentrale, Ingelheim, Germany, for his continued interest and generous support.

It should not go unnoticed that the Dr. D. Steinkopff-Verlag, Darmstadt, Germany, a subsidiary of the Springer-Verlag, Berlin – Heidelberg – New York, has been a most helpful and understanding partner in publishing this series of books. In particular we thank Ms. Sabine Ibkendanz for her continued interest and help.

Regarding the topic of this volume a brief introductory note is in order:

Recently, the possibilities to study human myocardium, both normal, as well as in the failing state with and without hypertrophy, have led us to revise earlier concepts, primarily derived from animal experimentation. It could be shown that in the human myocardium a characteristic phenotyp prevails, which at a subcellular level may be quite different from the animal model. As a matter of fact in the state of hypertrophy and under the conditions of heart failure a very characteristic change of myocardial phenotype can be observed. This results from altered gene expression under the specific internal and external conditions of the failing human heart, which increases wall tension under the conditions of altered contractile geometry and tissue composition, as well as an activation of the sympatho-adrenal system, the renin-angiotensin system, and the nitric oxide-endothelin system. As a consequence of myocardial regeneration or growth myocyte hypertrophy, sometimes hypoplegia and fibroblast growth with connective tissue development occurs. The altered gene expression under these conditions leads primarily to an alteration of the structures of excitation-contraction coupling. To a lesser extent the contractile apparatus may show certain alterations. In the center of functional consequences of myocardial phenotype change is an alteration of calcium homeostasis. This may characteristically lead to diastolic as well as to systolic dysfunction. In particular in the presence of maintained Frank-Starling mechanism, the force-frequency relationship (Bowditch Treppe phenomenon) is altered. While unter normal conditions with any increase in heart rate the force of contraction increases, this effect is attenuated or reversed in hypertrophy and heart failure. It could be shown that primarily the sarcoplasmic calcium ATPase pumping of calcium into the sarcoplasmic reticulum is reduced, therefore, rendering SR-calcium stores insufficient. This will lead to an attenuation of the force of contraction with increasing heart rates, i.e., with shortening of diastole, the time for pumping available to the sarcoplasmic calcium ATPase. Here the renin-angiotensin system seems to play the decisive role together with altered tension conditions of the working myocardium. If this were the only change, then diastolic dysfunction would have to be expected due to increased diastolic calcium content in the cytosol. This, however, is not the case. The explanation rests with a concomitant or subsequent up-regulation of the sarcolemmal sodium-calcium exchanger. A component of the myocardial phenotype change which is probably brought about due to chronic activation of the sympatho-adrenergic system.

All variations of systolic and/or diastolic dysfunction can be seen as a consequence of the specific alteration of these two proteins and their function. As a consequence of these alterations an increased sodium content in the cytosol can be anticipated. This is indeed the case and can be held responsible for a wide spectrum of ventricular arrhythmias and a propensity to develop life-threatening arrhythmias under these conditions. In addition, specific alterations of the responsiveness of the myocyte to sympathetic innervation is seen. This alteration may be considered protective to myocyte integrity and function, especially from an energetic point of view. Furthermore, the cardiac endothelin system seems to be activated. The consequences of this phenomenon are, however, not yet defined.

The improved methodology and the availability of normal myocardium and of myocardial specimen from end-stage failing human hearts, obtained at the time of transplantation, has uncovered these alterations, specific to the human myocardium. A further clarification of the subsequent subcellular changes of structure and function can be considered a major advancement in the understanding of the state of heart failure and will lead to improved therapeutic techniques and to new drugs. In fact a paradigmatic change to the treatment of congestive heart failure can be foreseen: While in the sixties the retention of sodium and water was considered a main problem in heart failure, diuretics and digitalis glycosides were used. With better understanding of myocardial mechanics the principal of unloading to the heart was then developed in the seventies. Here the introduction of vasodilators into the treatment was effected. In the eighties and nineties, however, it became increasingly clear that neurohumoral changes are very basic to the condition of heart failure and that their interception or correction can be utilized to the greatest advantage to the failing human heart. The introduction of renin-angiotensin system blockers, the ACE inhibitors, and more recently the angiotensin II-receptor antagonists were developed as well as the introduction of the beta-receptor blockade. Currently, we are expecting a group of new drugs interfering with the endothelin system.

We consider the contribution of this volume to the understanding of the failing human myocardium as another step forward, prompting yet new studies and new discussions in order to further deepen and clarify our understanding of the complex nature of the clinically significant syndrome of heart failure.

Freiburg, January 1998   Prof. Dr. H. Just

REFERENCES

1. Just H, Holubarsch Ch, Scholz H (1989) Inotropic stimulation and myocardial energetics. Steinkopff Verlag Darmstadt, Springer-Verlag New York
2. Holtz J, Drexler H, Just H (1992) Cardiac adaptation in heart failure. Steinkopff Verlag Darmstadt, Springer-Verlag New York
3. Hasenfuss G, Holubarsch Ch, Just H, Alpert NR (1992) Cellular and molecular alterations in the failing human heart. Steinkopff Verlag Darmstadt, Springer-Verlag New York
4. Zehender M, Meinertz T, Just H (1994) Myocardial ischemia and arrhythmia. Steinkopff Verlag Darmstadt, Springer-Verlag New York

Contents

Preface and Introduction   V

Ca transport during contraction and relaxation in mammalian ventricular
muscle
Bers, D. M.   1

Sites of regulatory interaction between calcium ATPases and phospholamban
MacLennan, D. H., T. Toyofuku, Y. Kimura   17

The relative phospholamban and SERCA2 ratio: a critical determinant
of myocardial contractility
Koss, K. L., I. L. Grupp, E. G. Kranias   25

Phosphorylation and regulation of the Ca^{2+}-pumping ATPase in cardiac
sarcoplasmic reticulum by calcium/calmodulin-dependent protein kinase
Narayanan, N., A. Xu   39

Site-specific phosphorylation of a phospholamban peptide by cyclic
nucleotide- and Ca^{2+}/calmodulin-dependent protein kinases of cardiac
sarcoplasmic reticulum
Karczewski, P., M. Kuschel, L. G. Baltas, S. Bartel, E.-G. Krause   55

Sodium-calcium exchange: Recent advanves
Hryshko, L. V., K. D. Philipson   67

Expression and function of the cardiac Na^{+}/Ca^{2+} exchanger in postnatal
development of the rat, in experimental-induced cardiac hypertrophy, and
in the failing human heart
Studer, R., H. Reinecke, R. Vetter, J. Holtz, H. Drexler   77

Plasma membrane calcium pump: structure, function, and relationships
Carafoli, E.   85

Regulation of mRNA-expression of the sarcolemmal calmodulin-
dependent calcium pump in cardiac hypertrophy
Krain, B., A. Hammes, L. Neyses   89

Molecular mechanisms regulating the myofilament response to Ca^{2+}:
Implications of mutations causal for familial hypertrophic cardiomyopathy
Palmiter, K. A., R. J. Solaro   105

Ca^{2+}-dependent and Ca^{2+}-independent regulation of contractility in isolated human myocardium
Pieske, B., K. Schlotthauer, J. Schattmann, F. Beyersdorf, J. Martin,
H. Just, G. Hasenfuss   123

Calcium handling proteins in the failing human heart
Hasenfuss, G., M. Meyer, W. Schillinger, M. Preuss, B. Pieske, H. Just . . .   141

Role of cAMP in modulating relaxation kinetics and the force-frequency relation in mitral regurgitation heart failure
Mulieri, L. A., B. J. Leavitt, R. K. Wright, N. R. Alpert   153

Contributions of Ca^{2+}-influx via the L-type Ca^{2+}-current and Ca^{2+}-release from the sarcoplasmic reticulum to [Ca^{2+}]$_i$-transients in human myocytes
Beuckelmann, D. J.   169

Molecular and cellular aspects of re-entrant arrhythmias
Kleber, A. G., V. Fast   179

Subject Index   195

Ca transport during contraction and relaxation in mammalian ventricular muscle

D. M. Bers

Department of Physiology, Loyola University School of Medicine, Maywood, USA

Abstract

During relaxation of cardiac muscle four Ca transport systems can compete to remove Ca from the myoplasm. These are 1) the SR Ca-ATPase, 2) the sarcolemmal Na/Ca exchange, 3) the sarcolemmal Ca-ATPase, and 4) the mitochondrial Ca uniporter. Isolated ventricular myocytes loaded with the intracellular fluorescent Ca indicator indo-1 were used to study $[Ca]_i$ decline during relaxation. By selective inhibition of the various Ca transporters above the dynamic interaction of these systems during relaxation was evaluated. Quantitatively the SR Ca-ATPase and Na/Ca exchange are clearly the most important (accounting for > 95 % of Ca removal). However, the balance of Ca fluxes between these systems vary in a species dependent manner. For example, the SR is much more strongly dominant in rat ventricular myocytes, where ~ 92 % of Ca removal is via SR Ca-ATPase and only 7 % via Na/Ca exchange during a twitch. In other species (rabbit, ferret, cat, and guinea-pig) the balance is more in the range of 70–75 % SR Ca-ATPase and 25–30 % Na/Ca exchange. Ferret ventricular myocytes also exhibit a unusually strong sarcolemmal Ca-ATPase. During the normal steady state cardiac contraction-relaxation cycle the same amount of Ca must leave the cell as enters over a cardiac cycle. This implies that 25–30 % of the Ca required to activate contraction must enter the cell at each cardiac cycle. Experiments using voltage clamp to measure both Ca current and Na/Ca exchange current demonstrate that this amount of Ca may be supplied by the L-type Ca current.

The ability of the SR Ca-ATPase to reduce $[Ca]_i$ may also be modified both acutely (e.g. by catecholamines) as well as chronically (e.g. during cardiac hypertrophy and heart failure). Using tissue cultured neonatal rat ventricular myocytes, we studied the effect of chronic arrest or stimulation with phorbol esters (to stimulate protein kinase C). Verapamil-induced arrest increased the SR Ca-ATPase at the level of mRNA, protein expression and functional ability to lower $[Ca]_i$ in intact cells. Conversely, stimulation or protein kinase C reduced SR Ca-ATPase at all three of these levels.

Key words Rat – rabbit – ferret – shortening – fluorescence – cardiac myocyte – sarcoplasmic reticulum – cardiac hypertrophy

Introduction

For the activation of cardiac ventricular muscle contraction a large amount of Ca must enter the cytosol, resulting in an increase in cytoplasmic [Ca] ($[Ca]_i$) and Ca binding to troponin C (thereby activating the myofilaments). During the cardiac action potential Ca influx occurs via L-type Ca channels and some amount of Ca influx may also be expected via Na/Ca exchange (1). In several species sufficient Ca can enter the cell during the action potential to activate substantial contraction even in the absence of a functional sarcoplasmic reticulum (SR, e.g. rabbit and guinea-pig), while in rat this does not seem to be the case (2, 3). Furthermore, under normal conditions the quantity of Ca entry via Na/Ca exchange is probably small compared to that which enters via Ca current (I_{Ca}), although Ca influx via Na/Ca exchange can be greatly increased when intracellular [Na] ($[Na]_i$) is elevated (e.g. 4, 5).

Nevertheless, when the SR is functional in mammalian ventricular myocytes most of the activating Ca is released from the SR during excitation-contraction (E-C) coupling. While it is clear that L-type I_{Ca} can trigger SR Ca release via Ca-induced Ca-release (6, 7). Ca entry via Na/Ca exchange can also trigger SR Ca release under certain conditions (8–10). The physiological importance of Na/Ca exchange in triggering SR Ca release remains to be clarified.

For ventricular relaxation to occur $[Ca]_i$ must be lowered by transporting Ca out of the cytosol, allowing Ca to dissociate from troponin C. There are four Ca transport systems which compete for cytosolic Ca in cardiac myocytes: 1) the SR Ca-ATPase, 2) the sarcolemmal Na/Ca exchange, 3) the sarcolemmal Ca-ATPase, and 4) the mitochondrial Ca uniporter (11–13). Indeed, in the steady state, the amount of Ca which enters the cytosol (from the extracellular space or the SR) must be restored between beats to prevent net shifts in Ca content. This implies an intrinsic link between Ca fluxes involved in activation of contraction and relaxation under steady state conditions.

There is substantial evidence that during the course of cardiac hypertrophy and heart failure, there are chronic changes in relaxation (slowing) and down-regulation of the SR Ca-ATPase (for review see 14). Cultured neonatal rat ventricular myocytes have also been a valuable tool to study alterations of gene expression accompanying myocyte hypertrophy in a more controlled setting (e.g. 15).

In this paper, I will describe collaborative work with Drs. R. A. Bassani, J. W. M. Bassani, L. M. D. Delbridge, M. Qi and A. M. Samarel in which we have: 1) quantitatively characterized the relative contributions of the 4 Ca transport systems contributing to relaxation during the normal twitch contraction in various mammalian species, 2) compared the amount of Ca entry via Ca current to the amount extruded via Na/Ca exchange, and 3) evaluated changes in SR Ca-ATPase expression and function in conditions that alter hypertrophic state in cultured neonatal rat ventricular myocytes.

Methods

Individual freshly dissociated ventricular myocytes were studied in a chamber on the stage of an inverted microscope equipped for epifluorescence measurement of $[Ca]_i$

using the indicator indo-1, cell shortening using a video edge detector and ionic currents using whole cell voltage clamp and incorporating a rapid solution switching device. The details of the experimental methods are described more completely in the individual papers from which the figures below and the data discussed were obtained (11, 12, 16–19). Most of the experiments described were done with a default rate of stimulation (0.5 Hz), at 23 °C and modified normal Tyrode's (NT) solution containing (in mM): 140 NaCl, 6 KCl, 1 MgCl$_2$, 2 CaCl$_2$ (1 in rat experiments), 10 glucose and 5 HEPES at pH 7.40.

Results and discussion

Rapid cooling contractures and relaxation

We have previously used rapid cooling contractures (RCCs) in two different ways to evaluate the competition between the SR Ca-pump and the Na/Ca exchange in cardiac relaxation (20, 21). Rapid cooling to ~ 0 °C causes release of SR Ca and the cold inhibits Ca transport. One strategy was to prevent Na/Ca exchange by replacing the extracellular solution with Na-free, Ca-free (0Na, 0Ca) solution during the cold and upon rewarming. Then when the muscle is rewarmed to reactivate Ca transport, the Na/Ca exchange cannot compete with the SR Ca-pump. In rabbit ventricular muscle this slowed the $t_{1/2}$ of relaxation by about 30 % (20). Similarly, inclusion of 10 mM caffeine during the cold and rewarming prevents SR Ca reuptake (due to the activation of the SR Ca release channel). This slowed relaxation by ~ 75 % and when both the SR Ca-pump and Na/Ca exchange were simultaneously inhibited (0Na, 0Ca solution with caffeine), relaxation was dramatically slowed (i.e., by more than 1000 %). This result indicates that the SR Ca-pump and to a lesser extent sarcolemmal Na/Ca exchange can produce cardiac relaxation. It also shows that other systems (such as the sarcolemmal Ca ATPase or mitochondrial Ca uptake) are too slow to account for cardiac relaxation. There was also no voltage dependence of relaxation by the SR, whereas relaxation attributed primarily to Na/Ca exchange was slowed by depolarization, as expected for this electrogenic exchanger.

RCCs were also used in a different way to assess this competition in guinea-pig ventricular myocytes (21) and rabbit ventricular myocytes and muscle (22). In those experiments paired RCCs were performed where Ca extrusion via Na/Ca exchange was prevented during the rewarming relaxation of the first RCC. This resulted in no change in the amplitude of RCC or the associated Ca$_i$ transients. This indicated that when the Na/Ca exchange was inhibited, virtually all of the Ca released by the SR was taken back up by the SR. On the other hand, if the Na/Ca exchange was allowed to function during relaxation of the first RCC, then the second RCC was 23 ± 3 % smaller than the first in rabbit and 36 % in guinea-pig ventricular myocytes (and comparable results, 27 % were found in multicellular rabbit ventricular muscle, 22). These results indicate that the Ca responsible for 23–36 % of relaxation in these cells is extruded by Na/Ca exchange.

Ca removal during relaxation of caffeine contractures and twitches in rabbit and rat myocytes

Large contractions and Ca_i transients are produced by rapid application of 10 mM caffeine (which appears to release all of the SR Ca). Maintenance of caffeine exposure during the time that $[Ca]_i$ is declining also prevents Ca accumulation into the SR (but unlike RCCs does not prevent Ca transport by other mechanisms). By studying the $[Ca]_i$ decline and relaxation during such caffeine-induced contractures (CafC) information can be obtained about the other Ca removal systems (Na/Ca exchange, sarcolemmal Ca-ATPase and mitochondrial uniporter).

In a series of experiments summarized in Fig. 1, we measured relaxation of twitch vs CafC in rabbit ventricular myocytes where one or more of the other Ca transport systems were inhibited by changing the extracellular solution (11). That is, Na/Ca exchange was inhibited by 0Na, 0Ca solution (with EGTA), mitochondrial Ca uptake was inhibited by exposure to the protonophore uncoupler, FCCP (1 µM, which is expected to dissipate the mitochondrial membrane potential) and Ca extrusion via the sarcolemmal Ca-ATPase was limited by elevating $[Ca]_o$ after pre-depletion of $[Na]_i$ (by superfusion for 5 min in 0Na, 0Ca solution). Pre-depletion of $[Na]_i$ in this situation is necessary to prevent Ca entry via Na/Ca exchange when $[Ca]_o$ was increased during the CafC in the absence of $[Na]_o$.

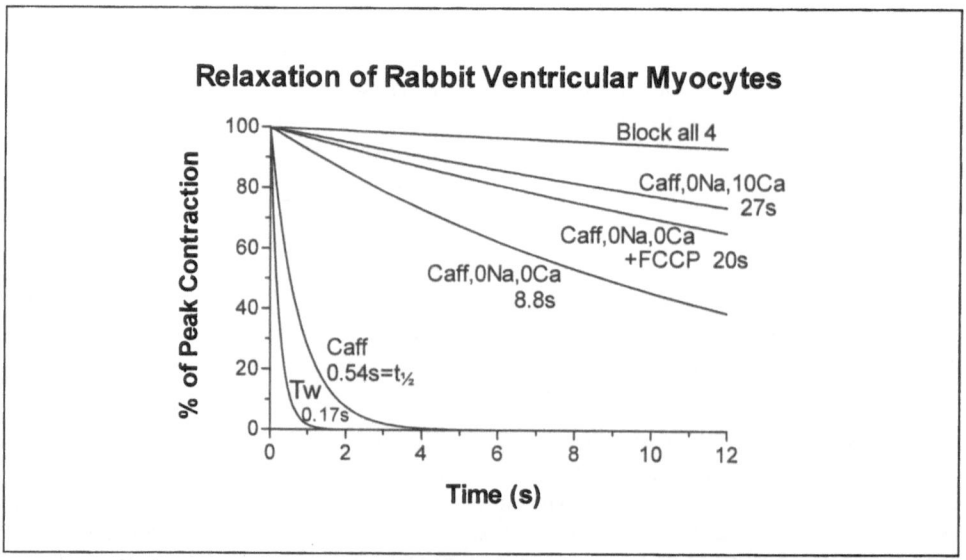

Fig. 1. Normalized cell relaxation in single rabbit ventricular myocytes. The conditions were either 1) having all Ca transporters functional during a steady state twitch (Tw), 2) preventing SR Ca uptake during a caffeine-induced contracture (CafC) in NT (Caff), 3) Additionally inhibiting Na/Ca exchange in 0Na, 0Ca solution (Caff, 0Na, 0Ca) and a) either inhibiting mitochondrial Ca uptake with 1 µM FCCP + 1 µM oligomycin so only sarcolemmal Ca-ATPase was functional (Caff, 0Na, 0Ca + FCCP) or b) additionally inhibiting the sarcolemmal Ca-pump by elevating $[Ca]_o$ to 10 mM after predepletion of $[Na]_i$, so that only mitochondrial Ca uptake was functional (Caff, 0Na, 10Ca). All four Ca removal systems were also blocked by combining the caffeine application with 0Na, 10Ca and FCCP. The traces are based on mean $t_{1/2}$ values (shown along the traces) for relaxation measured in experiments described by Bassani et al. (11).

In Fig. 1 it can be seen that inhibition of SR Ca uptake during the CafC slows relaxation by three-fold ($t_{1/2}$ increases from 170 ± 30 ms to 540 ± 70 ms). When both SR Ca uptake and Na/Ca exchange are inhibited (Caff, 0Na, 0Ca) relaxation is slowed almost another 20-fold ($t_{1/2} = 8.8 \pm 1.0$ sec). When either the mitochondrial system or the sarcolemmal Ca-ATPase were also inhibited relaxation was slowed another two- to three-fold. When all four Ca removal systems were simultaneously blocked (top trace in Figs. 1 and 4A) relaxation and $[Ca]_i$ decline were almost completely abolished, although the cells relaxed promptly when caffeine was removed and $[Na]_o$ returned. This demonstrates that the Ca transport systems were effectively blocked and that there does not appear to be the need to be concerned about additional Ca removal systems.

Based on a simplistic comparisons of the $t_{1/2}$ values for relaxation, we concluded that with respect to the Na/Ca exchange, the SR Ca uptake was two- to three-fold faster and the sarcolemmal Ca-ATPase and mitochondrial Ca transport was 37 to 50 times slower respectively (11). Even at this superficial level of analysis this might suggest that two-thirds to three-fourths of the Ca during relaxation in rabbit goes to the SR, with most of the rest extruded via Na/Ca exchange.

Further studies by Bassani et al. (12, 13) explored this issue more quantitatively and also examined possible species differences in this aspect of Ca regulation. Fig. 2B shows the normalized relaxation of a CafC in rabbit and rat ventricular myocytes. In the upper traces the Na/Ca exchange is also inhibited by 0Na, 0Ca solution, immediately before and during the CafC. The relaxation was not appreciably different in rat vs rabbit cells ($t_{1/2} = 9$–10 s). This indicated that the combined function of the slow systems (sarcolemmal Ca-ATPase and mitochondria uptake) were comparable in these species.

When the Na/Ca exchanger was allowed to function during CafC in control solution (Fig. 2B lower traces), the rabbit myocytes relaxed much faster than rat (almost four-fold), possibly reflecting a stronger Na/Ca exchange in rabbit myocytes. When all four Ca removal systems were allowed to participate in $[Ca]_i$ decline during a twitch (Fig. 2A), the situation reversed, such that relaxation in the rat myocytes was about twice as fast as in rabbit. This may indicate a faster SR Ca accumulation in the rat, which more than compensates for the slower Na/Ca exchange. Similar results were observed for Ca_i transients in these cells (12). This is also consistent with comparative SR Ca transport measurements in a more isolated system, where SR Ca transport rate was $\sim$ two times faster in rat ventricular myocytes than rabbit (23).

A limitation with the type of experiments in Figs. 1 and 2 is that twitches are being compared with CafC. Thus we developed experimental protocols where either the SR Ca-ATPase or the sarcolemmal Na/Ca exchange could be selectively blocked during a normal twitch activated by an action potential (12). Figure 3 shows Ca_i transients during twitches in rabbit and rat myocytes before and after selective inhibition of the SR Ca-ATPase by thapsigargin (but with normal SR Ca load at the time of each twitch). The experimental protocol for this is the following. After steady state stimulation cells were incubated for 5 min in 0Na, 0Ca solution, with 2.5 μM thapsigargin included during the last 2 min just before switching back to NT and stimulation of a twitch. This specific protocol allowed the SR Ca load to remain at the normal level, but also produces complete inhibition of SR Ca uptake (as tested by attempts to reload the SR after Ca depletion, 24). Of course only one test twitch can be given and after much longer rest times in thapsigargin solution, the SR Ca content gradually declines, even in 0Na, 0Ca (25).

There are two key features of note in Fig. 3. First, the Ca_i transients are larger after the SR Ca-pump is blocked. This is consistent with the idea that rapid Ca transport by the SR Ca-pump normally limits the peak of the Ca_i transient and this seems to be true for both rabbit and rat myocytes. Second, the time constant (τ) of $[Ca]_i$ decline is prolonged in the presence of thapsigargin. In rabbit the $[Ca]_i$ decline is only slowed by a factor of 2 (τ increases from 0.496 ± 0.034 s to 0.978 ± 0.120 s), where in rat myocytes thapsigargin slows $[Ca]_i$ decline by a factor of 9 (τ increases from 0.181 ± 0.008 s to 1.66 ± 0.30 s). This is certainly consistent with the foregoing results suggesting that SR Ca uptake is stronger in rat.

Similar experiments were done with selective inhibition of the Na/Ca exchange. In this case cells were first depleted of $[Na]_i$ by superfusion for 5–7 min in 0Na, 0Ca solution to allow the Na-pump to extrude Na and prevent Ca influx via Na/Ca exchange when $[Ca]_o$ is subsequently elevated (even to 100 mM) in the continued absence of $[Na]_o$. Twitches in this case were activated in Na-free solution with Li in place of Na so

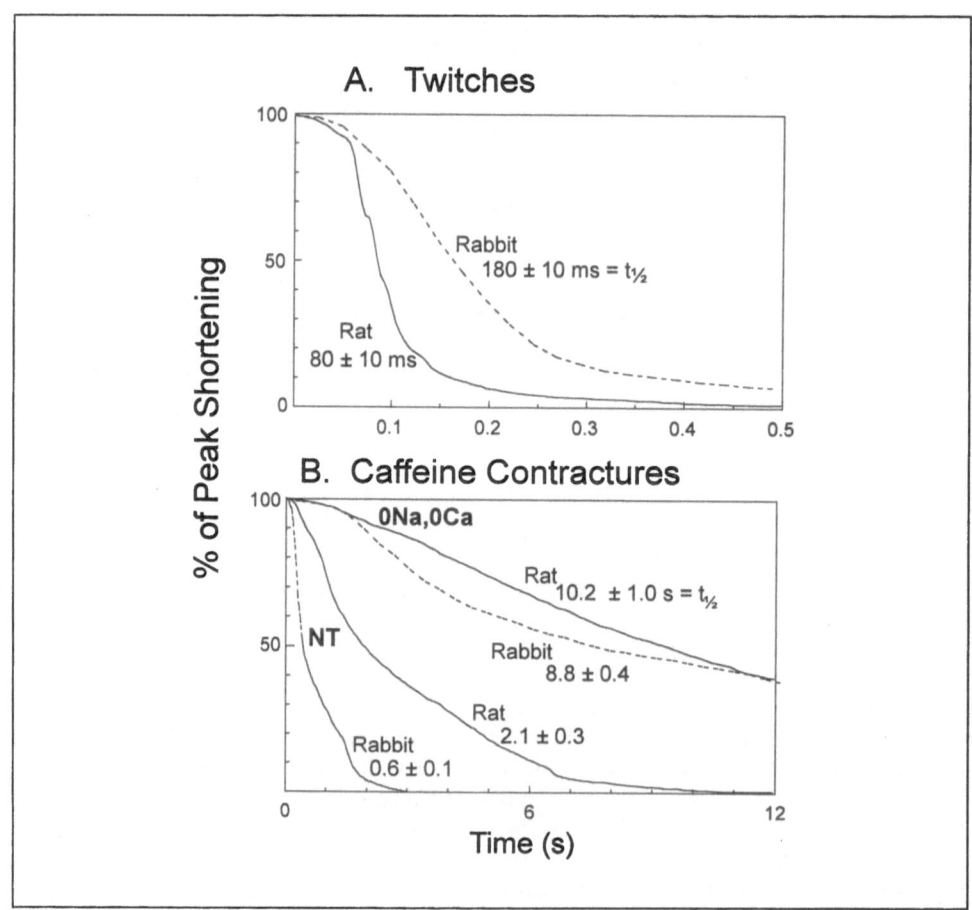

Fig. 2. Normalized mechanical relaxation of (**A**) stedy-state twitches and (**B**) caffeine contractures in control and 0Na, 0Ca solution recorded in rat and rabbit ventricular myocytes. Mean $t_{1/2}$ values for each type of contraction are also indicated (modified after Bassani et al. (12)).

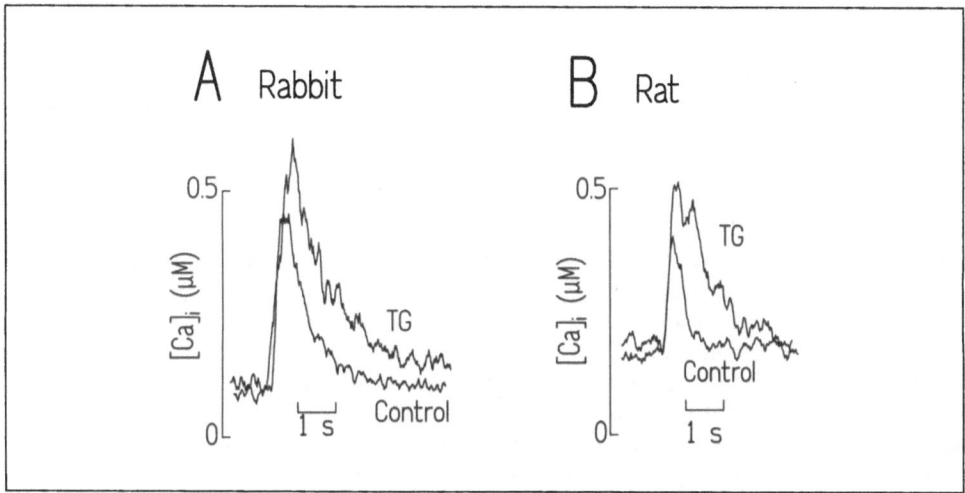

Fig. 3. [Ca]$_i$ transients recorded during electrically-stimulated twitches in rabbit (**A**) and rat (**B**) ventricular myocytes before (Control) and after treatment with 2.5 μM thapsigargin (TG). Stimulation was applied 10 s after switching to control solution (after 5–7 min pre-perfusion with 0Na, 0Ca solution). TG treatment (2 min exposure) was performed during this pre-perfusion period and SR Ca load was maintained despite complete block of the SR Ca-pump (from Bassani et al. (12) with permission).

that the measured action potentials were essentially normal and Na/Ca exchange in either direction was completely prevented. For rabbit cells this produced qualitatively similar results to those for thapsigargin in Fig. 3, although the effect of Na/Ca exchange inhibition was smaller than for SR Ca-pump inhibition. That is, the amplitude of the Ca$_i$ transient was still increased, but the τ of [Ca]$_i$ decline was prolonged by only 45 % (from 406 ± 28 ms to 588 ± 54 ms). For rat the effects of Na/Ca exchange inhibition were very modest. There was no significant increase in the amplitude of the Ca$_i$ transient and there was only a 20 % slowing of [Ca]$_i$ decline (consistent with voltage clamp results in rat ventricular myocyte, 26). These results indicate that the Na/Ca exchanger is considerably more important in rabbit than rat myocytes as inferred above.

When the two procedures above were combined to produce simultaneous block of both the Na/Ca exchange and the SR Ca-ATPase, the rate of [Ca]$_i$ decline in both rabbit and rat myocytes was greatly slowed, but was the same in both species (τ ~ 12 s). This is also the same τ measured for the [Ca]$_i$ decline during CafC in 0Na, 0Ca in these same cells. However, the amplitude of the Ca$_i$ transients during twitches with the SR Ca-pump and Na/Ca exchanger blocked is only about half of that observed during CafC with the Na/Ca exchanger blocked. This may well be because only about half of the SR Ca content is released during a normal twitch (24, 27).

Sarcolemmal Ca-ATPase in ferret ventricular myocytes is vigorous

We previously evaluated the contribution of the sarcolemmal Ca-ATPase and the mitochondrial uniporter to the slow decline of [Ca]$_i$ observed during CafC in 0Na,

0Ca in rabbit ventricular myocytes (see Fig. 1, ref. (11)). Using high $[Ca]_o$ (after $[Na]_i$ depletion) to limit Ca extrusion via the sarcolemmal Ca-pump and FCCP to inhibit mitochondrial Ca uptake, we demonstrated that about half of the slow Ca flux went through each of these systems (with the sarcolemmal Ca-pump being slightly faster). Furthermore, when all four Ca transport systems were inhibited during a CafC in 0Na, 10 mM $[Ca]_o$ and FCCP, relaxation and $[Ca]_i$ decline in rabbit ventricular myocytes was virtually abolished. This can be seen in the trop trace in Fig. 4A. This type of experiment made it convincing that these were the only 4 Ca transport systems which are important to consider in relaxation and that our inhibitory approaches seem to work (at least in rabbit ventricle).

Figure 4B shows that when we extended this approach to ferret ventricular myocytes we were surprised to find that relaxation of CafC in 0Na, 0Ca was remarkably fast ($t_{1/2} \sim 1.8$ s vs 9–10 s in rabbit and rat, 12, 13). In addition, the protocol which virtually abolished relaxation in rabbit ventricular myocytes (CafC in 0Na, 10 mM $[Ca]_o$ and FCCP) only increased the $t_{1/2}$ of relaxation or $[Ca]_i$ decline in ferret myocyte to ~ 4 s (13 and see top $[Ca]_i$ curve in Fig. 4B). We first ruled out the possibility that this rapid relaxation in ferret was due to incomplete inhibition of SR Ca uptake, Na/Ca exchange, mitochondrial Ca uptake or any other saturable internal pool (13). The likeliest explanation then seemed that the thermodynamic approach which we used

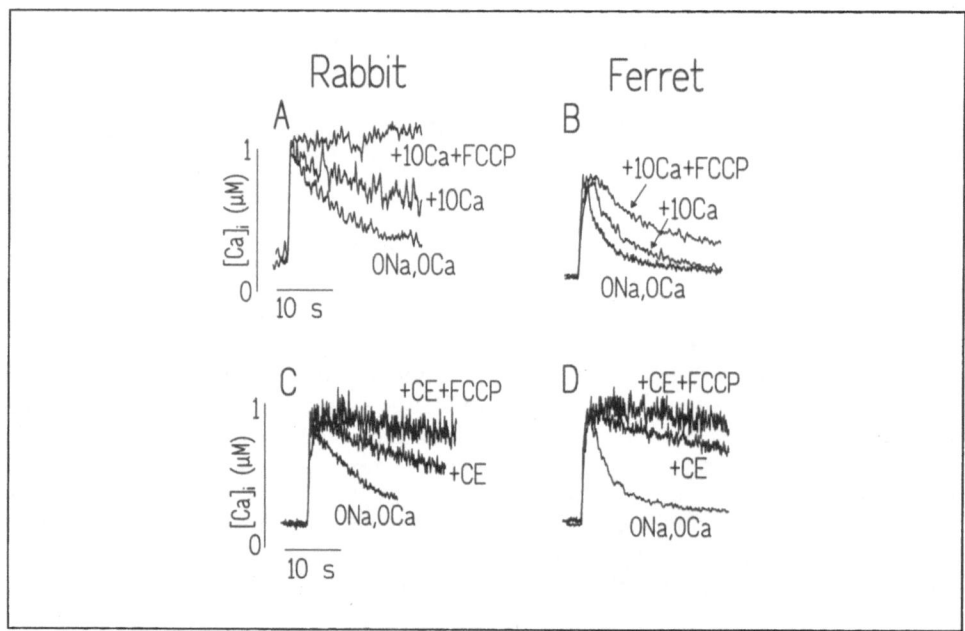

Fig. 4. $[Ca]_i$ transients in rabbit (A and C) and ferret ventricular myocytes (B and D) obtained during SR Ca release by 10 mM caffeine in Na-free solution. The control conditions in each panel were a CafC in 0Na, 0Ca solution containing 10 mM EGTA (0Na, 0Ca). In A and B CafC were repeated during inhibition of the sarcolemmal Ca-ATPase with 10 mM Ca (+ 10 Ca) and after additional inhibition of mitochondrial Ca uptake by FCCP (+ 10 Ca + FCCP). In C and D the CafC were repeated after carboxyeosin loading to inhibit the sarcolemmal Ca pump (+ CE) and after additional inhibition of the mitochondrial Ca uptake by FCCP (+ CE + FCCP) (from Bassani et al. (19) with permission).

to limit the sarcolemmal Ca-ATPase (increasing $[Ca]_o$ even to 100 mM), which appeared to work well in the rabbit and rat, was not able to suppress this system in ferret.

Recently, Gatto and coworkers (28, 29) demonstrated that the plasma membrane Ca pump is strongly inhibited by several fluorescein analogues, among them eosin (tetrabromofluorescein) and carboxyeosin (at μM levels). We used carboxyeosin as an alternative means to inhibit the sarcolemmal Ca-ATPase, loading it into myocytes by incubation with a cell permeant esterified form of carboxyeosin, which can be trapped in cells in the same way as the familiar Ca indicator acetoxymethylesters. Figure 4C shows that loading rabbit ventricular myocytes with carboxyeosin produced similar effects to elevating $[Ca]_o$ to 10 mM during CafC $\pm$ FCCP (e.g., compare Fig. 4A and 4C, ref. (19)). In ferret myocytes carboxyeosin produced the same effects as either high $[Ca]_o$ or carboxyeosin did in rabbit myocytes ($\pm$ FCCP, compare Figs. 4C and 4D). Thus, the sarcolemmal Ca-pump seems likely to be responsible for the much faster relaxation observed in ferret cells after block of SR Ca accumulation and Na/Ca exchange transport. Since the thermodynamic [Ca] gradient was less effective in limiting Ca extrusion in the ferret myocytes, the sarcolemmal Ca-pump in these cells may also have different fundamental characteristics from that in rabbit ventricular myocytes. Indeed, the more powerful sarcolemmal Ca-ATPase in ferret can be appreciated by the larger difference between the 0Na, 0Ca and + CE curves in Figs. 4C vs 4D.

Quantitative analysis of Ca fluxes during relaxation

Using data from experiments like those described above and in Figs. 3 and 4 allow us to go a step further in quantitative analysis of the dynamic interplay among the Ca transport systems (12, 13). First, the free $[Ca]_i$ can be converted to total cytoplasmic [Ca] ($[Ca]_t$), using the passive myoplasmic buffering characteristics measured by Hove-Madsen and Bers (30) and assuming that this buffering is in rapid equilibrium. Then differentiation of $[Ca]_t$ with respect to time ($d[Ca]_t/dt$) provides the rate of Ca transport from the myoplasm during relaxation. This transport rate must be the sum of the individual transport rates given by

$$d[Ca]_t/dt = J_{SR} + J_{Na/CaX} + J_{Slow} - L \qquad (1)$$

where the J terms refer to flux through the SR Ca-ATPase, Na/Ca exchange and the combined slow transporters respectively and L is a constant Ca leak into the cytoplasm (assumed to be small compared to other fluxes during $[Ca]_i$ decline). For simplicity J_{SR}, $J_{Na/CaX}$ and J_{Slow} can be empirically described as simple [Ca] dependent fluxes of the form

$$J_x = \frac{V_{max}}{1 + (K_m/[Ca]_i)^n} \qquad (2)$$

We first fit J_{slow} by using the decline of $[Ca]_i$ during a twitch in 0Na, 0Ca + TG (or a caffeine-induced contracture in 0Na, 0Ca) where J_{SR} and J_{NaCaX} are zero. In other words, we plot $d[Ca]_t/dt$ as a function of $[Ca]_i$ and fit it to Eq. (2). Then the determined V_{max}, K_m and n for J_{Slow} are held constant to determine the set of parameters which best describe either J_{SR} or J_{NaCaX} (using a twitch $[Ca]_i$ transient in either 0Na or TG respectively) leaving out the appropriate term in Eq. (1). Finally, we can simulate the action of all system working simultaneously during a normal twitch by using the free $[Ca]_i$ during that twitch to calculate the instantaneous individual fluxes through each system. This also provides an internal check that this strategy describes the Ca_i transient. Additionally, integration of the fluxes during a normal twitch Ca_i transient allows the calculation of how the individual systems contribute to the total Ca flux during twitch relaxation.

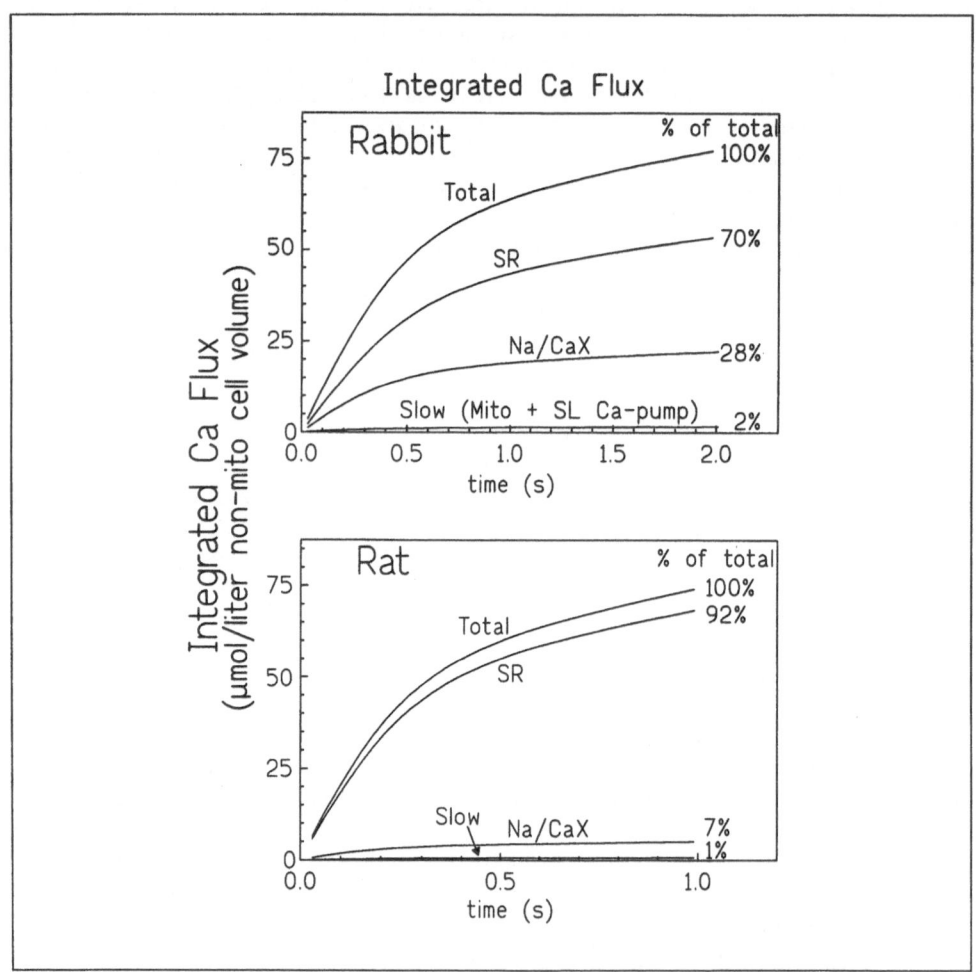

Fig. 5. Integrated Ca flux during a normal twitch in rabbit and rat myocytes. Free $[Ca]_i$ during relaxation of a normal twitch was used as a driving function so that Ca flux via each system could be integrated over time using the $[Ca]_i$ dependence, $J_x = V_{max}/\{1 + (K_m/[Ca]_i)^n\}$ derived as described in the text for J_{SR}, J_{NaCaX} and J_{Slow}. Independent values obtained for J_{SR}, J_{NaCaX} and J_{Slow} respectively were: V_{max} (in $\mu mol \cdot l$ non-mitochondrial volume$^{-1} \cdot s^{-1}$) = 81, 46 and 3.9 for rabbit and 207, 27 and 4 for rat; K_m (in nM) = 264, 316, and 362 in rabbit and 184, 257 and 268 in rat; n = 3.7, 3.7, 3.2 in rabbit and 3.9, 3.4 and 3.5 in rat. To convert values in units of $\mu mol \cdot liter$ non-mitochondrial volume^{-1} to units of $\mu mol \cdot kg$ wet wt^{-1}, the V_{max} values (and buffer concentrations) should be divided by 2.5, 42 (after Bassani et al. (12) with permission).

Figure 5 shows the results of such calculations based on measured Ca_i transients. It can be seen that during a normal twitch the fractions of Ca transported by the SR, Na/Ca exchange and slow systems are 70, 28 and 2 % respectively in rabbit and 92, 7 and 1 % in rat myocytes. This 28 % estimate of Ca flux by Na/Ca exchange in rabbit agrees with previous estimates described above (22). The 7 % value for rat agrees with similar experimental results in that species by Negretti et al. (31), but is smaller than previous indirect estimates based on time constants of relaxation or $[Ca]_i$ decline (26, 32).

Steady state cellular Ca balance

So far Ca extrusion from the myoplasm during relaxation has been the focus of the quantitative analysis discussed. However, in the steady state, the total amount of Ca extruded across the sarcolemmal membrane during each cardiac cycle must be the same as the amount which enters the cell over a cardiac cycle. Otherwise, there would be a progressive net change in cellular Ca and this would not correspond to a true steady state. Thus, if 28 % of the cytosolic Ca removed during relaxation leaves the rabbit ventricular cell via Na/Ca exchange, then this same amount of Ca must enter the cell. That is, 28 % of the amount of Ca responsible for activating contraction must enter the cell during a steady state twitch.

Figure 6 shows the experimental protocol of Delbridge et al. (18) using voltage clamp in rabbit ventricular myocytes to assess this tissue. A series of conditioning vol-

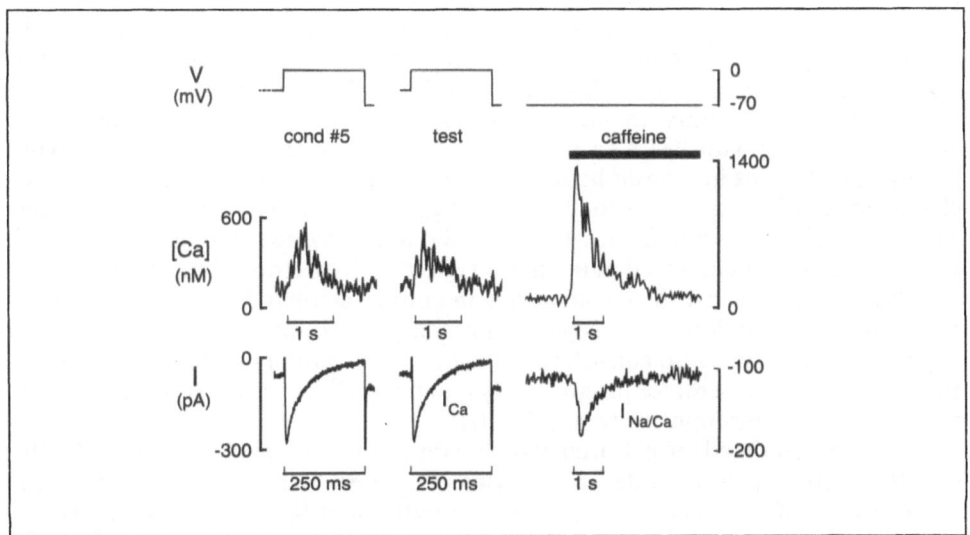

Fig. 6. $[Ca^{2+}]_i$ transients and inward currents (I_{Ca} and Na/Ca exchange current, $I_{Na/Ca}$) in a rabbit ventricular cardiomyocyte (dialysed with 50 μM indo-1). During the last of five conditioning voltage clamp pulses, during the test clamp (to 0 mV) and during rapid caffeine (10 mM) application (holding potential −70 mV) (from Delbridge et al. (18) with permission).

tage clamp pulses to 0 mV loads the SR to a steady state level. The last conditioning pulse and the test pulse are shown and both the Ca_i transient and Ca current (I_{Ca}) are also in steady state. The integral of the I_{Ca} was then used to assess the amount of Ca influx during a steady state twitch activated by depolarization from -40 to 0 mV (under conditions where Ca influx via Na/Ca exchange was limited by low $[Na]_i$). They also integrated the Na/Ca exchange current activated during a CafC to assess the SR Ca content. In doing so they also accounted for the 7 % of SR Ca release which is expected to be transported by the mitochondria and sarcolemmal Ca-ATPase under these conditions (with the SR uptake prevented, see Fig. 5A and ref. (12)). Assuming that 43 % of the SR Ca content was released during a steady state twitch (24), the Ca current contributed 23 ± 2 % of the activating Ca. This is in very good agreement with the estimates described above concerning the amount of Ca extruded via Na/Ca exchange during a steady state twitch. Considering the shorter action potential in rat ventricular myocytes, it is quite possible that less Ca enters in this species, consistent with the smaller Ca extrusion seen in Fig. 5.

An interesting side note is that the less direct conclusions drawn from contraction/ relaxation and RCC studies agree surprisingly well with more direct detailed analysis of $[Ca]_i$ transients even in quantitative terms. This may make some initial types of experiments possible with simpler technology. It also indicates that Ca removal from the myoplasm is a very important rate limiting step in the process of myocardial relaxation.

Changes in SR Ca-ATPase expression and function with chronic activation or arrest

There is considerable evidence that the expression of the SR Ca-ATPase mRNA and protein can change during cardiac hypertrophy and heart failure in animals and man (14, 33, 34). Cultured neonatal rat ventricular myocytes provide a controlled and rapidly responding setting where we can study the effects of chronic arrest of cell contraction (using verapamil) or chronic stimulation (e.g., with phorbol esters like phorbol 12-myristate 13-acetate or PMA (16, 17). The cellular Ca transport can also be studied by methods similar to those discussed above (16). Indeed, activation of such cutured myocytes with PMA or α-adrenergic activation can lead to cellular hypertrophy and changes in myosin heavy chain isoform and SR Ca-ATPase expression characteristic of pressure overload induced hypertrophy *in vivo* (14, 15, 17, 33–36). Thus this cell culture model may be beneficial in analyzing some of the important regulatory pathways involved in the pathogenesis of hypertrophy and heart failure.

The neonatal rat ventricular myocytes in culture actually have a balance of Ca fluxes during relaxation which is more like that in adult rabbit than rat ventricular myocytes (16). This is also consistent with studies of developmental changes where the SR Ca-ATPase increases progressively and the Na/Ca exchanger decreases progressively during development (e.g. (37–39)).

When we stimulated the cultured neonatal rat ventricular myocytes with PMA (for as little as 30 min) to activate protein kinase C, there was a dramatic decrease in expression of SR Ca-ATPase after 2 days at both the mRNA and protein level (to about 50 % of control, see Fig. 7A and ref. (17)). This down-regulation of SR Ca-ATPase was also paralleled by a 50 % decrease in the rate of $[Ca]_i$ decline during twitch contractions where the Na/Ca exchange was inhibited (so $[Ca]_i$ decline was almost exclusively due to the SR Ca-ATPase). In another series of experiments, we arrested the normally spontaneous cells by inclusion of 10 μM verapamil in the cultures (16). In verapamil arrested cells there was a marked increase (∼ 65 %) in SR Ca-ATPase mRNA and protein levels (Fig. 7B). Again this was paralleled by a 74 % increase in the rate of $[Ca]_i$ decline attributed to the SR Ca-ATPase. Thus the changes of SR Ca-ATPase with these interventions seems to show excellent correlations between message, protein and function in the intact cell.

Interestingly, despite these marked changes in SR Ca-ATPase induced by verapamil arrest, no changes were detected in the Na/Ca exchanger at the mRNA, protein

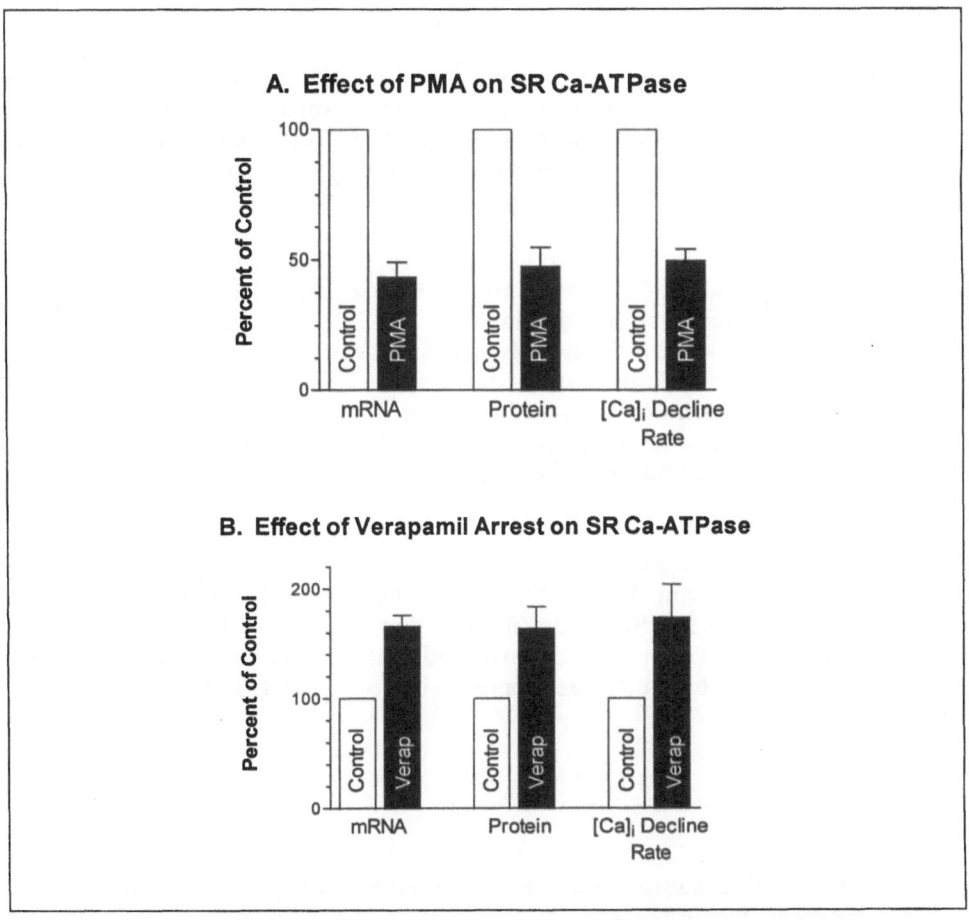

Fig. 7. Expression of SR Ca-ATPase and the functional rate of $[Ca]_i$ decline in intact single cells. Neonatal rat ventricular myocytes in culture were treated with either 200 nM PMA (**A**) or 10 μM verapamil for 48–72 h (**B**) with parallel controls in both cases. Then SR Ca-ATPase mRNA was measured by densitometric scans of Northern blots using a cDNA probe specific for SR Ca-ATPase, where glyceraldehyde phosphate dehydrogenase (GAPDH) mRNA was used as a standard. SR Ca-ATPase protein levels were measured by Western blots using a SR Ca-ATPase specific antibody. The rates of $[Ca]_i$ decline are based on the reciprocals of the $t_{1/2}$ values of $[Ca]_i$ decline for contractions where Na/Ca exchange was prevented (so that $[Ca]_i$ decline is almost exclusively due to the SR Ca-ATPase). The SERCA2 specific cDNA and antisera were gifts from Drs. Ronald Hartung and Wolfgang Dillman, University of California San Diego. The data presented are from Bassani et al. (16) and Qi et al. (17).

or functional level. Thus these systems are not necessarily co-regulated although it would not be surprising to see compensatory regulatory changes between these two important proteins involved in removal of cytoplasmic Ca (as seems to occur during development). Indeed, there have been recent reports that Na/Ca exchange mRNA and protein levels are elevated in human idiopathic dilated cardiomyopathy where the SR Ca-ATPase expression is also reduced (34, 41, 42).

Conclusions

In conclusion, we have evaluated the dynamic interaction of the four key Ca transport systems which are responsible for relaxation in cardiac muscle. In mammalian ventricular myocytes it seems clear that SR Ca uptake is the dominant Ca removal process. However, this dominance differs in different species. For example, in rabbit (ferret and neonatal rat) ventricular myocytes the SR Ca-pump transports only 2.5 times the amount transported by the Na/Ca exchange, whereas in adult rat ventricular myocytes this value is closer to 14. Furthermore, this difference is probably due to differences in both the SR Ca-ATPase and Na/Ca exchange. Among the slower systems involved in Ca removal, the sarcolemmal Ca-ATPase is particularly powerful in ferret ventricular myocytes. We have also shown that in rabbit ventricular myocytes where $\sim 25\%$ of the activating Ca is extruded by the Na/Ca exchange, a similar fraction of the activating Ca enters the cells via the Ca current. Finally, there may be important long-term changes in the balance of Ca fluxes between the SR Ca-ATPase and Na/Ca exchange that occur during normal development as well as during cardiac pathogenesis.

Acknowledgments   The author is pleased to acknowledge the central contributions of Drs. Rosana A. Bassani, José W. M. Bassani, Leanne M. D. Delbridge, Ming Qi and Allen M. Samarel for direct contributions to the body of work described here. Ms. Melanie Robinson, Christina Zakavec and Beth Tumilty also provided valuable technical assistance. This study was supported by grants from the USPHS, HL30077 and HL52478.

REFERENCES

1. Bers DM (1991) Excitation-contraction coupling and cardiac contractile force. Kluwer Academic Press, Dordrecht, Netherlands, pp 1–258
2. Sutko JL, Willerson JT (1980) Ryanodine alteration of the contractile state of rat ventricular myocardium. Comparison with dog, cat and rabbit ventricular tissues. Circ Res 46: 332–343
3. Bers DM (1985) Ca influx and SR Ca release in cardiac muscle activation during postrest recovery. Amer J Physiol 248: H366–H381
4. Bers DM (1987) Mechanisms contributing to the cardiac inotropic effect of Na-pump inhibition and reduction of extracellular Na. J Gen Physiol 90: 479–504
5. Bers DM, Christensen DM, Nguyen TX (1988) Can Ca entry via Na-Ca exchange directly activate cardiac muscle contraction? J Molec Cell Cardiol 20: 405–414
6. Beuckelmann DJ, Wier WG (1988) Mechanism of release of calcium from sarcoplasmic reticulum of guinea pig cardiac cells. J Physiol 405: 233–255

7. Fabiato A (1985) Time and calcium dependence of activation and inactivation of calcium-induced release of calcium from the sarcoplasmic reticulum of a skinned canine cardiac Purkinje cell. J Gen Physiol 85: 247–290
8. Leblanc N, Hume JR (1990) Sodium current-induced release of calcium from cardiac sarcoplasmic reticulum. Science 248: 372–376
9. Levi AJ, Spitzer KW, Kohmoto O, Bridge JHB (1994) Depolarization-induced Ca entry via Na-Ca exchange triggers SR release in guinea pig cardiac myocytes. Amer J Physiol 266: H1422–H1433
10. Kohmoto O, Levi AJ, Bridge JHB (1994) Relation between reverse sodium-calcium exchange and sarcoplasmic reticulum calcium release in guinea pig ventricular cells. Circ Res 74: 550–554
11. Bassani RA, Bassani JWM, Bers DM (1992) Mitochondrial and sarcolemmal Ca transport can reduce [Ca]$_i$ during caffeine contractures in rabbit cardiac myocytes. J Physiol 453: 591–608
12. Bassani JWM, Bassani RA, Bers DM (1994) Relaxation in rabbit and rat cardiac cells: Species-dependent differences in cellular mechanisms. J Physiol 476: 279–293
13. Bassani RA, Bassani JWM, Bers DM (1994) Relaxation in ferret ventricular myocytes: Unusual interplay among calcium transport systems. J Physiol 476: 295–308
14. Arai M, Matsui H, Periasamy M (1994) Sarcoplasmic reticulum gene expression in cardiac hypertrophy and heart failure. Circ Res 74: 555–564
15. Simpson P (1985) Stimulation of hypertrophy of cultured neonatal rat cardiac cells through an α_1-adrenergic receptor and induction of beating through an α_1- and β_1-adrenergic receptor interaction. Circ Res 56: 884–894
16. Bassani JWM, Qi M, Samarel AM, Bers DM (1994) Contractile arrest increases SR Ca uptake and SERCA2 gene expression in cultured neonatal rat hearts cells. Circ Res 74: 991–997
17. Qi M, Bassani JWM, Bers DM, Samarel AM (1996) Phorbol 12-myristate 13-acetate alters SR Ca^{2+}-ATPase gene expression in neonatal rat heart cells. Amer J Physiol 271: H1031–H1039
18. Delbridge LM, Bassani JWM, Bers DM (1996) Steady-state twitch Ca fluxes and cytosolic Ca buffering in rabbit ventricular myocytes. Amer J Physiol 270: C192–C199
19. Bassani RA, Bassani JWM, Bers DM (1995) Relaxation in ferret ventricular myocytes: role of the sarcolemmal Ca ATPase. Pflügers Archiv 430: 573–579
20. Bers DM, Bridge JHB (1989) Relaxation of rabbit ventricular muscle by Na-Ca exchange and sarcoplasmic reticulum Ca-pump: Ryanodine and voltage sensitivity. Circ Res 65: 334–342
21. Bers DM, Bridge JHB, Spitzer KW (1989) Intracellular Ca transients during rapid cooling contractures in guinea-pig ventricular myocytes. J Physiol 417: 537–553
22. Hryshko LV, Stiffel VM, Bers DM (1989) Rapid cooling contractures as an index of SR Ca content in rabbit ventricular myocyte. Amer J Physiol 257: H1369–1377
23. Hove-Madsen L, Bers DM (1993) SR Ca uptake and thapsigargin sensitivity in permeabilized rabbit and rat ventricular myocytes. Circ Res 73: 820–828
24. Bassani JWM, Bassani RA, Bers DM (1993) Twitch-dependent SR Ca accumulation and release in rabbit ventricular myocytes. Amer J Physiol 265: C533–C540
25. Bassani RA, Bers DM (1995) Rate of diastolic Ca release from the sarcoplasmic reticulum of intact rabbit and rat ventricular myocytes. Biophys J 68: 2015–2022
26. Bers DM, Lederer WJ, Berlin JR (1990) Intracellular Ca transients in rat cardiac myocytes: Role of Na/Ca exchange in excitation-contraction coupling. Amer J Physiol 258: C944–C954
27. Bassani JWM, Yuan W, Bers DM (1995) Fractional SR Ca release is altered by trigger Ca and SR Ca content in cardiac myocytes. Amer J Physiol 268: 1313–1319
28. Gatto C, Milanick MA (1993) Inhibition of the red blood cell calcium pump by eosin and other fluorescein analogues. Am J Physiol 264: C1577–C1586
29. Gatto C, Hale CC, Milanick MA (1995) Eosin, a potent inhibitor of the plasma membrane Ca pump, does not inhibit the cardiac Na-Ca exchanger. Biochemistry 34: 965–972
30. Hove-Madsen L, Bers DM (1993) Passive Ca buffering and SR Ca uptake in permeabilized rabbit ventricular myocytes. Amer J Physiol 264: C677–C686
31. Negretti N, O'Neill SC, Eisner DA (1993) The relative contributions of different intracellular and sarcolemmal systems to relaxation in rat ventricular myocytes. Cardiovasc Res 27: 1826–1830
32. Crespo LM, Grantham CJ, Cannell MB (1990) Kinetics, stoichiometry and role of the Na-Ca exchange mechanism in isolated cardiac myocytes. Nature 345: 618–621
33. de la Bastie D, Levitsky D, Rappaport L, Mercadier J-J, Marotte F, Wisnewsky C, Brovkovich V, Schwartz K, Lompré A-M (1990) Function of the sarcoplasmic reticulum and expression of its Ca^{2+}-ATPase gene in pressure overload-induced cardiac hypertrophy in the rat. Circ Res 66: 554–564
34. Hasenfuss G, Reinecke H, Studer R, Meyer M, Pieske B, Holubarsch C, Posival H, Just H, Drexler H (1994) Relation between myocardial function and expression of sarcoplasmic reticulum Ca^{2+}-ATPase in failing and non-failing human myocardium. Circ Res 75: 434–442
35. Samarel AM, Engelmann GL (1991) Contractile activity modulates myosin heavy chain-β expression in neonatal rat heart cells. Am J Physiol 261: H1067–H1077

36. Toaldo G-L, Hefner CA, Bailey BA, Houser SR (1995) Reduced SERCA expression correlates with prolongation of the systolic Ca^{2+} transient in hypertrophy hypertrophied neonatal rat ventricular myocytes. Biophys J 68: A311

37. Boerth SA, Zimmer DB, Artman M (1994) Steady state mRNA levels of the sarcolemmal Na^+-Ca^{2+} exchanger peak near birth in developing rat and rabbit hearts. Cir Res 74: 354–359

38. Kaufman TM, Horton JW, White DJ, Mahony L (1990) Age-related changes in myocardial relaxation and sarcoplasmic reticulum function. Am J Physiol 259: H309–316

39. Artman M, Ichikawa H, Avkiran M, Coetzee WA (1995) Na^+/Ca^{2+} exchange current density in cardiac myocytes from rabbits and guinea-pigs during postnatal development. Am J Physiol 268: H1714–H1722

40. Studer R, Reinecke H, Bilger J, Eschenhagen T, Böhm M, Hasenfuss G, Just H, Holtz J, Drexler H (1994) Gene expression of the cardiac Na^+-Ca^{2+} exchanger in end-stage human heart failure. Circ Res 75: 443–453

41. Kent RL, Rozich JD, McCollam PL, McDermott DE, Thacker UF, Menick DR, McDermott PJ, Cooper G IV (1993) Rapid expression of the Na^+-Ca^{2+} exchanger in response to cardiac pressure over-load. Am J Physiol 265: H1024–H1029

42. Fabiato A (1983) Calcium-induced release of calcium from the cardiac sarcoplasmic reticulum. Amer J Physiol 245: C1–C14

Authors' address:
Donald M. Bers, PhD
Department of Physiology
Loyola University School of Medicine
2160 S. First Ave.
Maywood, IL 60153, USA

Sites of regulatory interaction between calcium ATPases and phospholamban

D. H. MacLennan, T. Toyofuku, Y. Kimura

Banting and Best Department of Medical Research, University of Toronto, Toronto, Canada

Abstract

In an effort to define the amino acids that are involved in functional interactions between phospholamban (PLN) and the Ca^{2+} ATPase of cardiac sarcoplasmic reticulum (SERCA2), we have coexpressed wild type and mutant forms of phospholamban with wild type and mutant forms of SERCA2, isolated microsomal fractions and measured Ca^{2+} dependence of Ca^{2+} transport. We have found that both charged and hydrophobic residues in the cytoplasmic domains of both PLN and SERCA2 make up the cytoplasmic interaction site. In SERCA2, this site is the linear sequence Lys-Asp-Asp-Lys-Pro-Val^{402}: In PLN, the site is more diffuse and complex. Function was retained if the net charge over the first 20 amino acids was +1 or +2, but function was lost if the net charge was −3, −2, 0 or +3. Function was also lost if the long alkyl side chains of Val^4, Leu^7 or Ile^{12} were replaced with the methyl group of Ala. We have also obtained evidence that a site of functional interaction is present in the transmembrane domains of PLN and SERCA2.

Key words Phospholamban – calcium ATPases, sarcoplasmic reticulum, phosphorylation

Introduction

The era of investigation of the regulation of cardiac Ca^{2+} pumps began when Tada et al. (27) found that Ca^{2+} transport by cardiac sarcoplasmic reticulum was stimulated about three fold when protein kinase A catalyzed the phosphorylation of a 22000 Da membrane protein which they named phospholamban (PLN). Plots of the Ca^{2+} dependency of Ca^{2+} transport (see Fig. 1) for the cardiac Ca^{2+} pump, now known as SERCA2 (sarco- or endo-plasmic reticulum Ca^{2+} ATPase 2), were shifted to a lower apparent Ca^{2+} affinity in the presence of PLN and to higher apparent affinity in the presence of phospho PLN (26).

Phospholamban has been shown to be a pentamer of 6000 Da subunits, which is located in the sarcoplasmic reticulum of cardiac, slow-twitch and smooth muscles. It contains 52 amino acids which are organized into three physical and functional domains (5, 6, 24). Domain Ia, consisting of residues 1–20, largely in an α-helical conformation, and domain Ib, consisting of residues 21–30, likely existing as a random coil, constitute the cytoplasmic sector. Domain Ia has a net positive charge, with acidic residues at positions 2 and 19 and basic residues at positions 3, 9, 13 and 14. Ser^{16}, however, can be phosphorylated by protein kinase A, and Thr^{17} can be phosphorylated by calmodulin kinase (24), shifting the net charge from positive to neutral or even negative. Domain Ib is polar and positively charged, with Gln at positions 22, 23, 26 and 29, Asn at positions 27 and 30 and Arg at position 25. Domain II is the transmembrane domain, made up solely of uncharged residues, Asn, Met, Val, Phe, Cys, Ile and Leu, probably in an α-helical conformation.

Sites of interaction between phospholamban and SERCA2

James et al. (11) crosslinked Lys^3 of PLN to Lys^{397} or Lys^{400} of SERCA2 under conditions where SERCA2 was inhibited. Crosslinking did not occur in the presence of saturating levels of Ca^{2+} or when PLN was phosphorylated. These results suggested that there is a physical interaction between PLN and SERCA2 to inhibit the rate of Ca^{2+} transport and that this physical interaction is broken up by phosphorylation of PLN or by the availability to SERCA2 of higher levels of Ca^{2+}. The addition of other highly charged molecules can also disrupt the interaction between PLN and SERCA2 (4, 32), suggesting that electrostatic interactions are important in the functional association between PLN and SERCA2. An antibody against residues 7–16 of PLN mimics phosphorylation of PLN in its activation of the Ca^{2+} ATPase (2, 21). Thus residues in PLN domain Ia are critical to interaction between SERCA2 and PLN.

Several investigators have attempted to reconstitute purified PLN (12) with purified SERCA2 (10, 13, 22, 23, 25). Reconstitution has also been used to study the interaction of PLN domains with SERCA2 (9, 22, 23). In general, high concentrations of PLN have been required to achieve functional interaction. Reddy et al. (22) reported reconstitution with an eight fold excess of PLN. Sasaki et al. (23) reported that reconstitution of SERCA2 with a synthetic hydrophilic domain peptide (PLN^{1-31}) at 400 μg/ml lowered V_{max}. The addition of a synthetic transmembrane domain peptide (PLN^{28-47}) to SERCA2 altered its K_{Ca} from 0.52 to 1.33 mM, without affecting V_{max}, when applied in 100-fold molar excess. Hughes et al. (9) have reproduced the V_{max} inhibition with PLN_{1-25}, while Reddy et al. (22) used reconstitution with an eight fold excess of PLN^{26-52} to decrease Ca^{2+} uptake at both pCa 5.4 and 6.8 without lowering Ca^{2+} ATPase activity. They proposed that PLN^{26-52} uncoupled Ca^{2+} uptake from Ca^{2+} ATPase. These studies illustrate that reconstitution experiments are difficult to perform and reproduce and that the ratio between the interacting proteins is far from physiological.

Phospholamban-Ca^{2+} ATPase interactions in proteins expressed in heterologous cell culture

A major goal in our laboratory is to define the sites of molecular interaction between PLN and SERCA2. When we initiated our studies of interactions between PLN and SERCA2, we recognized that reconstitution of the interactions with purified proteins would be difficult, because the interaction does not survive solubilization in detergent. Moreover, reconstitution is limited to either purified native proteins or synthetic peptides, which are expensive to prepare.

Accordingly, it was important to explore the possibility that we could achieve reconstitution by coexpressing PLN and SERCA2 in a heterologous cell culture system (7, 8, 20, 29–31). In our first experiments, we demonstrated that we could express PLN cDNA in COS-1 cells (7). In our next series of experiments, we coexpressed PLN with SERCA2 (8). When we compared the Ca^{2+} dependence of Ca^{2+} uptake by SERCA2 coexpressed with or without PLN, we found that PLN shifted the full curve of Ca^{2+} dependence so that the apparent Ca^{2+} affinity was lowered by about 0.3 pCa units. In later experiments (29), we demonstrated that this effect of PLN on apparent Ca^{2+} affinity was reversible. If we phosphorylated PLN with added PKA, the full curve of Ca^{2+} dependence was shifted about 0.3 pCa units to a higher affinity. Thus we could reproduce the essential measures of PLN-SERCA2 interaction using microsomes from a transfected, heterologous cell culture system. This system provides an excellent alternative to in vitro reconstitution systems.

Use of chimeric SERCA proteins to define regions of PLN interaction

In early studies, we cloned cDNAs encoding three isoforms of the Ca^{2+} ATPase: SERCA1, the fast twitch isoform (1); SERCA2, the cardiac/slow twitch isoform (18) which, in an alternatively spliced form, is ubiquitously expressed in non-muscle tissues (15); and SERCA3, a widely expressed isoform with specialized function (3). In more recent studies (16, 28), we expressed SERCA1, SERCA2a, SERCA2b and SERCA3 and found that SERCA3 has an apparent Ca^{2+} affinity, as measured by Ca^{2+} dependence of Ca^{2+} transport, about 0.6 pCa units lower than the apparent Ca^{2+} affinity of SERCA1 or SERCA2. When we coexpressed PLN with SERCA1 or SERCA2, we found that apparent Ca^{2+} affinity was lowered. When we coexpressed PLN with SERCA3, we saw little effect on apparent Ca^{2+} affinity of SERCA3 (29).

These observations led us to try to localize the regions in the different ATPases responsible for the differences in apparent Ca^{2+} affinity (28). We made chimeras between SERCA2 and SERCA3 by inserting the same restriction endonuclease sites into corresponding sequences of the two DNA molecules and swapping four domains; the NH$_2$-terminal transmembrane and β strand domain; the phosphorylation domain; the nucleotide binding/hinge domain; and the COOH-terminal transmembrane domain. We found high apparent Ca^{2+} affinity to be linked to the inclusion of the nucleotide binding/hinge domain of SERCA2 in the chimeras. Attempts to subdivide this region in chimeras were unsuccessful.

We then coexpressed each of the 14 SERCA2/SERCA3 chimeras with PLN (29). We found that PLN would interact functionally only with those chimeras that had both the nucleotide binding/hinge domain of SERCA2 (which conferred high Ca^{2+} affinity to the chimera) and the phosphorylation domain of SERCA2 (which apparently contained the PLN interaction site). The phosphorylation domains of SERCA2 and SERCA3 were subdivided and two new chimeras were formed. We then found that a SERCA3 chimera containing residues 336–412 and 467–762 of SERCA2 would interact functionally with PLN, thereby defining the regions in SERCA2 essential for interaction with PLN.

Identification of amino acids in SERCA2 essential for PLN interaction

In our experiments using chimeras, function would only be affected if the amino acids involved in the interaction between the ATPase and PLN differed between the two proteins contributing to the chimera. Thus, we were confident of the existence of an essential site of interaction between ATPase residues 370 and 400, but we wanted to determine whether other residues essential to the interaction, but invisible because of their identity between SERCA2 and SERCA3 existed in this region. Accordingly, we mutated all of the charged residues and some of the uncharged residues in SERCA2 between Arg^{365} and Asp^{408}. Mutation affected functional interaction only for residues Lys^{397}, Asp^{398}, Asp^{399}, Lys^{400}, Pro^{401}, and Val^{402} (31). To prove that these were the essential interacting residues, we made a SERCA2 chimera containing the SERCA3 phosphorylation domain. This chimera did not interact functionally with PLN. If the SERCA3 sequence Gln-Gly-Glu-Gln-Leu-Val^{402} were substituted with the SERCA2 sequence Lys-Asp-Asp-Lys-Pro-Val^{402} or with the sequence Lys-Gly-Glu-Tyr-Pro-Val^{402}, function was restored (Fig. 1). These and other experiments demonstrated that the SERCA2 residues essential for PLN interaction are: at least one basic residue at positions 397 or 400; at least one acidic residue at positions 398 or 399; a Pro at position 401 and a long chain hydrophic residue at position 402 (31).

Cytoplasmic PLN residues essential for interaction with SERCA2

We have used our coexpression and mutagenesis system to evaluate the roles of amino acids 1 to 30 in domains Ia and Ib of PLN in the PLN-SERCA2 interaction (30). Our results were more complex than those with SERCA2. We found that mutation of positively charged residues Lys^{3}, Arg^{9}, Arg^{13} and Arg^{14}, of the negatively

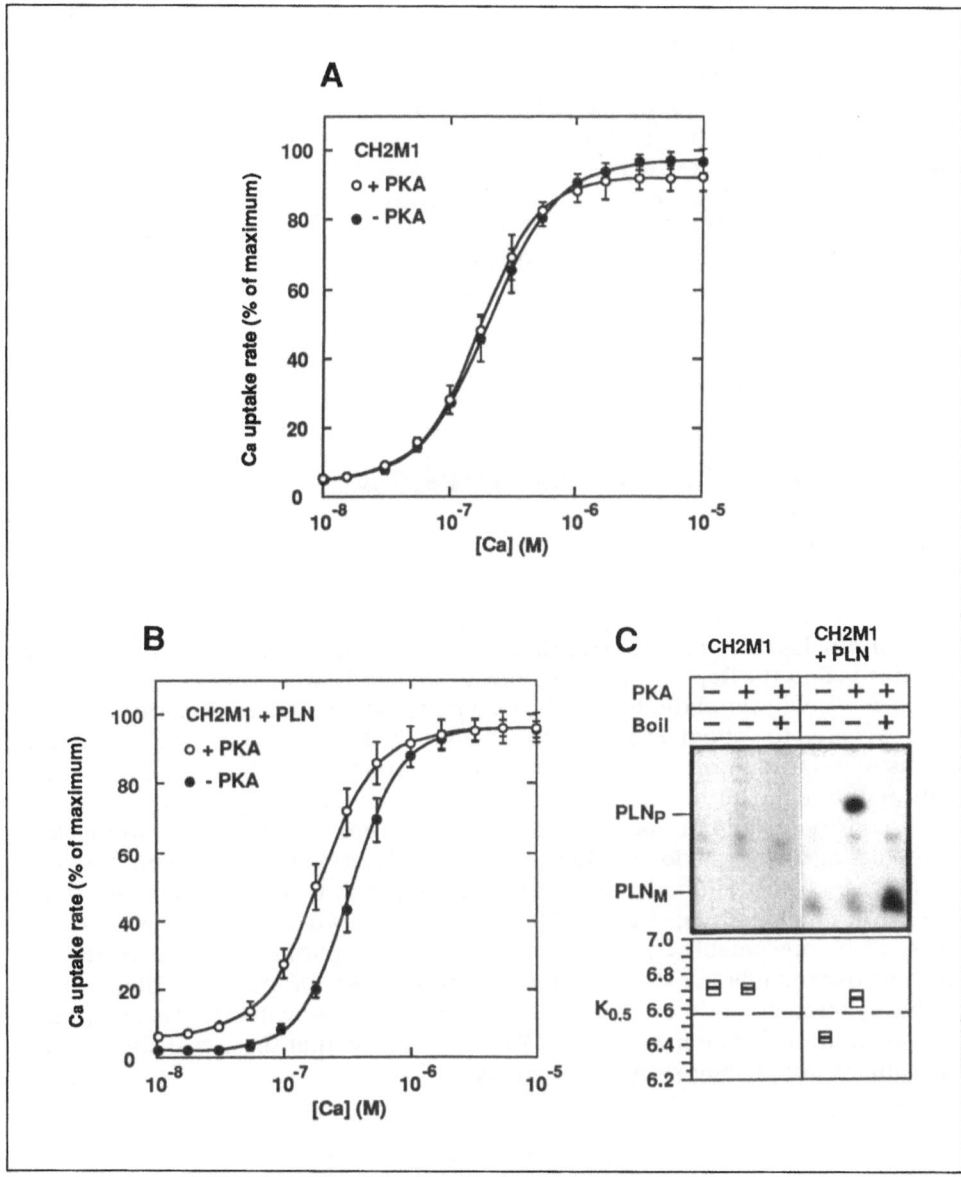

Fig. 1. Effects of cAMP-dependent protein kinase on phospholamban-dependent alterations in Ca^{2+} dependence of Ca^{2+} transport by chimeric Ca^{2+}-ATPase molecule. The chimeric molecule CH2M1 was constructed in two steps. It was a SERCA2 molecule substituted with residues 336–412 of SERCA3. The sequence QGEQL[401] was further substituted with the corresponding SERCA2 sequence, KDDKP[401]. Ca^{2+} dependence of the Ca^{2+} uptake rate was measured using microsomes from cDNA transfected HEK-293 cells. Microsomes were preincubated with (open circles) and without (closed circles) 25 units of the catalytic subunit of cAMP-dependent protein kinase (PKA). Panels A and B show the effects of PKA on Ca^{2+} dependence of Ca^{2+} uptake rates for CH2M1. Each point with a bar represents the mean ± S.D. obtained from three experiments. In panel C, microsomes prepared from HEK-293 cells were preincubated with $[\gamma$-$^{32}P]ATP$ in the absence and presence of PKA. Phosphorylated microsomes were subjected to SDS-polyacrylamide gel electrophoresis in 13.5 % polyacrylamide, with or without boiling. The effects of PKA on $K_{0.5}$ for Ca^{2+} dependence of Ca^{2+} transport are summarized. Boxes represent the mean (central vertical line) and S.D. (right and left edges of box). (Reprinted from ref. (29), with permission from the Journal of Biological Chemistry).

charged residue Glu^2, of hydrophobic residues Val^4, Leu^7, Ala^{11}, Ile^{12}, Ala^{15} and Ile^{18} and of phosphorylation residues Ser^{16} and Ser^{17}, in domain Ia of PLN, all affected functional interaction with SERCA2. Charge appeared to be an important element in the interaction. If residues 2 to 18 had a net charge of $+1$ or $+2$, the molecule was functional. If the net charge were 0, -2, -3, or $+3$, function was lost. Hydrophobic interactions also appeared to be critical. Function was lost if the long alkyl side chains of Val^{14}, Leu^7 or Ile^{12} were replaced by the methyl group of Ala. Thus there is evidence, both in the SERCA2 interaction site sequence and in the PLN interaction site sequence, that electrostatic and hydrophobic interactions are critical. We found no functional role for residues 21–30 in domain Ib.

Demonstration of a transmembrane PLN/SERCA2a interaction site

In recent experiments, we have expressed SERCA2 with a variety of PLN constructs in which the NH_2-terminal cytoplasmic domains were either deleted or replaced (14). Deletions included domain Ia (residues 1–20), domain Ib (residues 21–30) or both domains Ia and Ib. Replacements of domains Ia and Ib were with HA, Myc or Flag epitopes. PLN lowered the K_{Ca} by 0.3 pCa units, while domain II (residues 31–52), alone, lowered K_{Ca} about 0.15 pCa units. Although all three epitope-labelled domain II constructs lowered K_{Ca}, the HA-domain II construct "supershifted" K_{Ca} by 0.6 pCa units and the domain Ib-deleted construct supershifted K_{Ca} by at least 1 pCa unit. These constructs did not uncouple Ca^{2+} ATPase from Ca^{2+} transport. Monoclonal antibodies against PLN domain Ia reversed the inhibition by the domain Ib-deleted construct and Flag antibodies reversed the inhibition by the Flag-domain II construct. All domain II constructs inhibited SERCA3, which does not interact with native PLN, presumably because SERCA3 lacks cytoplasmic interaction sites, but contains transmembrane sequence interaction sites. We propose that there are two inhibitory interaction sites between PLN and SERCA2, one in cytoplasmic domains and one in transmembrane domains. We also propose that these two sites regulate each other through long-range interactions.

Conclusion

In our studies of structure/function relationships in sarcoplasmic reticulum proteins, we have cloned cDNA encoding relevant proteins, mutagenized the cDNA, expressed or coexpressed the mutated cDNAs in heterologous cell culture systems, and assayed the altered function. Our studies of SERCA1 have allowed us to define the catalytic domain in the cytoplasmic sector of the Ca^{2+} pump, the Ca^{2+} binding and translocation domain in the transmembrane sequences, and specific residue scattered throughout the pump that are involved with conformational changes. With this information, we have been able to propose a straight forward model for ATP dependent Ca^{2+} transport, which involves longrange interactions between a cytoplasmic catalytic site and a transmembrane Ca^{2+} binding and translocation site (17, 19).

We have also been able to study the interaction between SERCA2 and PLN by coexpression of the two molecules. This strategy is superior to attempts at reconstitution of purified components, since detergents, which complicate reconstitution systems, are avoided and interactions can be observed with more physiological ratios of the interacting components. With this system, combined with mutagenesis and measurement of function, we have been able to define a relatively few residues in both SERCA2 and PLN that are involved in the cytoplasmic interaction between these two proteins. We have also been able to demonstrate a second, functional site of PLN-SERCA2 interaction in the transmembrane domains of the two proteins. We suggest that long range interactions between the cytoplasmic and transmembrane interaction sites in PLN and SERCA2 may have analogies with the long range interactions that we have defined within SERCA1.

Acknowledgments   We thank the many colleagues who participated in the work from our laboratory that is described in this review. Research grants supporting original work from our laboratory were from the Medical Research Council of Canada (MRCC), The National Institutes of Health (USA), The Heart and Stroke Foundation of Ontario and The Human Frontier Science Program Organization. Dr. T. Toyofuku was a postdoctoral fellow of the MRCC: Dr. Y Kimura was a postdoctoral fellow of the Pharmaceutical Roundtable and the Heart and Stroke Foundation of Canada.

REFERENCES

1. Brandl CJ, Green NM, Korczak B, MacLennan DH (1986) Two Ca^{2+} ATPase genes: Homologies and mechanistic implications of deduced amino acid sequences. Cell 44: 597–607
2. Briggs FN, Lee KF, Wechsler AW, Jones LR (1992) Phospholamban expressed in slow-twitch and chronically stimulated fast-twitch muscle minimally affects calcium affinity of sarcoplasmic reticulum Ca^{2+} ATPase. J Biol Chem 267: 26056–26061
3. Burk SE, Lytton J, MacLennan DH, Shull GE (1989) cDNA cloning, functional expression, and mRNA tissue distribution of a third organellar Ca^{2+} pump. J Biol Chem 264: 18561–18568
4. Chiesi M, Schwaller R (1989) Involvement of electrostatic phenomena in phospholamban-induced stimulation of Ca uptake into cardiac sarcoplasmic reticulum. FEBS 244: 241–244
5. Fujii J, Kadoma M, Tada M, Tada H, Sakiyama F (1986) Characterization of structural unit of phospholamban by amino acid sequencing and electrophoretic analysis. Biochem and Biophys Res Commun 138: 1044–1050
6. Fujii J, Ueno A, Kitano K, Tanaka S, Kadoma M, Tada M (1987) Complete complementary DNA-derived amino acid sequence of canine cardiac phospholamban. J Clin Invest 79: 301–304
7. Fujii J, Maruyama K, Tada M, MacLennan DH (1989) Expression and sitespecific mutagenesis of phospholamban. Studies of residues involved in phosphorylation and pentamer formation. J Biol Chem 264: 12950–12955
8. Fujii J, Maruyama K, Tada M, MacLennan DH (1990) Co-expression of slow-twitch/cardiac muscle Ca^{2+}-ATPase (SERCA2) and phospholamban. FEBS 273: 232–234
9. Hughes G, East JM, Lee AG (1994) The hydrophilic domain of phospholamban inhibits the Ca^{2+} transport step of the Ca^{2+}-ATPase. Biochem J 303: 511–516
10. Inui M, Chamberlain BK, Saito A, Fleischer S (1986) The nature of the modulation of Ca^{2+} transport as studied by reconstitution of cardiac sarcoplasmic reticulum. J Biol Chem 261: 1794–1800
11. James P, Inui M, Tada M, Chiesi M, Carafoli E (1989) Nature and site of PLB regulation of the Ca^{2+} pump of sarcoplasmic reticulum. Nature 342: 90–92

12. Jones LR, Simmerman HKB, Wilson WW, Gurd FRN, Wegener AD (1985) Purification and characterization of phospholamban from canine cardiac sarcoplasmic reticulum. J Biol Chem 260: 7721–7730
13. Kim HW, Steenaart NAE, Ferguson, DG, Kranias EG (1990) Functional reconstitution of the cardiac sarcoplasmic reticulum Ca^{2+} ATPase with phospholamban in phospholipid vesicles. J Biol Chem 265: 1702–1709
14. Kimura Y, Kurzydlowski K, Tada M, MacLennan DH (1996) Phospholamban regulates the Ca^{2+}-ATPase through intramembrane interactions. J Biol Chem 271: 21726–21731
15. Lytton J, MacLennan DH (1988) Molecular cloning of cDNAs from human kidney coding for two alternatively spliced products of the cardiac Ca^{2+}-ATPase gene. J Biol Chem 263: 15024–15031
16. Lytton J, Westlin M, Burk SE, Shull GE, MacLennan DH (1992) Functional comparisons between isoforms of the sarcoplasmic or endoplasmic reticulum family of calcium pumps. J Biol Chem 267: 14483–14489
17. MacLennan DH (1990) Molecular tools to elucidate problems in excitation-contraction coupling. Biophys J 58: 1355–1365
18. MacLennan DH, Brandl CJ, Korczak B, Green NM (1985) Sequence of a Ca^{2+} + Mg^{2+} dependent ATPase from rabbit muscle sarcoplasmic reticulum, deduced from its complementary DNA sequence. Nature 316: 696–700
19. MacLennan DH, Clarke DM, Loo TW, Skerjanc I (1992a) Site-directed mutagenesis of the Ca^{2+} ATPase of sarcoplasmic reticulum. Acta Physiol Scand 146: 141–150
20. MacLennan DH, Toyofuku T, Lytton J (1992b) Structure-function relationships in sarcoplasmic or endoplasmic reticulum type Ca^{2+} pumps. Ann NY Acad Sci 671: 1–10
21. Morris GL, Cheng H-C, Colyer J, Wang JH (1991) Phospholamban regulation of cardiac sarcoplasmic reticulum $(Ca^{2+}-Mg^{2+})$-ATPase. Mechanism of regulation and site of monoclonal antibody interaction. J Biol Chem 266: 11270–11275
22. Reddy LG, Jones LR, Cala SE, O'Brian JJ, Tatulian SA, Stokes DL (1995) Functional reconstitution of recombinant phospholamban with rabbit skeletal Ca^{2+}-ATPase. J Biol Chem 270: 9390–9397
23. Sasaki T, Inui M, Kimura Y, Kuzuya T, Tada M (1992) Molecular mechanism of regulation of Ca^{2+} pump ATPase by phospholamban in cardiac sarcoplasmic reticulum. Effects of synthetic phospholamban peptides on Ca^{2+} pump ATPase. J Biol Chem 267: 1674–1679
24. Simmerman HKB, Collins JH, Thiebert JL, Wegener AD, Jones LR (1986) Sequence analysis of phospholamban: Identification of phosphorylation sites and two major structural domains. J Biol Chem 261: 13333–13341
25. Szymanska G, Kim HW, Cuppoletti J, Kranias EG (1992) Regulation of the skeletal sarcoplasmic reticulum Ca^{2+}-pump by phospholamban in reconstituted vesicles. Membrane Biochem 9: 191–202
26. Tada M, Katz AM (1982) Phosphorylation of the sarcoplasmic reticulum and sarcolemna. Ann Rev Physiol 44: 401–423
27. Tada M, Kirchberger MA, Katz AM (1975) Phosphorylation of a 22,000-dalton component of the cardiac sarcoplasmic reticulum by adenosine 3'-5'-monophosphate-dependent protein kinase. J Biol Chem 250: 2640–2647
28. Toyofuku T, Kurzydlowski K, Lytton J, MacLennan DH (1992) The nucleotide binding/hinge domain plays a crucial role in determining isoform specific Ca^{2+} dependence of organellar Ca^{2+} ATPases. J Biol Chem 267: 14490–14496
29. Toyofuku T, Kurzydlowski K, Tada M, MacLennan DH (1993) Identification of regions in the Ca^{2+} ATPase of sarcoplasmic reticulum that affect functional association with phospholamban. J Biol Chem 268: 2809–2815
30. Toyofuku T, Kurzydlowski K, Tada M, MacLennan DH (1994a) Amino acids Glu^2 to Ile^{18} in the cytoplasmic domain of phospholamban are essential for functional association with the Ca^{2+} ATPase of sarcoplasmic reticulum. J Biol Chem 269: 3088–3094
31. Toyofuku T, Kurzydlowski K, Tada M, MacLennan DH (1994b) Amino acids Lys-Asp-Asp-Lys-Pro-Val^{402} in the Ca^{2+}-ATPase of cardiac sarcoplasmic reticulum are critical for functional association with phospholamban. J Biol Chem 269: 22929–22932
32. Xu Z-C, Kirchberger MA (1989) Modulation by polyelectrolytes of canine cardiac microsomal calcium putake and the possible relationship of phospholamban. J Biol Chem 264: 16644–16651

Authors' address:
Dr. David H. MacLennan
Banting and Best Department of Medical Research
University of Toronto
Charles H. Best Institute
112 College St.,
Toronto, Ontario, Canada M5G1L6

The relative phospholamban and SERCA2 ratio: a critical determinant of myocardial contractility

K. L. Koss, I. L. Grupp[1], E. G. Kranias[1]

Dept. of Molecular and Cellular Physiology, University of Cincinnati College of Medicine, Cincinnati, USA
[1] Dept. of Pharmacology and Cell Biophysics, University of Cincinnati College of Medicine, Cincinnati, USA

Abstract

Phospholamban is a regulatory phosphoprotein which modulates the active transport of Ca^{2+} by the cardiac sarcoplasmic reticular Ca^{2+}-ATPase enzyme (SERCA2) into the lumen of the sarcoplasmic reticulum. Phospholamban, which is a reversible inhibitor of SERCA2, represses the enzyme's activity, and this inhibition is relieved upon phosphorylation of phospholamban in response to β-adrenergic stimulation. In this way, phospholamban is an important regulator of SERCA2-mediated myocardial relaxation during diastole. This report centers on the hypothesis that the relative levels of phospholamban: SERCA2 in cardiac muscle plays an important role in the muscle's overall contractility status. This hypothesis was tested by comparing the contractile parameters of: a) murine atrial and ventricular muscles, which differentially express phospholamban, and b) murine wild-type and phospholamban knock-out hearts. These comparisons revealed that atrial muscles, which have a 4.2-fold lower phospholamban: SERCA2 ratio than ventricular muscles, exhibited rates of force development and relaxation of tension, which were three-fold faster that these parameters for ventricular muscles. Similar comparisons were made via analyses of left-ventricular pressure development recorded for isolated, work-performing hearts from wild-type and phospholamban knock-out mice. In these studies, hearts from phospholamban knock-out mice, which were devoid of phospholamban, exhibited enhanced parameters of left-ventricular contractility in comparison to wild-type hearts. These results suggest that the relative phospholamban: SERCA2 ratio is critical in the regulation of myocardial contractility and alterations in this ratio may contribute to the functional deterioration observed during heart failure.

Key words Phospholamban – SERCA2 – atrium – ventricle – gene-targeting

Introduction

Phospholamban is a regulatory phosphoprotein of cardiac sarcoplasmic reticulum membrane, which is phosphorylated *in vivo* in response to β-adrenergic agonist stimulation (1). This relatively small phosphoprotein, which is 6080 D in size, modulates the active transport of Ca^{2+} into the cardiac sarcoplasmic reticulum via reversible regulation of the sarcoplasmic reticular Ca^{2+}-ATPase enzyme (SERCA2) (2, 3, 4). In the dephosphorylated sate, phospholamban inhibits Ca^{2+}-ATPase activity by decreasing the affinity of the enzyme for Ca^{2+} (5). Such inhibition of the Ca^{2+}-ATPase enzyme by phospholamban increases the EC_{50} of the enzyme for Ca^{2+} resulting in decreased Ca^{2+}-uptake into the cardiac sarcoplasmic reticulum, ultimately prolonging myofibrillar relaxation time (6). Inversely, phosphorylation of phospholamban, in response to β-adrenergic stimulation, relieves this inhibition, producing an increase in the affinity of the enzyme for Ca^{2+} and increasing the rate of myofibrillar relaxation (7). Therefore, the phosphorylation status of phospholamban is a primary determinant of calcium sequestration and of myocardial relaxation.

Recently, it has been demonstrated that phospholamban is not only a regulator of myocardial relaxation, but it is also an important regulator of the basal cardiac contraction cycle and that phosphorylation of phospholamban in intact hearts is a major regulatory pathway involved in the heart's responses to β-adrenergic stimulation. To determine the regulatory role of phospholamban in basal myocardial contractility, mice were generated in which the phospholamban gene was ablated using gene-targeting methodologies (8). These phospholamban knock-out mice, which have disrupted phospholamban alleles, exhibited hyperdynamic cardiac function including increased rates of basal myocardial contraction as well as increased rates of basal myocardial relaxation (8–10), demonstrating the functional role of phospholamban in both the contractile and relaxational phases of the cardiac cycle. In addition, hearts from the phospholamban knock-out mice, when studied as isolated, work-performing preparations, were refractory to administration of isoproterenol (8, 9). These experiments were instrumental in the delineation of the important functional role of phospholamban in the myocardial β-adrenergic signaling pathway.

This report centers on the hypothesis that phospholamban is an important regulator of the basal cardiac contraction cycle and is founded on studies of the phospholamban knock-out mouse, which demonstrate that phospholamban is a potent repressor of both myocardial contractility and myocardial relaxation (9, 10). Furthermore, this hypothesis is supported by recent studies on the differential contractility parameters of murine atrial and ventricular muscles, which are correlated with the respective differential expression of phospholamban in the muscles (9, 11). Our data indicate that the relative levels of phospholamban: SERCA2 in cardiac muscle have a determinant function as to the muscle's overall contractility status. The basal contractility parameters for muscles with relatively high phospholamban: SERCA2 ratios, are lower in comparison to those for muscles with relatively low phospholamban: SERCA2 ratios (8–11). These studies suggest that variations in phospholamban expression levels, which alter sarcoplasmic reticular function, are associated with concomitant variations in myocardial contractility. Thus, the relationship between phospholamban expression levels and myocardial contractility may be an important aspect of myocardial loss-of-function during cardiomyopathic disease, as well as an important consideration for restoration-of-function in cardiomyopathic therapy.

Methods

In situ hybridization of cardiopulmonary tissue sections

Cardiopulmonary tissues were excised from young adult female mice, rinsed with PBS, fixed in 4 % paraformaldehyde, and cryopreserved as previously described (11). All solutions were prepared under RNase-free conditions as outlined by Sambrook et al. (12). Tissues were sectioned, mounted, and permeabilized as previously described (11) and were then hybridized with [^{35}S]-labeled riboprobes, which were synthesized as phospholamban cRNA products using a template consisting of a DNA polymerase chain reaction product, subcloned into PBS SK$^-$ (11). The cRNA sequence and hybridization procedure have been previously reported (11). Hybridized tissue sections were processed according to previously described methods (13, 14) and were photographed using the dark-field optics of an Olympus BHTU microscope.

Analysis of cardiac RNA

In preparation for dot blot quantitation, total RNA was extracted and spectrophotometrically quantitated from right and left atrial flaps (auricles), ventricular apices comprised of left and right ventricular muscle, and whole hearts as previously described (11). Three RNA pools were collected from total RNA extracts from 180 atrial flaps, 30 ventricular apices, and eight whole-hearts. Serial dilutions of RNA extracts were blotted, three consecutive times each, onto triplicate nylon membranes, and quantitation of phospolamban and SERCA2 mRNA transcripts, relative to α-MyHC mRNA were performed as previously described (11). The phospholamban oligonucleotide probes, utilized in these studies, were analyzed for specificity on both Southern and Northern blots prior to being used in dot blot hybridization (11).

Isometric contractility measurements for isolated, superfused atrial and ventricular muscles

Cardiac muscles were dissected from anesthetized, heparinized female FVB/N mice according to the method of Grupp and Grupp (15). For atrial measurements, the left atrial appendages (auricles) were utilized, as the right auricles had to be excluded due to automatic pacemaker activity. For ventricular measurements, muscle strips containing the ventricular out-flow tract were dissected from right ventricles, while the left ventricles were excluded due to size (11). The muscles were mounted in baths and superfused at 35 °C. This was accomplished by mounting two atrial or two ventricular muscles in the same bath using double-electrode clamp holders. One end of each muscle was clamped firmly on top of two electrodes, while the other end was connected via suture filament to the mechanical arm of a force transducer. The muscles were electrically stimulated as previously described (11). Great care was taken so that muscle orientation was identical between experiments as described by Koss et al.

(11). Resting tension was set via micrometer, and following equilibration, length-tension curves were established. Final equilibration was achieved close to maximum length-tension (L_{max}), and all muscles were normalized for loading conditions at L_{max} as previously described (11). Muscles were stimulated with isoproterenol as previously described (11). For each muscle, developed force, resting tension, the rate of force development ($+dF/dt$), and the rate of relaxation of tension ($-dF/dt$) were recorded via polygraph. Measurements of time-to-peak tension (TPT) and time to half-relaxation of tension ($RT_{1/2}$) were made by digital micrometer. These measurements were normalized to the developed force and are expressed as mean ms/mg $\pm$ S.E.M. Measurements of $+dF/dt$ and $-dF/dt$ are reported as mean mg/s $\pm$ S.E.M. Significance between paired comparisons was determined using paired t-test analyses.

Generation of phospolamban-deficient (phospholamban knock-out) mice

Phospholamban knock-out mice were generated using gene targeting methodologies as described by Luo et al. (8). Heterozygous mice carrying a phospholamban-ablated allele were bred to homozygosity, generating phospholamban knock-out mice (8). Wild-type, litter-mate mice of identical mixed-strain background were bred simultaneously for use in control experiments (8).

Contractility measurements for isolated, work-performing hearts from phospholamban knock-out and wild-type mice

Work-performing heart preparations were carried-out according to the methodology described by Grupp et al. (10). Measurements of developed left-ventricular pressure (DP), rate of left-ventricular pressure development ($+dP/dt$), and rate of pressure release ($-dP/dt$) were recorded as previously described (8, 10). These are reported as mean developed mm Hg/s $\pm$ S.E.M. under control conditions and at maximal isoproterenol stimulation, as previously described (8). The times to left-ventricular peak pressure development (TPP) and to half-relaxation of left ventricular pressure ($RT_{1/2}$) were measured via digital micrometer and normalized to DP. These are reported as mean ms/mm Hg $\pm$ S.E.M. under control conditions and during maximal isoproterenol stimulation, as previously described (8). Significance of paired comparisons was determined using paired t-test analyses.

Results

Phospholamban and SERCA2 transcript levels in atrial and ventricular muscles

In order to study the distribution of phospholamban gene transcripts in the murine heart, we performed *in situ* hybridization studies of murine cardiopulmonary sections (Fig. 1). Hybridization of these tissue sections with a phospholamban ribo-probe (antisense to the murine phospholamban gene) revealed a differential pattern of intensities of the phospolamban antisense hybridization signal between atrial and ventricular cardiac compartments (Fig. 1; left). The tissue-autoradiogram shown in Fig. 1, shows a higher intensity of phospholamban hybridization signal in the ventricle than in the atrium. This finding is similar to that which we have previously reported for other murine cardiac tissues, hybridized with radio-labeled phospholamban cRNA (11). Background hybridization for the phospolamban antisense cRNA probe is depicted in the lung tissue (Fig. 1; left). The degree of non-specific hybridization to the tissues was evaluated using a phospholamban sense riboprobe, which is demonstrated in the representative autoradiogram shown in Fig. 1 (right).

The differential pattern of phospholamban gene transcript expression observed between murine atrial and ventricular muscles in cardiac tissue sections, prompted us to extend our studies to include the relative *in vitro* quantitation of phospholamban mRNA in these muscles. Phospholamban gene transcripts were quantitated in RNA extracts from atrial and ventricular muscles, using previously described dot blot techniques (11). A 60-bp oligonucleotide, antisense to a portion of the murine phospolamban gene coding region, was used as a probe for this analysis. Prior to use on dot blots, the efficacy and specificity of this probe was demonstrated on Southern blots of murine genomic DNA and on Northern blots of murine cardiac RNA (11). A representative autoradiogram of a dot blot, probed for phospholamban mRNA is shown in Fig. 2. In addition to RNA extracts from atrial and ventricular muscles, RNA extracts from whole hearts were blotted onto the same membrane and served as standards for normalization of RNA loading onto the membranes. In addition, this provided for quantitation of relative expression levels of atrial and ventricular gene

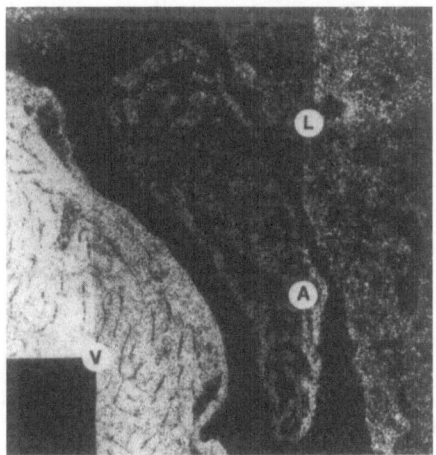 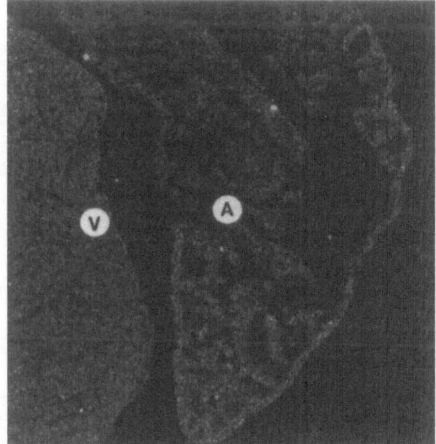

Fig. 1. Differential phospholamban gene transcript expression visualized by *in situ* hybridization of cardiopulmonary sections from the FVB/N mouse. Tissue sections from wild-type FVB/N mice were probed with either cRNA, antisense to the phospholamban gene (left) or phospholamban sense-strand cRNA (right) as a control. All photomicrographs were taken under dark-field illumination. The composite photomicrographs allow for visualization of phospholamban gene expression in murine atrium (A) and ventricle (V). Background hybridization of the antisense cRNA probe is depicted in the lung (L).

transcripts to the whole heart. Each blot also contained: 1) tRNA blotted at the same concentration as the cardiac RNA samples, serving as a negative control; and 2) the diluent (SSC) blotted as a blank, demonstrating no carry-over or contamination of the diluent in serial dilutions (Fig. 2). As previously described, the RNA samples were additionally probed for quantitation of alpha myosin heavy chain (α-MyHC) mRNA, and phospolamban gene transcripts were expressed relative to α-MyHC transcripts in order to normalize these measurements relative to cardiac muscle (11).

Quantitative results obtained from dot blot analyses indicate that phospholamban gene transcripts are significantly lower in atrial muscles than in ventricular muscles,

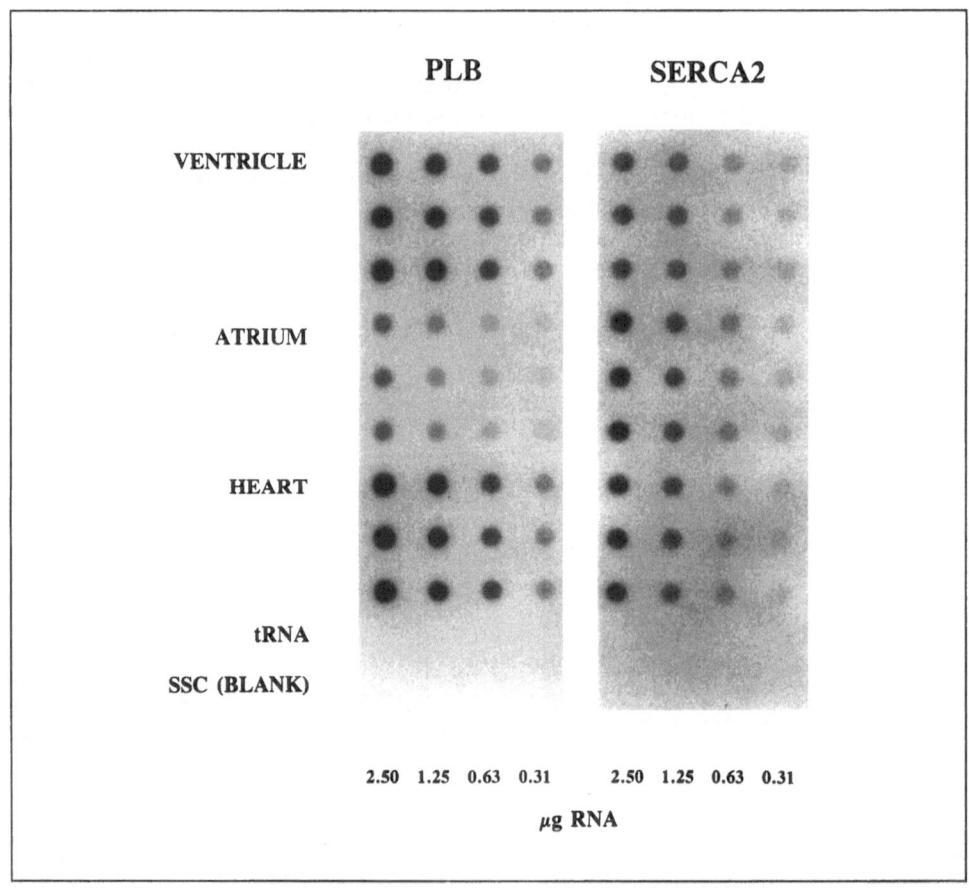

Fig. 2. Dot blot quantitation of phospholamban and SERCA2 gene transcripts in murine atrium and ventricle. Representative autoradiograms are shown in the photos depicting total cardiac RNA extracts, which were blotted onto nylon membranes and probed with [^{32}P]-end labeled DNA oligonucleotides. Blots were probed with either a 60-bp oligonucleotide, antisense to the murine phospholamban gene or a 60-bp oligonucleotide, antisense to the murine SERCA2 gene. Measurements of phospholamban and SERCA2 mRNAs were normalized to α-MyHC mRNA by blotting of the pooled RNA samples onto separate membranes, which were probed with an oligonucleotide, antisense to the murine α-MyHC gene. All dot blots were standardized for RNA membrane-loading via subsequent re-probing with a 60-bp oligonucleotide, antisense to the murine 18S gene.

when expressed relative to the whole heart (Fig. 2). Our data indicate that the relative ratio of phospholamban to α-MyHC was 3.2-fold higher in the murine ventricles as compared to murine atrial muscles (Fig. 3). This ratio is similar to that previously reported comparing murine ventricular phospholamban mRNA copy numbers to those of the atrium (11). That report showed ventricular mRNA to be 2.5-fold above atrial mRNA in measurements which were not normalized to a cardiac muscle indicator such as α-MyHC.

To determine whether SERCA2 is also differentially expressed between murine atrial and ventricular compartments, we similarly analyzed the transcript ratios of SERCA2 relative to α-MyHC mRNA, using dot blots of the same cardiac RNA samples used in the quantitation of phospholamban gene transcripts (Fig. 3). Blotted RNA was probed with a 60–bp oligonucleotide, antisense to a portion of the murine SERCA2 gene. The specificity of this probe was previously determined via hybridization of murine cardiac mRNA on Northern blots (data not shown). These results demonstrate that ventricular SERCA2 mRNA is 20 % below that found in atrial muscle (Fig. 2). Therefore, the relative ratio of phospolamban: SERCA2 is 4.2-fold higher in the murine ventricle than in the murine atrium.

Contractility measurements for atrial and ventricular muscle tissues

Since phospholamban is an important regulator of basal myocardial contractility in the mouse (8–10) and since it appears that phospholamban is differentially expressed between murine cardiac compartments (11), parameters of atrial and ventricular contractility were assessed for isolated, superfused atrial and ventricular muscles in

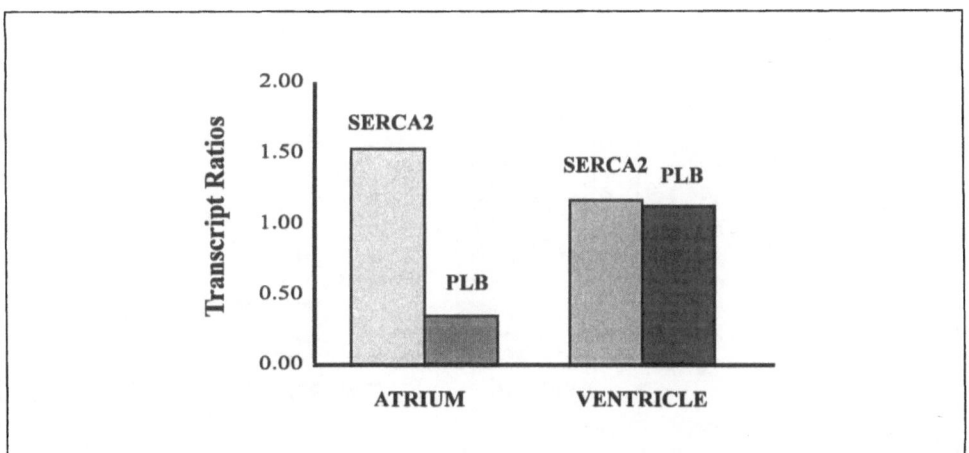

Fig. 3. Relative gene expression levels of phospholamban and SERCA2 gene transcripts to cardiac α-MyHC in murine atrium and ventricle. Atrial SERCA2 mRNA is 1.2-fold above that of ventricular muscle, while atrial phospholamban mRNA is three-fold below that of ventricular muscle. All mRNA levels were measured by phosphorimager analysis of hybridized RNA dot blots and reported relative to whole heart mRNA. Values represent the mean of six determinations.

order to determine whether there exists a correlation between varying levels of phospholamban and contractility for these muscles. For each isolated muscle, resting tension (mg), developed force (mg), rate of force development (+dF/dt in mg/s), and rate of relaxation of tension (−dF/dt in mg/s) were recorded. Each muscle was normalized for loading conditions to maximal length-tension (L_{max}) and isoproterenol responses were then recorded. Our findings demonstrate that at L_{max} under basal isometric stimulation, the atrial muscles exhibited on average a three-fold faster rate of contraction than did the ventricular muscles ($p < 0.05$) (Fig. 4). This relationship also held true for the rates of atrial vs. ventricular relaxation of tension, which on average were nearly three-fold faster for atria as compared to ventricles ($p < 0.05$) (Fig. 4). It is interesting to note that the slower rates of ventricular contraction and relaxation, which are three-fold slower than those observed for atrial muscles, correlate with the higher level of ventricular phospholamban transcript expression, which is three-fold higher in the ventricle than in the atrium (Figs. 3 and 4).

Contractile parameters for the time-to-peak tension (TPT) and the time to half-relaxation of tension ($RT_{1/2}$) were measured from atrial and ventricular recordings of developed force via digital micrometer for each muscle. These parameters were calculated in ms and were normalized to the extent of developed force (mg). Time parameters, reported as mean ms/mg are shown in Table 1. These data demonstrate that at L_{max}, the ventricular muscles exhibited significantly greater TPT and $RT_{1/2}$ values than did atrial muscles, indicating that these muscles required more time to develop a specific level of force as well as more time to relax following force development. This relationship also held true during isoproterenol stimulation of the muscles (Table 1). While isoproterenol significantly decreased TPT and $RT_{1/2}$ parameters for both muscles groups (Table 1), at maximal isoproterenol response, the ventricular muscles still required more time to contract and to relax than did the atrial muscles

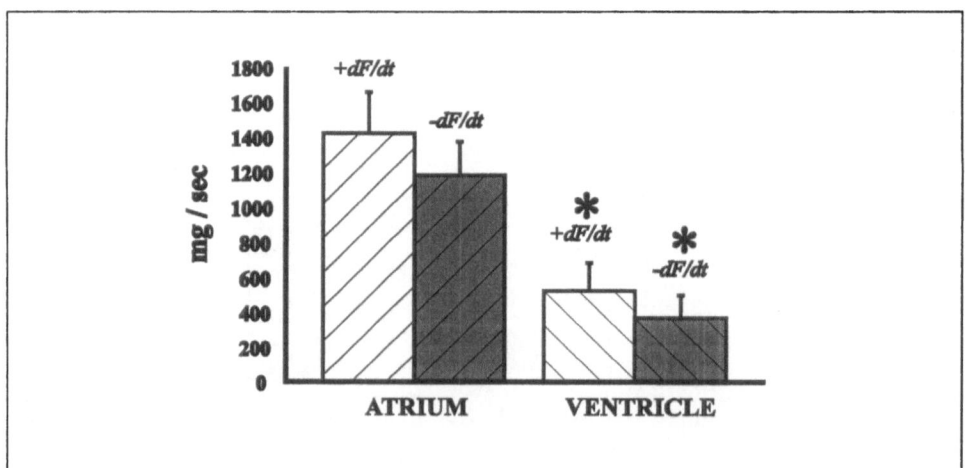

Fig. 4. Average rates of atrial and ventricular force development (+dF/dt) and relaxation of tension (−dF/dt). The rate of ventricular contraction (+dF/dt) is approx. three-fold slower than the rate of contraction for atrial muscle. Similarly, the rate of ventricular relaxation is nearly three times slower than the rate of atrial relaxation. Each average rate represents the mean ± S.E.M. for five to six individual muscles, recorded at maximal length-tension, which provided for normalization of the load on the muscles.

Table 1. Contractility parameters for isolated, superfused myocardial muscles. Reported as ms/mg developed force

	Atria (n = 7)	Ventricles (n = 4)	p Values* (df = 9)
TPT (L_{max})	0.66 ± 0.88	2.75 ± 0.50	0.0004
TPT (ISO-$_{max}$)	0.25 ± 0.03	0.85 ± 0.27	0.0136
p values**	0.0006	0.016	
$RT_{1/2}$ (L_{max})	0.41 ± 0.05	2.14 ± 0.34	0.0001
$RT_{1/2}$ (ISO-$_{max}$)	0.14 ± 0.02	0.52 ± 0.12	0.003
p values**	0.0006	0.004	

n indicates number of muscles; $RT_{1/2}$ is the time to half-relaxation; TPT is the time to peak-tension; df indicates degrees of freedom.
  * Assessed by *t*-test for paired comparisons between atrial and ventricular strips.
 ** Assessed by *t*-test for paired comparisons between basal and maximal for a given tissue.

(Table 1). Such greater time parameters for ventricular muscles as compared to atrial muscles correlate with the greater levels of phospholamban compared to SERCA2 gene expression in the ventricular muscles compared to atria (Figs. 1, 2 and 3).

Contractility measurements for isolated, work-performing hearts from phospholamban knock-out and wild-type mice

In order to determine the role of phospholamban in murine myocardial contractility, measurements of developed left-ventricular pressure (DP), rate of left-ventricular pressure development (+dP/dt), and rate of pressure release (−dP/dt) were recorded for isolated work-performing hearts from both wild-type and phospholamban knock-out mice. These studies demonstrate that in the absence of phospholamban, both the rate of left-ventricular pressure-development and the rate of left-ventricular pressure-release are significantly enhanced when compared to similar measurements for hearts from aged-matched, wild-type litter-mate mice (Fig. 5A). In addition, time parameters (in ms) of left-ventricular contractility were calculated from recordings of left-ventricular force development for each heart and were normalized to the extent of left-ventricular pressure development (in mm Hg) for that respective heart. These parameters, reported as mean ms/mm Hg are shown in Fig. 5B. In the phospolamban knock-out heart, both the TPP and $RT_{1/2}$ parameters are significantly shortened with respect to these parameters in wild-type hearts (Fig. 5B). These shortened parameters indicate that in the absence of phospholamban, the heart cannot only relax more quickly, but can also contract more quickly compared to hearts in which phospolamban is normally expressed.

Administration of isoproterenol via cumulative dosage failed to inotropically stimulate the phospholamban knock-out hearts, in contrast to wild-type hearts, which displayed enhanced contractility parameters for DP, +dP/dt, −dP/dt, TPP, and $RT_{1/2}$ (8–10). These parameters were not significantly affected, even at isoproterenol doses, which maximally stimulated the wild-type hearts (8–10). However, heart rate increased in both wild-type and phospholamban knock-out hearts during isoproterenol exposure (8). It is also interesting to note that the maximally stimulated contrac-

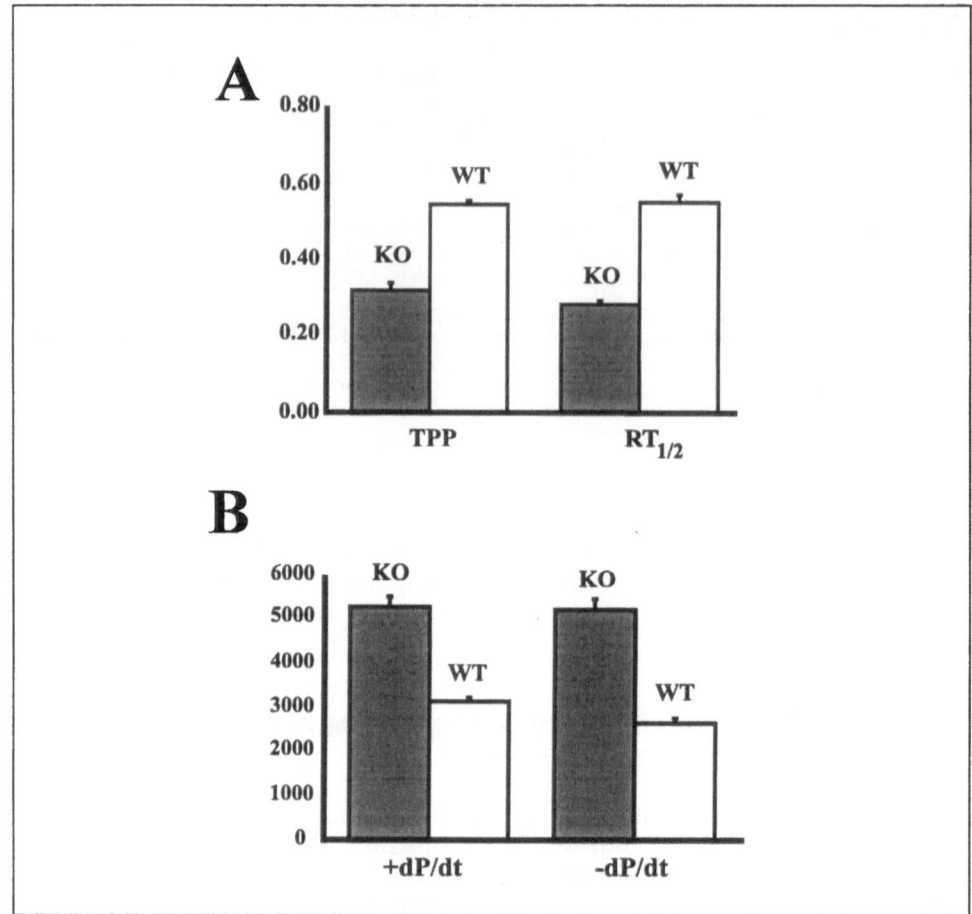

Fig. 5. Contractility parameters for isolated, perfused hearts from wild-type (WT) and phospholamban knock-out (KO) mice. The average time to left-ventricular peak pressure development (TPP) and average time to half-relaxation of developed pressure (RT$_{1/2}$) are represented in Fig. 5A as mean ms ± S.E.M., normalized to mm Hg of developed pressure (DP). The average rate of left-ventricular pressure development (+dP/dt) and rate of pressure release (−dP/dt) are depicted in Fig. 5B as mean mm Hg/ms ± S.E.M.

tile parameters in wild-type hearts were similar to the basal levels of these parameters in the phospholamban knock-out hearts (8–10).

Discussion

In this report, we suggest that the phospholamban: SERCA2 ratio is a critical regulator of contractility in cardiac muscle. This suggestion is based on our findings in murine atrial and ventricular muscles and in phospholamban knock-out hearts.

Murine atrial muscles, which have relatively low phospholamban: SERCA2 ratios, have faster rates of contraction and relaxation, as well as shorter times to peak tension development than do ventricular muscles, which have a higher phospholamban: SERCA2 ratio (11). Our data demonstrate that while SERCA2 expression is similar between atrial and ventricular muscles, phospholamban is differentially expressed between these two muscles with the ventricle having three-fold greater phospholamban than the atrium. This differential phospholamban gene expression gives rise to the different phospholamban: SERCA2 ratios observed for these muscles. While it is clear that the relatively low phospholamban: SERCA2 ratio is not the only factor affecting differences between atrial and ventricular contractility, the suggestion that this low ratio is an important determinant of enhanced atrial contractility is consistent with observations recently reported for hearts from hyperthyroid rats which displayed decreased levels of phospholamban and enhanced sarcoplasmic reticular Ca^{2+}-uptake (17). However, effects due to other atrial factors such as: 1) shortened action potential duration, 2) abbreviated calcium currents, or 3) differential myosin light-chain expression may also have a role in the enhanced contractility of atrial muscles as compared to ventricles (11).

Comparative association of the enhanced contractile properties of atrial muscles to ventricular muscles with the relatively lower phospholamban content of atrial muscle, is in keeping with our recent observations on enhanced myocardial contractility in a phospholamban knock-out mouse (8–10). Hearts from these mice, which are devoid of phospholamban, express a Ca^{2+}-ATPase enzyme, which is unregulated by phospholamban (8–10). Measurements of left-ventricular contractility made from isolated, work-performing heart preparations, demonstrated that the phospholamban knock-out hearts displayed greatly enhanced contractile parameters in comparison to hearts from wild-type mice. The increased inotropic characteristics of the phospholamban knock-out hearts includes shortened times to left-ventricular peak pressure development, shortened times to half-relaxation of tension, enhanced rates of pressure development, and enhanced rates of pressure release (8–10). In addition, these hearts exhibited no chronotropic differences in comparison to wild-type controls (8). Consistent with these observations on the critical role of the phospholamban: SERCA2 ratio in contractility, recent studies in our laboratory indicated that phospholamban over-expression in the murine heart results in an increased phospholamban: SERCA2 ratio and decreses in the contractile parameters (unpublished observations). Furthermore, it is interesting to note that hearts from phospholamban knock-out mice were refractory to the inotropic effects of isoproterenol, which was effective in stimulating wild-type hearts (8, 9). The lack of isoproterenol response in phospholamban knock-out hearts suggests that phosphorylation of phospholamban is a major signaling pathway through which the β-adrenergic stimulus is transduced in murine myocardium. A second explanation for the lack of isoproterenol stimulation of phospholamban knock-out hearts may simply be the fact that these hearts exist in a maximally-stimulated inotropic state, which is incapable of further enhancement. While measurements of both right and left wild-type ventricles displayed marked inotropic enhancement in response to isoproterenol (8–11), it is interesting to note that isoproterenol also had a marked inotropic effect on wild-type atrial muscle, despite the fact that phospholamban levels in this muscle were three-fold below those of the ventricles (11).

The mechanism through which murine phospholamban gene expression is differentially regulated in murine atrium and ventricle is at present, unknown. Our recent studies on phospholamban and SERCA2 gene transcript expression in these cardiac compartments indicates that the expression of these genes is not regulated in a coordinate manner (11). This assertion is supported by reports in rat heart (17) and in rabbit heart (20), where hyperthyroidism and hypothyroidism affected the expression of phospholamban and SERCA2 in a dis-coordinate manner. Future studies using genetically altered, diseased, or aged animals will lend great insight as to the regulation of expression of these two cardiac sarcoplasmic reticular genes, which are so important in the regulation of myocardial contractility. In addition, molecular studies designed to isolate and express the phospholamban gene promoter will eventually lead to a greater understanding as to how the differential expression of this gene is regulated in cardiac compartments. This understanding will be an important tool for deciphering the role of altered phospholamban gene expression in cardiac disease.

Acknowledgments　This work was supported by National Institutes of Health Grants HL08901 (K.L.K.) and HL26057 and HL22619 (E.G.K.).

REFERENCES

1. Lindeman JP, Jones LR, Hathaway DR, Henry BG, Watanabe AM (1983) β-adrenergic stimulation of phospholamban phosphorylation and Ca^{2+}-ATPase activity in guinea pig ventricles. J Biol Chem 258: 464–471
2. Kranias EG (1985) Regulation of Ca^{2+} transport by cyclic $3':5'$-AMP-dependent and calcium-calmodulin dependent phosphorylation of cardiac sarcoplasmic reticulum. Biochim Biophys Acta 844: 193–199
3. Kranias EG (1986) Regulation of Ca^{2+} transport by phosphoprotein phosphatase activity associated with cardiac sarcoplasmic reticulum. J Biol Chem 260: 11006–11010
4. Edes I, Kranias EG (1989) Regulation of the cardiac sarcoplasmic reticulum function by phospholamban. Membr Biochem 7: 175–192
5. Mundina de Weilenmann C, Vittone L, de Cingolani G et al. (1987) Dissociation between contraction and relaxation: The possible role of phospholamban phosphorylation. Basic Res Cardiol 82: 507–516
6. Kranias EG, Garvey JL, Srivastava RD et al. (1985) Phosphorylation and functional modifications of sarcoplasmic reticulum and myofibrils in isolated rabbit hearts stimulated with isoprenaline. Biochem J 226: 113–121
7. Talosi L, Edes I, Kranias EG (1993) Intracellular mechanisms mediating the reversal of β-adrenergic stimulation in intact beating hearts. Am J Physiol 264: H791–H797
8. Luo W, Grupp IL, Doetschman T, Ponniah S, Harrer J, Zhou Z, Kranias EG (1994) Targeted ablation of the phospholamban gene is associated with markedly enhanced myocardial contractility and loss of β-agonist stimulation. Circ Res 75: 401–409
9. Luo W, Kiss E, Koss KL, Grupp IL, Harrer J, Edes I, Jones WK, Kranias EG (1995) Cardiac remodeling by alterations in phospholamban protein levels. Heart Hypertrophy and Failure. Dhalla NS, Pierce GN, Panagia V, Blamish RE (eds). Kluwer Academic Press, Boston, MA (in press)
10. Grupp IL, Kranias EG, Kiss E, Harrer JM, Slack J, Koss KL, Lui W, Grupp G (1995) The contribution of phospholamban, a sarcoplasmic reticulum phosphoprotein, to myocardial contractility in health and disease. Heart Failure 11: 48–61
11. Koss KL, Ponniah S, Jones WK, Grupp IL, Kranias EG (1995) Differential expression of the phospholamban gene in murine cardiac compartments: Molecular and physiological analyses. Circ Res 77: 342–353
12. Sambrook J, Fritsch EF, Maniatis T (1989) Molecular Cloning. New York, NY: Cold Spring Harbor Laboratory Press
13. Cox KH, DeLeon DV, Angerer LM, Angerer RC (1984) Detection of mRNAs in sea urchin embryos by *in situ* hybridization using asymmetric RNA probes. Dev Biol 101: 485–502
14. Jones WK, Sanchez A, Robbins JR (1994) The murine pulmonary myocardium: developmental analysis of cardiac gene expression. Dev Dyn 200: 117–128

15. Grupp IL, Grupp G (1984) Isolated heart preparations perfused or superfused with balanced salt solutions. Methods in Pharmacol 5: 111–128
16. Toyofuku T, Zak R (1991) Characterization of cDNA and genomic sequences encoding a chicken phospholamban. J Biol Chem 266: 5375–5383
17. Kiss E, Jakab G, Kranias EG, Edes I (1994) Thyroid hormone-induced alterations in phospholamban protein expression: regulatory effects on sarcoplasmic reticulum Ca^{2+} transport and myocardial relaxation. Circ Res 75: 245–251
18. Garvey J, Kranias EG, Solaro RJ (1988) Phosphorylation of C-protein, troponin I, and phospholamban in isolated rabbit hearts. Biochem J 245: 709–714
19. Presti CF, Jones LR, Lindemann JP (1991) Isoproterenol-induced phosphorylation of a 15-kilodalton sarcolemmal protein sarcolemmal protein in intact myocardium. J Biol Chem 266: 11126–11130
20. Arai M, Otsu K, MacLennan DH, Alpert NR, Periasamy M (1991) Effect of thyroid hormone on the expression of mRNA encoding sarcoplasmic reticulum proteins. Circ Res 69: 266–276

Authors' address:
Evangelia G. Kranias, PhD
Dept. of Pharmacology and Cell Biophysics
University of Cincinnati College of Medicine
231 Bethesda Ave.
Cincinnati, Ohio 45267-0575, USA

Phosphorylation and regulation of the Ca^{2+}-pumping ATPase in cardiac sarcoplasmic reticulum by calcium/calmodulin-dependent protein kinase

N. Narayanan, A. Xu

Department of Physiology, Medical Sciences Building, University of Western Ontario, London, Canada

Abstract

In cardiac muscle, a membrane-associated Ca^{2+}/calmodulin-dependent protein kinase (CaM kinase) phosphorylates the Ca^{2+}-pumping ATPase in addition to its previously characterized substrates, phospholamban and Ca^{2+}-release channel (ryanodine receptor). The phosphorylated amino acid in the Ca^{2+}-ATPase has been identified as serine. Posphorylation of the Ca^{2+}-ATPase is rapid and is reversible by a membrane-associated protein phosphatase. Ca^{2+}-ATPase purified from cardiac SR underwent phosphorylation by exogenous CaM kinase, and the phosphorylated enzyme displayed twofold greater catalytic activity without alteration in its Ca^{2+}-sensitivity. The phosphorylation of the Ca^{2+}-ATPase was found to be isoform-specific in that the cardiac and slow-twitch skeletal muscle isoform (SERCA 2), but not the fast-twitch skeletal muscle isoform (SERCA 1), underwent phosphorylation by CaM kinase. Studies using SERCA 1 and SERCA 2 isoforms and their mutants expressed in a heterelogous cell system have resulted in i) confirmation of the isoform specificity of Ca^{2+}-ATPase phosphorylation by CaM kinase, ii) identification of Ser^{38} as the site in SERCA 2 phosphorylated by CaM kinase, and iii) demonstration of phosphorylation-induced increase in Vmax of Ca^{2+} transport by the SERCA 2 enzyme. These observations suggest that in cardiac and slow-twitch skeletal muscle direct phosphorylation of the SR Ca^{2+}-ATPase by the membrane-bound CaM kinase may serve to stimulate Ca^{2+} sequestration and therefore, the speed of muscle relaxation.

Key words Cardiac muscle – sarcoplasmic reticulum – calcium ATPase – CaM kinase

Introduction

By regulating the concentration of cytosolic free Ca^{2+}, the sarcoplasmic reticulum (SR) plays a central role in the contraction-relaxation cycle of heart muscle. Excitation of cardiac muscle cells leads to the release of Ca^{2+} from the SR through a Ca^{2+} release channel (the ryanodine receptor), and the consequent increase in cytoplasmic Ca^{2+} produces myofilament activation and muscle contraction (1–4). Subsequently, active sequestration of Ca^{2+} back into the SR lumen by a Ca^{2+}-pumping

ATPase (Ca^{2+}-ATPase) in the SR lowers the cytoplasmic Ca^{2+}, thus promoting muscle relaxation (2, 3, 5). The Ca^{2+}-pumping function of this ATPase is well known to be regulated by another cardiac SR-specific protein, phospholamban (2, 6–9). Evidence from several studies suggest that non-phosphorylated phospholamban interacts with the ATPase and exerts an inhibitory effect on the Ca^{2+} pump and that phosphorylation of phospholamban by cAMP-dependent protein kinase (PKA) or Ca^{2+}/calmodulin-dependent protein kinase (CaM kinase) results in disruption of the ATPase-phospholamban interaction leading to removal of inhibition and consequent activation of the Ca^{2+} pump (6–14). In cardiac SR, the Ca^{2+}-release channel also undergoes phosphorylation by CaM kinase (15, 16), and this may result in stimulation of Ca^{2+} release from the SR (15). Recently, we have found that in cardiac SR, a membrane-associated CaM kinase phosphorylates the Ca^{2+}-ATPase, in addition to Ca^{2+} channel and phospholamban (17, 18). Phosphorylation of the Ca^{2+}-ATPase occurring at a serine residue, resulted in the stimulation of Ca^{2+}-dependent ATP hydrolysis and Ca^{2+} transport. Thus, phosphorylation of the Ca^{2+}-ATPase by the CaM kinase may provide an additional mechanism for the regulation of SR Ca^{2+} pump function. In this chapter, we review the studies demonstrating the phosphorylation and activation of the cardiac SR Ca^{2+}-ATPase by a membrane-associated CaM kinase.

Ca^{2+}/calmodulin-dependent phosphorylation of cardiac SR Ca^{2+}-ATPase

Findings, originally reported from our laboratory (19–22) and subsequently confirmed by others (23, 24) have described the presence of two distinct cytosolic proteins in heart muscle capable of modulating the Ca^{2+} uptake and release functions of the SR. One of these proteins, with an apparent molecular mass of 43 kDa, inhibits ATP-dependent Ca^{2+} uptake by SR membrane vesicles *in vitro* (19–24) and promotes Ca^{2+} release from the SR (21, 23, 24); the other, with an apparent molecular mass of 64 kDa, reverses the effects of 43 kDa protein (20, 22, 23). Recently, we found that calmodulin potentiated the action of 64 kDa protein in reversing the inhibition of SR Ca^{2+} uptake produced by the 43 kDa protein (25). However, the 64 kDa protein did not bind calmodulin, and it did not undergo phosphorylation by CaM kinase. In this, context, in attempting to understand the mechanism of action of calmodulin, we examined calmodulin-dependent protein phosphorylation in the SR membrane. Surprisingly, we found that when SR vesicles isolated from rabbit heart ventricles were incubated in a phosphorylation assay medium, a protein of approximate molcular mass 105 kDa underwent strong Ca^{2+} and calmodulin-dependent phosphorylation, in addition to phospholamban (6–9, 26) and Ca^{2+} channel (15, 16), the two previously characterized substrates for CaM kinase (Fig. 1). Western immunoblotting analysis and immunoprecipitation experiments using a Ca^{2+}-ATPase-specific antibody confirmed that the 105 kDa band undergoing phosphorylation represented the Ca^{2+}-pumping ATPase of SR. It was also established that the observed phosphorylation of the Ca^{2+}-ATPase is not due to the formation of the acylphoshate (aspartyl phosphate) intermediate of the Ca^{2+}-ATPase (27), since a) no phosphorylation occurred in the presence of Ca^{2+} without calmodulin (Fig. 1); b) acylphosphate does not survive the alkaline conditions of SDS-polyacrylamide gel electrophoresis (28); c) phosphorylation is fully resistant to hydroxylamine (0.8 M) treatment (29); and d) phosphoamino acid analysis revealed that the major amino acid residue undergoing phosphorylation is serine (17), unlike the case of phospholamban, where CaM kinase phosphorylates a threonine residue (30).

Isoform-specificity of Ca^{2+}-ATPase phosphorylation and identification of the phosphorylation site

The cardiac and slow-twitch skeletal muscle express the same Ca^{2+}-ATPase isoform (SERCA 2), which is distinct from that expressed in fast-twitch skeletal muscle

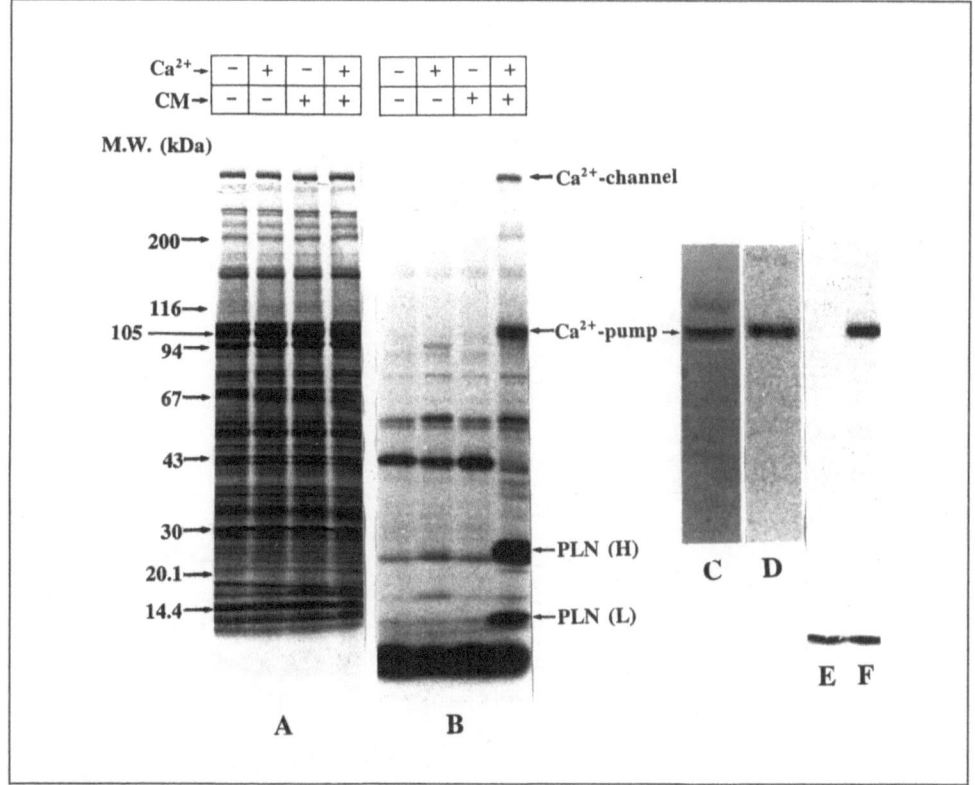

Fig. 1. Phosphorylation of Ca^{2+} channel and phospholamban (PLN; H, high molecular weight form; L, low molecular weight form) in rabbit cardiac SR by membrane-associated CaM kinase. **A)** Coomassie Blue-stained SDS-polyacrylamide gel showing SR protein profile. **B)** autoradiogram of the same gel. **C)** Western immunoblot of the 105-kDa phosphorylated peptide band excised from the gel showing immunoreactivity with SR Ca^{2+}-ATPase-specific antibody. **D)** autoradiogram of the Western immunoblot. Lanes E and F, autoradiogram of proteins fractionated on SDS polyacrylamide gel after subjecting phosphorylated SR to immuniprecipitation protocol in the absence (E) and presence (F) of Ca^{2+}-ATPase-specific antibody. The phosphorylation reaction was carried out for 3 min in the presence or absence of Ca^{2+} and calmodulin (CM) as indicated. (From Xu et al. (17), reprinted with permission.)

(SERCA 1) (31–34). These two isoforms show about 84 % sequence homology (32, 33), similar transmembrane topologies and tertiary structures (35–37), and qualitatively similar enzymatic properties (38) all of which likely reflect the uniformity in their function, viz., active Ca^{2+} transport. On the other hand, the limited structural differences among the Ca^{2+}-ATPase isoforms may signify subtle variations in their intrinsic functional properties and differences in the mechanisms by which their function is regulated physiologically. Some variation in the intrinsic functional properties between SERCA 1 and SERCA 2 isoforms has been suggested by observations demonstrating a) the inability of the cardiac, as opposed to the fast-twitch muscle enzyme, to utilize GTP as a substrate for Ca^{2+}-dependent phosphoenzyme formation and Ca^{2+} transport (39), and b) the susceptibility of the Ca^{2+}-induced conformation of the cardiac but not the fast-twitch muscle enzyme to inhibition by fluoride (40, 41). In cardiac and slow-twitch muscle SR, the Ca^{2+}-ATPase is subject to regulation

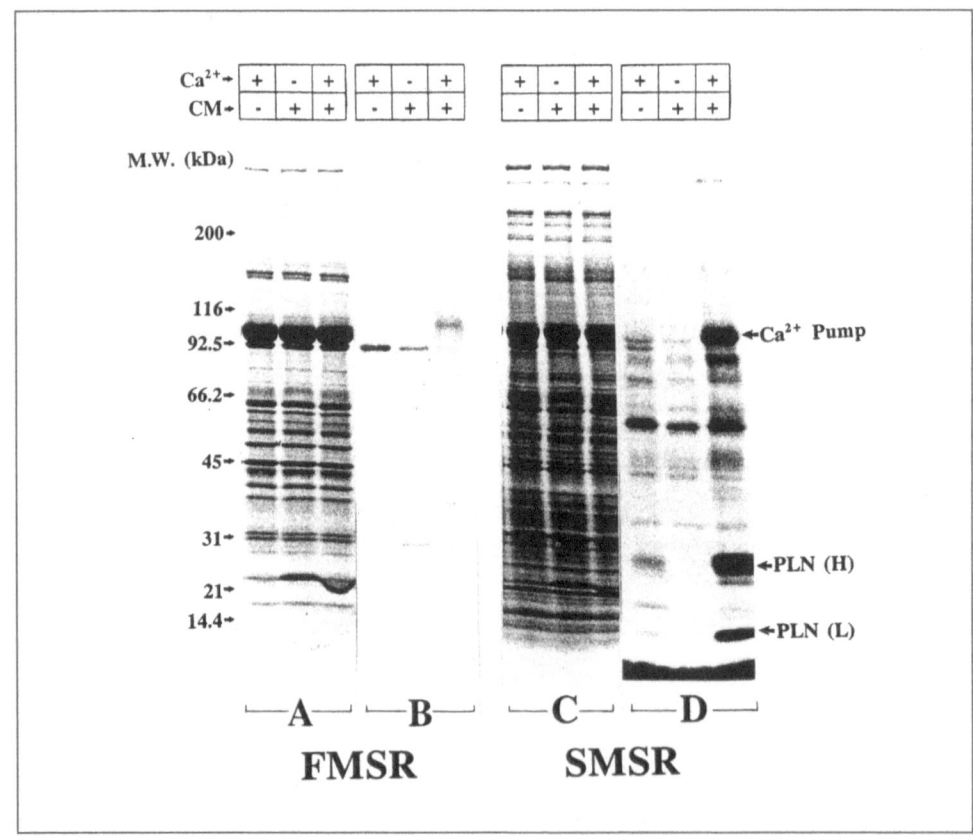

Fig. 2. Comparison of Ca^{2+}/calmodulin dependent protein phosphorylation in rabbit fast-twitch skeletal muscle (*adductor magnus*) SR (FMSR) and rabbit slow-twitch skeletal muscle (*soleus*) SR (SMSR). Panels A and C show Coomassie Blue-stained SDS-polyacrylamide gels showing SR protein profiles and Panels B and D show the corresponding autoradiograms. The phosphorylation reactions were carried out for 3 min in the presence or absence of Ca^{2+} and calmodulin (CM) as indicated. (Modified from Hawkins et al. (18).)

by the intrinsic membrane protein, phospholamban (2, 6–9). We examined whether the CaM kinase-mediated phosphorylation of the SR Ca²⁺-ATPase is cardiac muscle-specific or common to other muscle types. Studies using SR membranes isolated from slow-twitch (*soleus*) and fast-twitch (*adductor magnus*) skeletal muscles of the rabbit showed Ca²⁺/calmodulin-dependent phosphorylation of the Ca²⁺-ATPase in slow-twitch muscle SR but not in fast-twitch muscle SR (Fig. 2). Thus, an endogenous CaM kinase capable of phosphorylating the Ca²⁺-ATPase is present in cardiac and slow-twitch muscle SR. Exogenously added α-CaM kinase II stimulated the phosphorylation of the Ca²⁺-ATPase in cardiac and slow-twitch muscle SR (Fig. 3) but failed to induce phosphorylation of the Ca²⁺-ATPase in fast muscle SR (18). Therefore, the absence of an appropriate CaM kinase does not account for the inability of the fast-twitch muscle SR Ca²⁺-ATPase isoform (SERCA 1) to undergo phosphorylation.

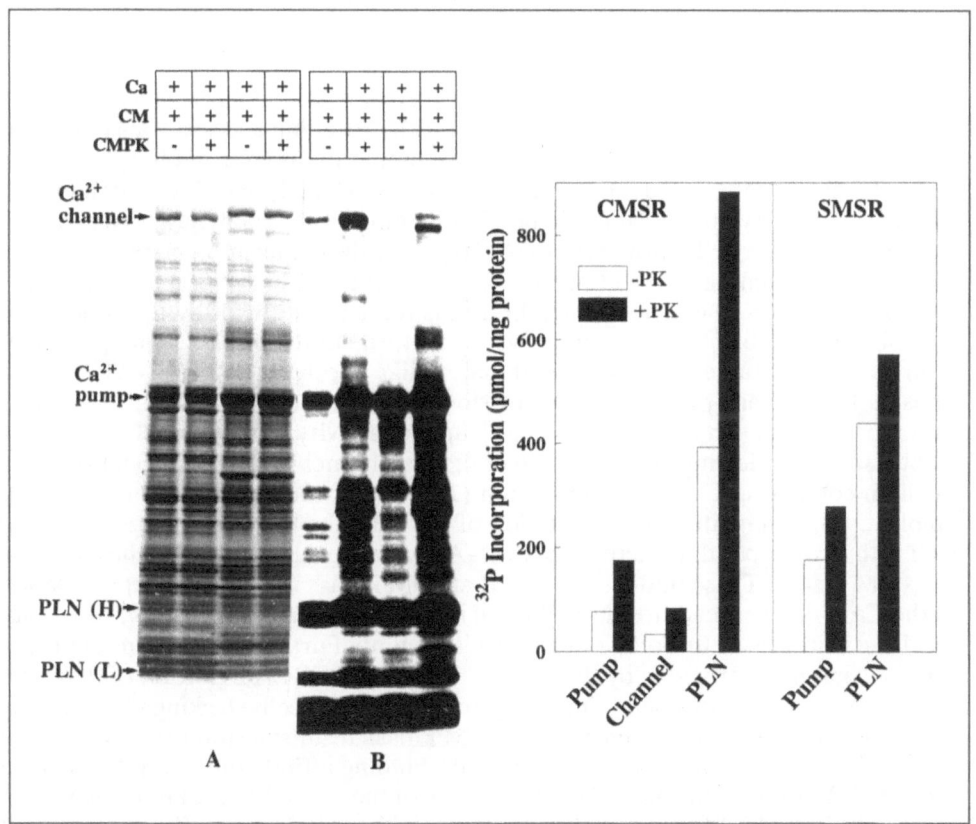

Fig. 3. Stimulation of protein phosphorylation in rabbit cardiac SR and slow-twitch muscle SR by exogenous CaM kinase. Panel A shows Coomassie Blue-stained SDS-polyacrylamide gel showing protein profiles of cardiac SR (first two lanes from the left) and slow-twitch muscle SR (last two lanes from the right) and Panel B shows autoradiogram of the same gel. The bar graph depicts quantification of ³²P incorporation into the peptide bands corresponding to the Ca²⁺ pump, Ca²⁺ channel and phospholamban. The phosphorylation reaction was carried out for 3 min in the presence of Ca²⁺ and calmodulin (CM) with or without CaM kinase II (CMPK) as indicated. (From Narayanan (29), reprinted with permission.)

The cardiac/slow-twitch muscle SR Ca^{2+}-ATPase isoform (SERCA 2) contains three serine residues in its primary structure (in positions 38, 167 and 531) (32) that have minimal consensus sequence (R-X-X-S/T) for phosphorylation by CaM kinase (42). Site-directed mutagenesis studies have led to the identification of Ser^{38} as the residue subject to phosphorylation by CaM kinase (43). The SERCA 1 isoform expressed in the fast-twitch muscle lacks a phosphorylatable serine or threonine residue in position 38, and the amino acid sequence upstream of this site shows several substitutions, at least some of which are nonconservative (32). These structural differences may explain the inability of SERCA 1 to undergo phosphorylation by CaM kinase (43).

Effect of serine phosphorylation on Ca^{2+}-ATPase function

The impact of Ser^{38} phosphorylation on Ca^{2+}-ATPase function has been assessed by determining the effect of phosphorylation on the catalytic and ion transport functions of the ATPase. In purified Ca^{2+}-ATPase preparations (free of phospholamban and other membrane components) from cardiac SR (Fig. 4) and slow-twitch muscle SR (18) phosphorylation resulted in nearly twofold greater catalytic activity (rate of Ca^{2+}-stimulated ATP hydrolysis) of the enzyme without any appreciable change in $K_{0.5}$ for Ca^{2+}. Analysis of the effect of Ca^{2+}-ATPase phosphorylation on its Ca^{2+} ion transport function in native SR membranes is rendered difficult by the concurrent phosphorylation of phospholamban, which in turn stimulates Ca^{2+} pump activity. However, some studies have suggested that, unlike in cardiac SR, Ca^{2+}-ATPase and phospholamban are poorly coupled in slow-twitch muscle SR (44, 45). We have observed marked stimulation of the Ca^{2+} uptake activity of slow-twitch muscle SR (rabbit *soleus*) following preincubation of the membranes in a phosphorylation assay medium containing Ca^{2+} and calmodulin (18). Under the experimental conditions employed, the magnitude of stimulation of Ca^{2+} uptake by SR could be correlated well with a corresponding increase in Ca^{2+}-ATPase phosphorylation by the endogenous CaM kinase. These findings suggest that CaM kinase mediated phosphorylation of the Ca^{2+}-ATPase leads to stimulation of its enzymatic and ion transport functions, resulting in increased turnover rate of the Ca^{2+} pump. Further evidence in support of this view has been provided by the finding that when SERCA 2 isoform of the Ca^{2+}-ATPase is expressed in a heterologous system (HEK 293 cells) lacking phospholamban, phosphorylation of the enzyme by CaM kinase results in stimulation of V_{max} of Ca^{2+} transport without alteration in the Ca^{2+} binding affinity of the ATPase (Fig. 5 and ref (43)). Our finding that phosphorylation of the Ca^{2+}-ATPase alters the V_{max} of ATP hydrolysis (17, 18) and Ca^{2+} transport (43) without influencing $K_{0.5}$ for Ca^{2+} is of particular interest. Activation of the Ca^{2+}-ATPase by phosphorylation of phospholamban is thought to involve mainly a decrease in the enzyme's $K_{0.5}$ for Ca^{2+} (44, 46, 47), but an increase in V_{max} may also occur (13). Thus, the positive V_{max} effect of phosphorylation of the Ca^{2+}-ATPase and the positive $K_{0.5}$ effect of phosphorylation of phospholamban may provide a powerful, mutually complementary mechanism for the stimulation of Ca^{2+} pumping in cardiac and slow-twitch skeletal muscle SR. Such a mechanism would be of particular physiological significance in these slow-contracting muscle types where myofilament activation and contraction result from binding of Ca^{2+} to a single Ca^{2+}-specific site on troponin C (4). This site has much lower affinity for Ca^{2+} than the Ca^{2+} binding sites on the Ca^{2+}-ATPase (4). Given the higher intrinsic affinity of the Ca^{2+}-ATPase for Ca^{2+} (even when associated with phospholamban, the apparent affinity of the Ca^{2+}-ATPase for Ca^{2+} is at least 25 times higher than that of the Ca^{2+}-specific site on cardiac troponin C (c.f. refs. 4, 38), it is

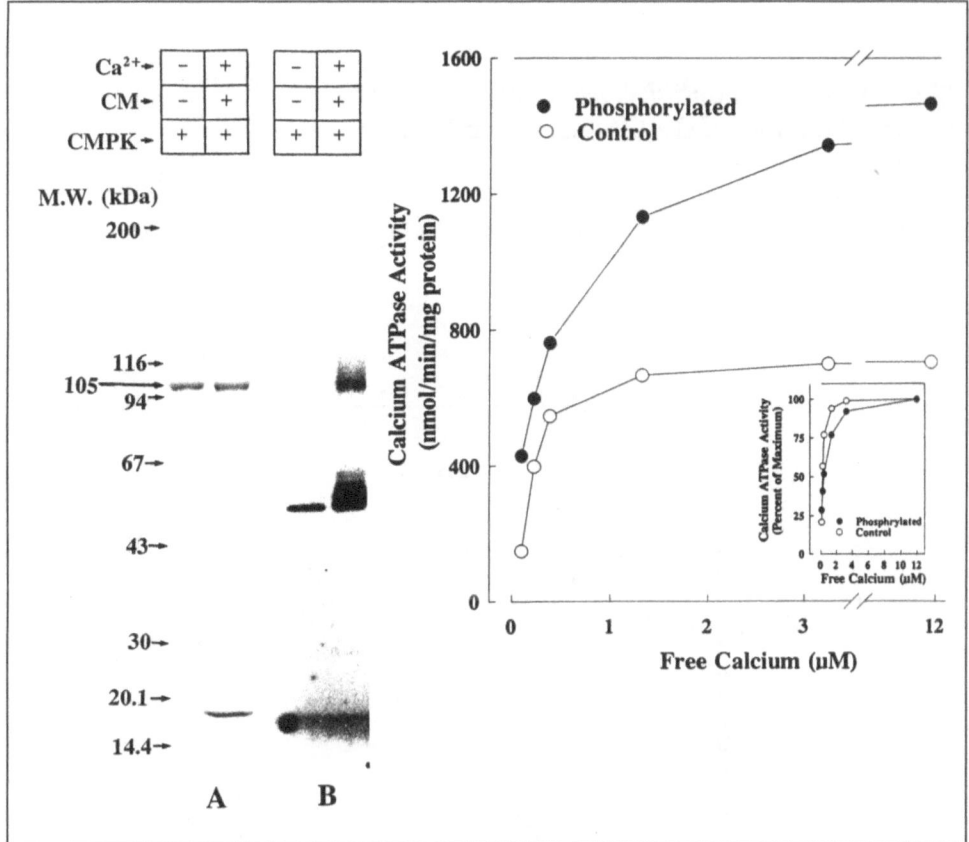

Fig. 4. Phosphorylation and stimulation of purified rabbit cardiac SR Ca^{2+}-ATPase by exogenous CaM kinase. Left panel: Phosphorylation of purified cardiac SR Ca^{2+}-ATPase (Ca^{2+} pump) by exogenous CaM kinase. **A)** Coomassie Blue-stained polycarylamide gel. **B)** autoradiogram of the same gel. Phosphorylation of the purified Ca^{2+}-ATPase was performed for 3 min in the presence of exogenous CaM kinase II (CMPK) at a concentration of 0.25 μM with or without Ca^{2+} and calmodulin (CM) as indicated. Following phosphorylation, the samples were subjected to SDS-polyacrylamide gel electrophoresis (A) and autoradiography (B). Right panel: Effect of CaM kinase-catalyzed phosphorylation of cardiac SR Ca^{2+}-ATPase on its enzymatic function. Ca^{2+}-ATPase purified from cardiac SR, was allowed to undergo phosphorylation as described above in the presence of exogenous CaM kinase, Ca^{2+} and calmodulin (CM) with nonradioactive ATP (0.8 mM) instead of [γ-^{32}P] ATP) as substrate. Ca^{2+}-ATPase subjected to the same incubation protocol in the absence of CaM kinase, Ca^{2+}, and calmodulin served as control (unphosphorylated enzyme) for this experiment. Aliquots of phosphorylated ATPase were transferred to an ATPase reaction medium to determine Ca^{2+}-stimulated ATPase activity. The assays were performed at varying concentrations of free Ca^{2+} as indicated. (From Xu et al. (17), reprinted with permission.)

unlikely that an increase in Ca^{2+} affinity alone would be sufficient to cause a large increase in the rate of Ca^{2+} uptake (and therefore relaxation rate) in the presence of systolic levels of cytoplasmic Ca^{2+} concentrations. It would, however, allow the SR to accumulate more Ca^{2+} for future release. When complemented with an increase in V_{max}, the two would form a powerful mechanism for the cell to increase both the rate and amount of Ca^{2+} uptake into SR; this, in turn, would facilitate augmentation of both heart rate (due to faster mechanical restitution) and contractility (due to greater SR Ca^{2+} load available for release).

Characteristics of Ca^{2+}-ATPase phosphorylation and identification of the SR-associated CaM kinase

Phosphorylation of the Ca^{2+}-ATPase by the endogenous CaM kinase occurs rapidly in both cardiac (Fig. 6) and slow-twitch muscle (18) SR and reaches maximum within

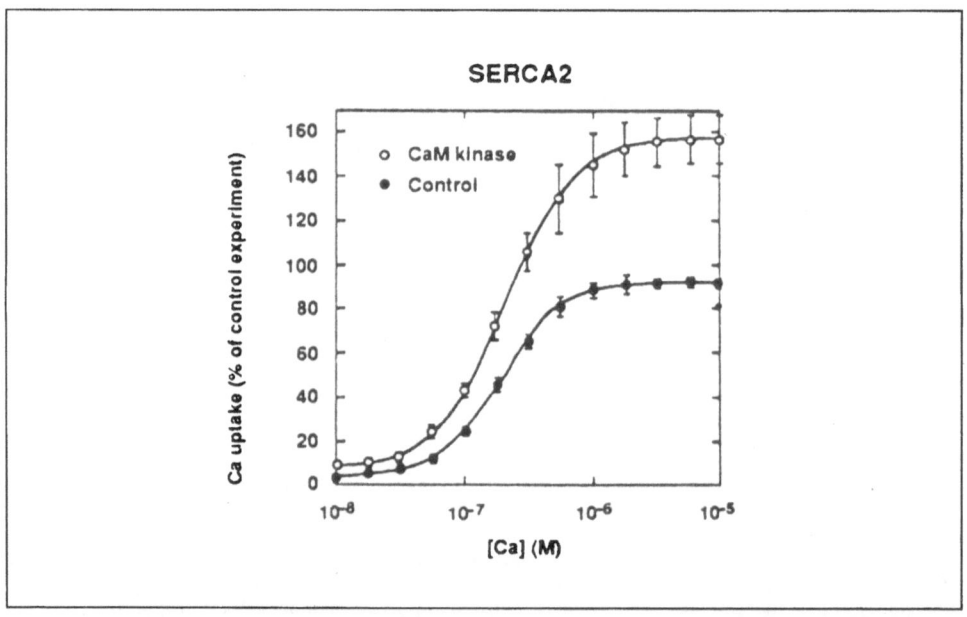

Fig. 5. Stimulation of Ca^{2+} uptake by SERCA 2 upon its phosphorylation by CaM kinase. SERCA 2 was expressed in HEK-293 cells. Microsomes containing the SERCA 2 enzyme were harvested from these cells and subjected to phosphorylation by exogenous α-CaM kinase II. The phosphorylated and unphosphory-lated (control) microsomes were then assayed for Ca^{2+} uptake activity at varying free Ca^{2+} concentrations as indicated. The Ca^{2+} uptake rate (nmol/min/mg of microsomal protein) of phosphorylated microsomes was normalized to the activity of control microsomes and is shown as a percentage of the control Ca^{2+} uptake rate. In these experiments phosporylation of SERCA 2 by CaM kinase was localized to Ser[38]. (From Toyofuku et al. (43), reprinted with permission.)

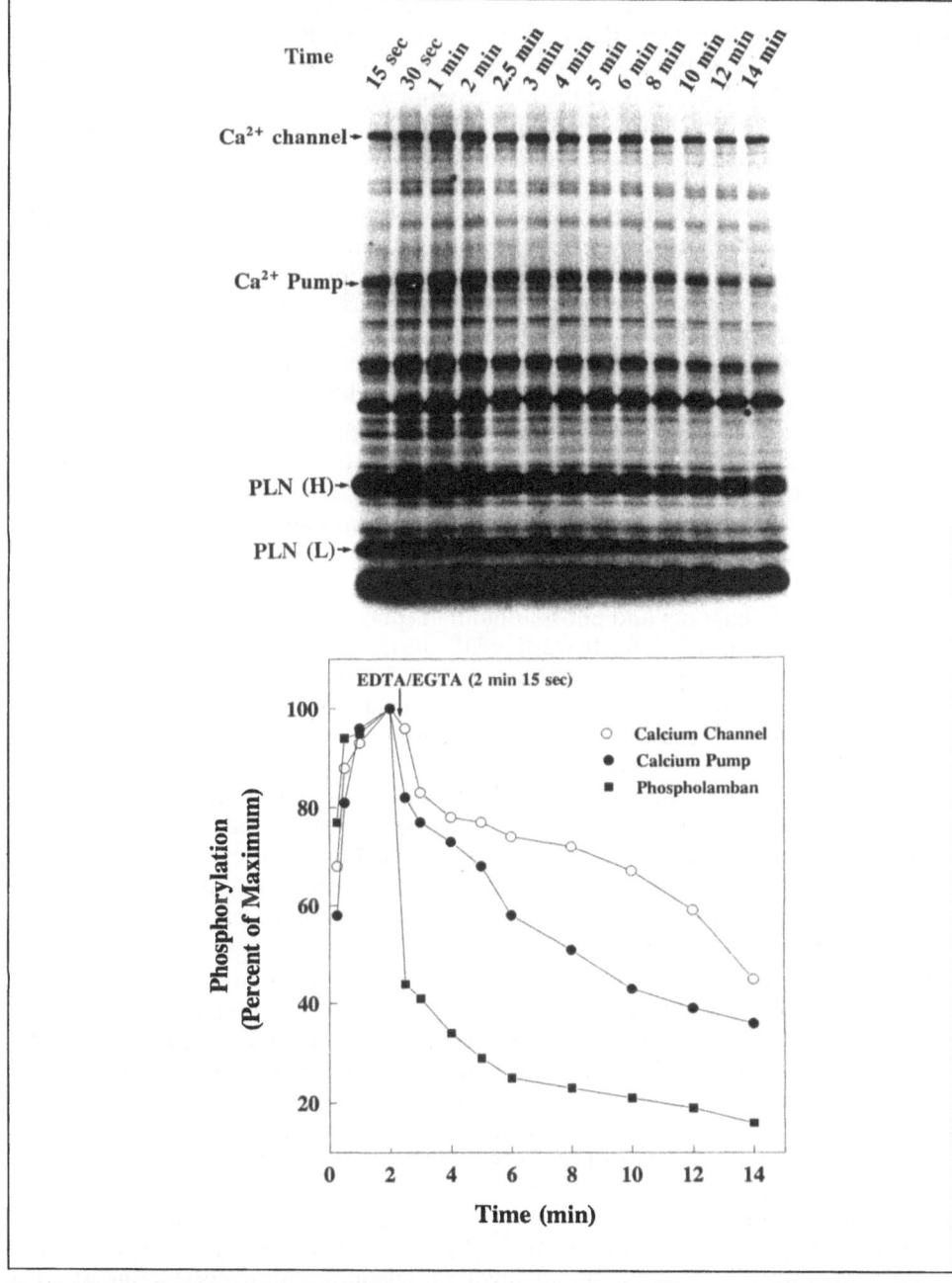

Fig. 6. Time-course of phosphorylation and dephosphorylation of Ca^{2+} pump, Ca^{2+} cannel and phospholamban in rabbit cardiac SR. The SR membranes were incubated in a phosphorylation assay medium in the presence of Ca^{2+} and calmodulin and the time-course of phosphorylation was monitored by removing aliquots at the various time intervals indicated. The time-course of dephosphorylation was monitored similarly after the addition (at 2 min 15s) of a mixture of EDTA/EGTA to chelate Mg^{2+} and Ca^{2+}. The left panel shows an autoradiogram depicting the time-dependent changes in phosphorylation of SR proteins fractionated on SDS-polyacrylamide gel; the right panel shows quantification of phosphorylation in the peptide bands corresponding to Ca^{2+} pump, Ca^{2+} channel and phospholamban. (From Xu et al. (17), reprinted with permission.)

2 min at 37 °C. The time-course of phosphorylation of the Ca^{2+}-ATPase is similar to that seen for phospholamban and Ca^{2+} release channel. Phosphorylation is strongly pH-dpendent, increasing six- to seven-fold with an increase in pH from 6.5 to 9 (pH optimum 8.5–9.0) (18). The striking pH-dependence of Ca^{2+}-ATPase phosphorylation by CaM kinase correlates with the pH-dependent alterations in SR Ca^{2+}-ATPase function. For example, a) in isolated SR vesicles, acidification results in depression of Ca^{2+}-ATPase activity and Ca^{2+} sequestration (48, 49); b) in skinned cardiac cells, Ca^{2+} loading of the SR declines with decreasing (7.4–6.2) pH (50); and c) intracellular acidosis is accompained by a decrease in the rates of muscle relaxation (51 and references therein). Since phosphorylation results in increased turnover rates of the Ca^{2+}-ATPase (17, 18, 43), the observed pH-dependent changes in Ca^{2+}-ATPase phosphorylation imply that the SR Ca^{2+} pump activity will be depressed at lower pH (due to relatively low level of Ca^{2+}-ATPase phosphorylation) and enhanced at higher pH (due to the high level of Ca^{2+}-ATPase phosphorylation).

In cardiac and slow-twitch muscle SR, phosphorylation of the Ca^{2+}-ATPase by CaM kinase increases with increasing temperature up to 30 °C with no further change at higher temperatures up to 40 °C (18). Phosphorylation is maximal with 0.2 μM calmodulin and is half-maximal with ~ 35–50 nM calmodulin (29).

In isolated SR vesicles from cardiac muscle and slow-twitch skeletal muscle, the extent of Ca^{2+}-ATPase phosphorylation by CaM kinase was found to be intermediate between the Ca^{2+} channel and phospholamban (phospholamban > Ca^{2+}-ATPase > Ca^{2+} channel: c.f. Figs. 1–3, 6). In cardiac SR, the ratio of ^{32}P incorporation into Ca^{2+} channel: Ca^{2+}-ATPase: phospholamban has been estimated to be about 0.5:1.5. The molar ratio of phospolamban to Ca^{2+}-ATPase in the SR membrane has not been clearly established (13); a ratio of one mole of phospholamban per mole of Ca^{2+}-ATPase has been suggested for cardiac SR (52). Since phospholamban is a homopentamer (53, 54) with each monomer having one phosphorylation site (Thr^{17}) for CaM kinase (30), a five-fold greater phosphorylation of phospholamban relative to Ca^{2+}-ATPase (with a single phosphorylation site at Ser^{38}) (43) is to be expected. The results with cardiac SR are in accordance with this expectation and suggest that CaM kinase phosphorylates one mole of Ca^{2+}-ATPase and one mole of phospholamban pentamer concurrently in this membrane.

Quantification of ^{32}P incorporation into Ca^{2+}-ATPase protein suggested that only a small proportion (< 20 %) of the Ca^{2+} pump units in the SR membrane underwent phosphorylation by CaM kinase under the experimental conditions employed in our studies (17, 18). The precise reasons for the low level of phosphorylation are not clear, but potential contributing factors include preexisting endogenous phosphorylation, incomplete inhibition of endogenous protein phosphatase activity, and heterogeneity in the sidedness of SR vesicles limiting the accessibility of phosphorylation sites to the substrate and exogenously added CaM kinase. It is also possible that membrane consituents may influence the extent of Ca^{2+} pump phosphorylation by exerting regulatory constraints on Ca^{2+} pump conformation. In purified Ca^{2+}-ATPase preparation, the maximum level of posphorylation corresponded to a stoichiometry of about 0.4 mole ^{32}P/mole of Ca^{2+}-ATPase (18). The inability to observe experimentally, the anticipated stoichiometry of 1 mole ^{32}P/mole of Ca^{2+}-ATPase is likely due to a combination of factors, including considerable inactivation of the ATPase during purification, susceptibility of the exogenous CaM kinase to inhibition by residual detergent present in purified ATPase preparation, and preexisting endogenous phosphorylation (18). The observed level of ^{32}P incorporation in purified Ca^{2+}-ATPase preparations suggested that about 40 % of the enzyme molecules were undergoing phosphorylation under the experimental conditions used. Since the same level of phosphorylation resulted in twofold greater catalytic activity of the ATPase (c.f. Fig. 4 and ref. 18), it appears that the maximum potential for the regulation of this enzyme by CaM kinase phosphorylation may be even greater than that which could be observed experimentally.

Besides pH, temperature and pre-existing endogenous phosphorylation, certain other factors were also found to influence greatly the phosphorylation of Ca^{2+}-ATPase and other SR proteins by CaM kinase. For example, we have found that when the phosphorylation assays are performed in the presence of potassium at a concentration approximating its intracellular level (120 mM), the phosphorylation of pospholamban is diminished ($\sim$ 60 %), whereas Ca^{2+}-ATPase and Ca^{2+} channel phosphorylation is unaffected (A. Xu and N. Narayanan, unpublished). On the other, addition of NaF (10 mM), a conventional protein phosphatase inhibitor, in the phosphorylation assay medium results in stimulation ($\sim$ 60 %) of phospholamban phosphorylation and inhibition ($\sim$ 40–50 %) of Ca^{2+}-ATPase and Ca^{2+} channel phosphorylation (55). Recently, fluoride has been shown to interact with and inhibit the Ca^{2+}-ATPase (40, 41, 56, 57); therefore, the inhibitory effect of fluoride on Ca^{2+}-ATPase phosphorylation may be due to fluoride-induced alteration in enzyme conformation. The critical dependence of Ca^{2+}-ATPase conformation on its ability to undergo phosphorylation by CaM kinase is demonstrated by the finding that creation of a CaM kinase phosphorylation site in SERCA 1, which mimicked the phosphorylation site (Ser^{38}) in SERCA 2, did not result in CaM kinase phosphorylation of SERCA 1 (43). In most previous studies, the presence of fluoride in the assay medium, may have contributed to the failure to detect substantial phosphorylation of the ATPase. It is noteworthy, however, that the autoradiograms presented in some studies using canine cardiac SR (16, 58, 59) did show appreciable phosphorylation of a petide in the molecular-size range 100–110 kDa, but no attempt was made to identify this substrate.

The phosphorylation of Ca^{2+}-ATPase, Ca^{2+} channel and phospholamban in cardiac and slow muscle SR could be readily stimulated by exogenously added α-CaM kinase II (Fig. 3 and refs. 17, 18). The nature of the endogenous, SR-associated CaM kinase, mediating the phosphorylation of the SR proteins is not yet clearly established. We have found that KN-62, a specific inhibitor of CaM kinase II (60), did not inhibit protein phosphorylation by SR-associated CaM kinase under conditions in which phosphorylation by exogenous α-CaM kinase II was completely inhibited (61). Recently, novel CaM kinase II isoforms have been identified in heart (62) and aorta (63), and it is possible that one or more unique CaM kinase isoforms may be involved in the Ca^{2+}/calmodulin-dependent protein phosporylation in cardiac and slow-twitch muscle SR.

Dephosphorylation of the Ca^{2+}-ATPase

The presence of protein phosphatase activity has been demonstrated in cardiac SR and some properties of the enzyme involved in the dephosphorylation of phospholamban have been described (59, 64, 65). We have observed that the SR-associated protein phosphatase(s) can also catalyze the dephosphorylation of Ca^{2+}-

ATPase (Fig. 6 and ref. 17). Under the experimental conditions employed in our studies, the rate of dephosphorylation of CaM kinase substrates in cardiac SR by membrane-associated phosphatase differed in the order, phospholamban > Ca^{2+}-ATPase > Ca^{2+} channel. The identity of the protein phosphatase mediating dephosphorylation of the Ca^{2+}-ATPase and the factors influencing protein dephosphorylation remain to be established.

Physiological implications of the phosphorylation of multiple substrates by SR-associated CaM kinase

The ability of the membrane-bound CaM kinase to phosphorylate the three major SR proteins (Ca^{2+}-ATPase, Ca^{2+} channel and phospholamban) involved in transmembrane Ca^{2+} cycling is indicative of a key role for this enzyme in the regulation of SR function. We have observed that, in contrast to the strong phosphorylation of the Ca^{2+}-ATPase by endogenous CaM kinase, exogenous PKA caused only weak phosphorylation of the Ca^{2+}-ATPase in cardiac and slow-twitch muscle SR (18). On the other hand, both kinases produce strong phosphorylation of phospholamban (18). These findings suggest that while PKA can produce stimulation of SR Ca^{2+} pump activity via phosphorylation of phospholamban, the membrane-bound CaM kinase can cause stimulation of SR Ca^{2+} pump activity via phospholamban phosphorylation as well as through direct phosphorylation of the Ca^{2+} pump. In cardiac SR, phosphorylation of Ca^{2+} channel by endogenous CaM kinase is about fivefold greater than that produced by PKA (18). Although the functional consequence of Ca^{2+} channel phosphorylation has not been clearly established, it has been demonstrated recently that in cardiac SR, CaM kinase mediated phosphorylation of the Ca^{2+} channel results in activation of Ca^{2+} release (15). Thus, it appears that the membrane-associated CaM kinase has a unique capacity to regulate the Ca^{2+} uptake as well as the Ca^{2+} release functions of the SR by virtue of its ability to phosphorylate Ca^{2+} pump, phospholamban and Ca^{2+} channel (see Fig. 7). However, in order to be physiologically effective, the function and activity of CaM kinase need to be coordinated with the events in muscle contraction and relaxation cycle. For example, CaM kinase-mediated phosphorylation and activation of the Ca^{2+} release channel would be fruitful if it were to occur coincident with or soon after the excitatory event involving membrane depolarization and the beginning of muscle contraction. Likewise, CaM kinase mediated phosphorylation of Ca^{2+} pump and phospholamban would be meaningful and effective if it were to occur coincident with or soon after cessation of contraction and the beginning of the relaxation phase. It is not known whether cardiac and slow-twitch muscle cells possess mechanisms to orchestrate timely and sequential targeting of the SR-bound CaM kinase to its specific substrates. In this regard, it is of considerable interest that a recent study reported membrane depolarization-dependent modulation of CaM kinase activity and consequent changes in transmembrane Ca^{2+} fluxes in cardiac sarcolemma (66). It is possible that depolarization of the SR membrane may favor Ca^{2+} channel phosphorylation and repolarization may favor Ca^{2+} pump phosphorylation by the SR-bound CaM kinase. Consis-

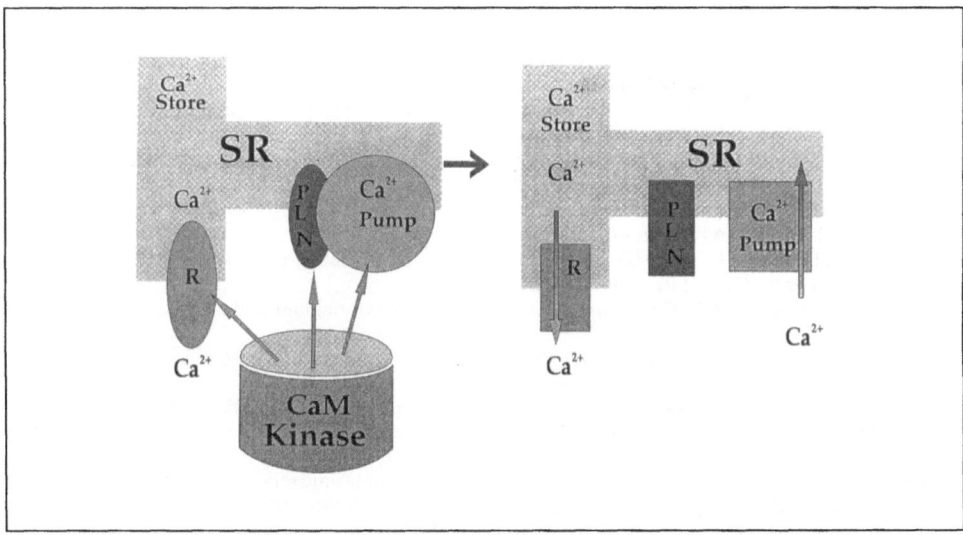

Fig. 7. Modulation of the Ca^{2+} uptake and release functions of cardiac SR through phosphorylation of multiple target proteins by membrane-associated CaM kinase. In cardiac SR, membrane-bound CaM kinase phosphorylates three major proteins *viz* phospholamban (PLN) Ca^{2+}-ATPase (Ca^{2+} pump) and Ca^{2+}-release channel (R, ryanodine receptor). Phosphorylation is accompanied by changes in protein conformation and function. In its unphosphorylated state, phospholamban associates with the Ca^{2+} pump and inhibits Ca^{2+} pumping. Phosphorylation of phospholamban results in disruption of the physical interaction between the two proteins and the stimulation of Ca^{2+} pumping, mainly due to an increase in the affinity of the Ca^{2+}-ATPase for Ca^{2+}. Direct phosphorylation of the Ca^{2+}-ATPase and consequent changes in enzyme conformation results in stimulation of Ca^{2+} pumping due to an increase in V_{max} of ATP hydrolysis and Ca^{2+} transport. Phosphorylation of the Ca^{2+} channel results in the activation of Ca^{2+} release, apparently due to an increase in the duration of the open state of the channel.

tent with the above possibility, we have obtained evidence suggesting that the "open state" but not the "closed state" conformation of the cardiac SR Ca^{2+}-release channel (ryanodine receptor) is subject to phosphorylation by the SR-associated CaM kinase (67). We have also observed that a 64 kDa cytosolic protein (P_{64} from heart muscle, which is capable of modulating Ca^{2+} transport across the SR *in vitro* (25), stimulates Ca^{2+} pump phosphorylation while producing concomitant inhibition of Ca^{2+} channel phosphorylation in cardiac SR by the membrane-associated CaM kinase (68). Perhaps, P_{64} may serve to target the SR-bound CaM kinase from the Ca^{2+} channel to the Ca^{2+} pump, and this may be facilitated by membrane repolarization. Verification of these conceptual possibilities and the functional roles of the SR-associated CaM kinase *in vivo* must be made by future studies.

Acknowledgements   The studies from the author's laboratory reported here were supported by a grant from the Medical Research Council of Canada.

REFERENCES

1. Fleisher S, Inui M (1989) Biochemistry and biophysics of excitation-contraction coupling. Annu Rev Biophys Chem 18: 333–364
2. Lytton J, MacLennan DH (1992) Sarcoplasmic reticulum. In: The Heart and Cardiovascular System (ed. Fozzard HA) Raven Press Ltd. New York, pp 1203–1222
3. Feher JJ, Fabiato A (1990) Cardiac sarcoplasmic reticulum: calcium uptake and release. In: Calcium and the Heart (ed. Langer GA) Raven Press Ltd. New York, pp 199–268
4. Thompson RB, Kimbrough DW, Potter JD (1990) Calcium at the myofibrils. In: Calcium and the Heart (ed. Langer, GA) Raven Press Ltd. New York, pp 127–165
5. Inesi G, Submilla C, Kirtley ME (1990) Relationships of molecular structure and function in Ca^{2+} transport ATPase. Physiol Rev 70: 749–760
6. Tada M, Katz AM (1982) Phosphorylation of sarcoplasmic reticulum and sarcolemma. Annu Rev Physiol 44: 401–423
7. Tada M, Kadoma M, Inui M, Fuji JI (1988) Regulation of Ca^{2+}-pump from cardiac sarcoplasmic reticulum. Methods Enzymol 157: 107–154
8. Davis BA, Edes I, Gupta RC, Young EF, Kim HW, Stewart NAE, Szymanska G, Kranias EG (1990) The role of phospholamban in the regulation of calcium transport by cardiac sarcoplasmic reticulum. Mol Cell Biochem 99: 83–88
9. Colyer J (1993) Control of the calcium pump of cardiac sarcoplasmic reticulum. A specific role for the pentameric structure of phospholamban? Cardiovasc Res 27: 1766–1771
10. Kirchberger MA, Borchman D, Kasinathan C (1986) Proteolytic activation of the canine cardiac sarcoplasmic reticulum calcium pump. Biochemistry 25: 5484–5492
11. Suzuki T, Wang JH (1986) Stimulation of bovine cardiac sarcoplasmic reticulum calcium pump and blocking of phospholamban phosphorylation by a phospholamban monoclonal antibody. J Biol Chem 261: 7018–7023
12. James P, Inui M, Tada M, Chiesi M, Carafoli E (1989) Nature and site of phospholamban regulation of the calcium pump of sarcoplasmic reticulum. Nature 342: 90–92
13. Sasaki T, Inui M, Kimura Y, Kuzuya T, Tada M (1992) Molecular mechanism of regulation of Ca^{2+} pump ATPase by phospholamban in cardiac sarcoplasmic reticulum. Effects of synthetic phospholamban peptides on Ca^{2+} pump ATPase. J Biol Chem 267: 1674–1679
14. Toyofuku T, Kurzydlowski K, Tada M, MacLennan DH (1993) Identification of regions in the Ca^{2+}-ATPase of sarcoplasmic reticulum that affect functional association with phospholamban. J Biol Chem 268: 2809–2815
15. Witcher DR, Kovacs RJ, Schulman H, Cefali DC, Jones LR (1991) Unique phosphorylation site on the cardiac ryanodine receptor regulates Ca^{2+} channel activity. J Biol Chem 266: 11144–11152
16. Takasago T, Imagawa T, Furukawa K, Ogurusu T, Shigekawa M (1991) Regulation of the cardiac ryanodine receptor by protein kinase-dependent phosphorylation. J Biochem (Tokyo) 1099: 163–170
17. Xu A, Hawkins C, Narayanan N (1993) Phosphorylation and activation of the Ca^{2+}-pumping ATPase of cardiac sarcoplasmic reticulum by a Ca^{2+}/calmodulin-dependent protein kinase. J Biol Chem 268: 8394–8397
18. Hawkins C, Xu A, Narayanan N (1994) Sarcoplasmic reticulum calcium pump in cardiac and slow twitch skeletal muscle but not fast twitch skeletal muscle undergoes phosphorylation by endogenous and exogenous Ca^{2+}/calmodulin-dependent protein kinase. Characterization of optimal conditions for calcium pump phosphorylation. J Biol Chem 269: 31198–31206
19. Narayanan N, Lee P, Newland M, Khandelwal RL (1982) Evidence for an endogenous protein inhibitor of sarcoplasmic reticulum calcium pump in heart muscle. Biochem Biophys Res Commun 108: 1158–1164
20. Narayanan N, Newland M, Neudorf D (1983) Inhibition of sarcoplasmic reticulum calcium pump by cytosolic protein(s) endogenous to heart and slow skeletal muscle but not fast skeletal muscle. Biochem Biophys Acta 735: 53–66
21. Narayanan N, Bedard P, Waraich T (1989) Effects of endogenous calcium transport inhibitor from heart muscle on the active calcium uptake and passive calcium release properties of sarcoplasmic reticulum. Can J Physiol Pharmacol 67: 999–1006
22. Donat ME, Su N, Narayanan N (1991) Ontogeny of cytosolic proteins capable of modulating sarcoplasmic reticulum calcium transport in heart muscle. Mol Cell Biochem 106: 41–48
23. Chiesi M, Geurini D (1987) Characterization of heart cytosolic proteins capable of modulating calcium uptake by sarcoplasmic reticulum. 1. Isolation of a protein with protective activity and its identification as muscle albumin. Eur J Biochem 162: 365–370
24. Chiesi M, Schwaller R (1987) Characterization of heart cytosolic proteins capable of modulating calcium uptake by sarcoplasmic reticulum. 2. Identification of actin isoforms with inhibitory activity. Eur J Biochem 162: 371–377

25. Xu A, Narayanan N (1994) Purification, amino-terminal sequence and functional properties of a 64 kDa cytosolic protein from heart muscle capable of modulating calcium transport across the sarcoplasmic reticulum in vitro. Mol Cell Biochem 132: 7–14

26. LePeuch CJ, Haiech J, Damaille JG (1979) Concerted regulation of cardiac sarcoplasmic reticulum calcium transport by cyclic adenosine monophosphate-dependent and calcium/calmodulin-dependent phosphorylations. Biochemistry 18: 5150–5157

27. Inesi G (1985) Mechanism of calcium transport. Annu Rev Physiol 47: 573–601

28. Buss JE, Stull JT (1983) Measurement of chemical phosphate in proteins. Methods Enzymol 99: 7–14

29. Narayanan N (1995) Multiple roles for the membrane-associated Ca^{2+}/calmodulin-dependent protein kinase in the regulation of sarcoplasmic reticulum function in heart muscle. In: Pathophysiology of Heart Failure (ed. Dhalla NS, Pierce GN, Panagia V) Kluwer Academic Publishers, Norwell (in press)

30. Simmemman HKB, Collins JH, Theibert JL, Wegener AD, Jones LR (1986) Sequence Analysis of Phospholamban. J Biol Chem 261: 13333–13341

31. MacLennan DH, Brandl CJ, Korezak B, Green NM (1985) Amino acid sequence of a $Ca^{2+} + Mg^{2+}$-dependent ATPase from rabbit muscle sarcoplasmic reticulum, deduced from its complementary DNA sequence. Nature 316: 696–700

32. Brandl CJ, Green NM, Korezak B, MacLennan DH (1986) Two Ca^{2+}-ATPase genes: Homologies and mechanistic implications of deduced amino acid sequences. Cell 44: 597–607

33. Brandl CJ, deLeon S, Martin DR, MacLennan DH (1987) Adult forms of the Ca^{2+}-ATPase of sarcoplasmic reticulum. Expression in developing skeletal muscle. J Biol Chem 262: 3768–3774

34. Zarain-Herzberg A, MacLennan DH, Periasamy M (1990) Characterization of rabbit sarco(endo)plasmic reticulum Ca^{2+}-ATPase gene. J Biol Chem 265: 4670–4677

35. MacLennan DH (1990) Molecular tools to elucidate problems in excitation-contraction coupling. Biophys J 58: 1355–1365

36. Inesi G, Kirtley ME (1992) Structural features of cation transport ATPases. J Bioenerg Biomembr 24: 271–283

37. MacLennan DH, Toyofuku T, Lytton J (1992) Structure-function relationships of endoplasmic reticulum type Ca^{2+} pumps. In: Ion-Motive ATPases: Structure, Function and Regulation (ed. Scarpa A, Carafoli E, Papa S) Vol 167, pp 1–10, The New York Academy of Sciences, New York

38. Lytton J, Westlin M, Burk SE, Shull GE, MacLennan DH (1992) Functional comparisons between isoforms of the sarcoplasmic or endoplasmic reticulum family of calcium pumps. J Biol Chem 267: 14483–14489

39. VanWinkle WB, Tate CA, Blick RJ, Entman ML (1981) Nucleotide triphosphate utilization by cardiac and skeletal muscle sarcoplasmic reticulum: Evidence for hydrolysis cycle not coupled to intermediate acylphosphate formation and calcium translocation. J Biol Chem 256: 2268–2274

40. Narayanan N, Su N, Bedard P (1991) Inhibitory and stimulatory effects of fluoride on the calcium pump of cardiac sarcoplasmic reticulum. Biochem Biophys Acta 1070: 83–91

41. Hawkins C, Xu A, Narayanan N (1994) Comparison of the effects of fluoride on the calcium pumps of cardiac and fast-twitch skeletal muscle sarcoplasmic reticulum: Evidence for tissue-specific qualitative difference in calcium-induced pump conformation. Biochem Biophys Acta 1191: 231–243

42. Pearson RB, Woodgett JR, Cohen P, Kemp BE (1985) Substrate specificity of a multifunctional calmodulin-dependent protein kinase. J Biol Chem 260: 14471–14476

43. Toyofuku T, Kurzydlowski K, Narayanan N, MacLenan DH (1994) Identification of the site in cardiac sarcoplasmic reticulum Ca^{2+}-ATPase that is phosphorylated by Ca^{2+}/calmodulin-dependent protein kinase. J Biol Chem 269: 26492–26496

44. Briggs FN, Lee KF, Wechsler AW, Jones JR (1992) Phospholamban expressed in slow-twitch and chronically stimulated fast-twitch muscles minimally affects calcium affinity of sarcoplasmic reticulum Ca^{2+}-ATPase. J Biol Chem 267: 26056–26061

45. Kirchberger MA, Tada M (1976) Effects of adenosine 3':5'-monophosphate-dependent protein kinase on sarcoplasmic reticulum isolated from cardiac and slow and fast contracting skeletal muscles. J Biol Chem 251: 725–729

46. Morris GL, Cheng HC, Colyer J, Wang JH (1991) Phospholamban regulation of cardiac sarcoplasmic reticulum (Ca^{2+}-Mg^{2+})-ATPase: Mechanism of regulation and site of monoclonal antibody interaction. J Biol Chem 266: 11270–11275

47. Toyofuku T, Kurzydlowski K, Lytton J, MacLennan DH (1994) Amino acids Glu^2 to Ile^{18} in the cytoplasmic domain of phospholamban are essential for functional association with the Ca^{2+}-ATPase of sarcoplasmic reticulum. J Biol Chem 269: 3088–3094

48. Nakamura Y, Schwartz A (1970) Possible role of intracellular calcium metabolism by [H^+] in sarcoplasmic reticulum of skeletal and cardiac muscle. Biochem Biophys Res Commun 41: 830–836

49. Mandel F, Kranias EG, DeGende AG, Sumidar M, Schwartz A (1982) The effect of pH on the transient state kinetics of Ca^{2+}-Mg^{2+}-ATPase of cardiac sarcoplasmic reticulum: A comparison with skeletal muscle sarcoplasmic reticulum. Circ Res 50: 310–317

50. Fabiato A (1985) Use of Aequorin for the appraisal of the hypothesis of the release of Calcium from the sarcoplasmic reticulum induced by a change of pH in skinned cardiac cells. Cell Calcium 6: 95–108

51. Orchrad CH, Kentish JC (1990) Effects of changes of pH on the contractile function of cardiac muscle. Am J Physiol 258: C967–C981

52. Tada M, Inui M, Yamada M, Kadoma M, Kuzuya T, Abe H, Kakiuchi S (1983) Effects of phospholamban phosphorylation catalyzed by adenosine 3':5'-monophosphate- and calmodulin-dependent protein kinases on calcium transport ATPase of cardiac sarcoplasmic reticulum. J Mol Cell Cardiol 15: 335–346

53. Wegener AD, Jones LR (1984) Phosphorylation-induced mobility shift in phospholamban in sodium dodecyl sulfate-polyacrylamide gels. J Biol Chem 259: 1834–1841

54. Fujii J, Kadoma M, Tada M, Toda H, Sakiyama F (1986) Characterization of structural unit of phospolamban by amino acid sequencing and electrophoretic analysis. Biochem Biophys Res Commun 138: 1044–1050

55. Xu A, Narayanan N (1994) Differential effects of fluoride on Ca^{2+}/calmodulin-dependent phosphorylation in cardiac sarcoplasmic reticulum. FASEB J 8: A162 (abstract)

56. Murphy AJ, Coll RJ (1992) Fluoride is a slow, tight-binding inhibitor of the Ca^{2+}-ATPase of sarcoplasmic reticulum. J Biol Chem 267: 5229–5235

57. Troullier A, Girardet JL, Dupont Y (1992) Fluoraluminate complexes are bifunctional analogues of phosphate in sarcoplasmic reticulum Ca^{2+}-ATPase. J Biol Chem 267: 22821–22829

58. Witcher DR, Strifler BA, Jones LR (1992) Cardiac-specific phosphorylation site for multifunctional Ca^{2+}/calmodulin-dependent protein kinase is conserved in the brain ryanodine receptor. J Biol Chem 267: 4963–4967

59. MacDougall LK, Jones LR, Cohen P (1991) Identification of the major protein phosphatases in mammalian cardiac muscle which dephosphorylate phospholamban. Eur J Biochem 196: 725–734

60. Tokumitsu H, Chijiwar T, Hagiwara M, Mizutani A, Terasawa M, Hidaka H (1990) KN-62, 1-[N,O-bis(1,5-isoquinolinesulfonyl)-N-methyl-N-methyl-L-tyrosyll}-4-phenylpiperazine, a specific inhibitor of Ca^{2+}/calmodulin-dependent protein kinase II. J Biol Chem 265: 4315–4320

61. Hawkins CE, Xu A, Narayanan N (1994) Evidence that the Ca^{2+}/calmodulin-dependent protein kinase intrinsic to cardiac sarcoplasmic reticulum is not CaM kinase II. Mol Cell Cardiol 26: CLXXX1X (abstract)

62. Edman CF, Schulman H (1994) Identification and characterization of δ_B-CaM kinase and δ_C-CaM kinase from rat heart, two new multifunctional Ca^{2+}/calmodulin-dependent protein kinase isoforms. Biochem Biophys Acta 1221: 89–101

63. Schworer CM, Rothblum LI, Thekkumkara TJ, Singer HA (1993) Identification of novel isoforms of δ subunit of Ca^{2+}/calmodulin-dependent protein kinase II. Differential expression in rat brain and aorta. J Biol Chem 268: 14443–14449

64. Kranias EG (1985) Regulation of calcium transport by protein phosphatase activity associated with cardiac sarcoplasmic reticulum. J Biol Chem 260: 11006–11010

65. Steenaart NAE, Ganin JR, DiSalvo J, Kranias EG (1992) The phospholamban phosphatase associated with cardiac sarcoplasmic reticulum is a type 1 enzyme. Arch Biochem Biophys 293: 17–24

66. Xiao RP, Cheng H, Lederer WJ, Suzuki T, Lakatta EG (1994) Dual regulation of Ca^{2+}/calmodulin-dependent protein kinase II activity by membrane voltage and by calcium influx. Proc Natl Acad Sci USA 91: 9659–9663

67. Netticadan T, Xu A, Narayanan N (1994) Ruthenium red inhibits Ca^{2+}/calmodulin-dependent phosphorylation of Ca^{2+}-release channel in cardiac sarcoplasmic reticulum. Can J Cardiol 10: 93A (abstract)

68. Hawkins C, Xu A, Narayanan N (1993) Divergent effects of a cytosolic protein on Ca^{2+}/calmodulin-dependent protein kinase (CaM kinase) mediated phosphorylation of calcium pump and calcium channel in cardiac sarcoplasmic reticulum (SR). Proc Can Fed Biol Soc 38: 81 (abstract)

Authors' address:
Dr. N. Narayanan
Department of Physiology
Medical Sciences Building
University of Western Ontario
London, Ontario, Canada, N6A 5C1

Site-specific phosphorylation of a phospholamban peptide by cyclic nucleotide- and Ca^{2+}/calmodulin-dependent protein kinases of cardiac sarcoplasmic reticulum

P. Karczewski, M. Kuschel, L. G. Baltas, S. Bartel, E.-G. Krause

Max Delbrück Center for Molecular Medicine, Berlin-Buch, Germany

Abstract

Phospholamban (PLB), the regulator of the cardiac sarcoplasmic reticulum (SR) Ca^{2+} pump is specifically phosphorylated at Ser^{16} and Thr^{17} by cAMP-dependent protein kinase (PKA) and Ca^{2+}/calmodulin-dependent protein kinase (CaMK), respectively. The regulation of this dual-site phosphorylation of amino acid residues in direct proximity is only poorly understood. In order to study the site-specific phosphorylation of PLB, we used a synthetic peptide (PLB-24) corresponding to the cytosolic part of the PLB monomer with the phosphorylation sites as a model substrate. PLB-24 possesses substrate properties as the native PLB as demonstrated by phosphorylation with exogenous, purified PKA, cGMP-dependent protein kinase (PKG) and a type II CaMK (CaMKII). In isolated vesicles of cardiac SR there was a rapid phosphorylation of the peptide by the endogenous PKA (SR-PKA) and CaMK (SR-CaMK), but not under conditions that activate PKG. Both SR-PKA and SR-CaMK incorporated the same amount of ^{32}P into PLB-24, 0.60 ± 0.01 nmol ^{32}P/mg SR protein and 0.61 ± 0.03 nmol ^{32}P/mg SR protein, respectively. Phosphorylation by SR-PKA was abolished by the specific PKA inhibitor ($IC_{50} = 0.2$ μM), whereas SR-CaMK phosphorylation was inhibited by calmidazolium ($IC_{50} = 1.6$ μM) and a CaMKII-specific inhibitor peptide ($IC_{50} = 2.5$ μM). Phosphorylation by SR-PKA was exclusively at Ser, whereas SR-CaMK phosphorylated only Thr. After simultaneous activation of both SR-kinases ^{32}P incorporation into PLB-24 was additive and occurred at Ser as well as at Thr. Sequential activation of SR-PKA and SR-CaMK also caused the additive phosphorylation of PLB-24 independently of which kinase was activated first. Thus, at the monomeric level of PLB the respective phosphorylation site appears to be accessible to its related SR protein kinase *in vitro* even when the adjacent site is phosphorylated.

Key words Phospholamban peptide – phosphorylation – cAMP-dependent protein kinase – Ca^{2+}/calmodulin-dependent protein kinase – cardiac sarcoplasmic reticulum

Introduction

Calcium transport by the cardiac sarcoplasmic reticulum (SR) is modulated through second messenger-specific phosphorylation of its calcium handling systems. Identified targets for protein kinases of different signaling pathways in the SR are phospholamban (27), the Ca^{2+}-pumping ATPase (32) and the Ca^{2+} release channel (6). Phospholamban is a small integral protein of SR membranes which in the dephosphorylated state inhibits the Ca^{2+} ATPase (12). Phosphorylation releaves this inhibition. Phospholamban is a pentameric protein consisting of identical subunits of 52 amino acids each carrying the complete set of phosphorylation sites (25). Each monomer has been predicted to consist of the cytosolic domain extending from the NH_2 terminus to residue 30, and the membrane-spanning domain with the remaining 20 amino acids (9). *In vitro* phospholamban is specifically phosphorylated by cyclic AMP-dependent protein kinase (PKA) at a serine residue that has been localized to position 16 (Ser^{16}) on the monomer and by Ca^{2+}/calmodulin-dependent protein kinase (CaMK) at a threonine residue identified as Thr^{17} (30). In cardiac SR preparations phospholamban is phosphorylated by cyclic GMP-dependent protein kinase (PKG) at about the same rate and at the same serine residue as by PKA (22). *In vitro* studies showed that PKA and CaMK can phosphorylate phospholamban independently of each other and that both phosphorylations stimulate SR Ca^{2+} uptake (26). Data on the action of the additive phosphorylation when both kinases are operating on SR Ca^{2+} uptake are controversial (2, 3). In the intact heart phospholamban is phosphorylated in response to β-adrenergic stimulation. Recent studies give strong evidence that phospholamban is the key mediator of catecholamine action on cardiac contractile function (19). Stimulation by the β-adrenergic agonist isoproterenol induces both cAMP-dependent phosphorylation and Ca^{2+}/calmodulin-dependent phosphorylation of phospholamban (11, 31). Interventions increasing intracellular Ca^{2+} independently on cAMP failed to induce phosphorylation of phospholamban (16). From these data it has been concluded that in the intact heart cAMP-dependent phosphorylation is a prerequisite for Ca^{2+}-dependent phosphorylation of phospholamban. Other authors reported on Ca^{2+}-induced phospholamban phosphorylation by cAMP-independent mechanisms (14). So the relative roles as well as the regulation of PKA- and CaMK-mediated phosphorylation of phospholamban are not clearly understood.

Synthetic peptides corresponding to the amino acid sequence of different parts of the phospholamban monomer have been widely used and proven to be a suitable tool to study the interaction with the SR Ca^{2+} ATPase and the effect of phosphorylation (7, 8, 24, 28, 31). In order to study the potency and dynamics of endogenous protein kinases in fractions of cardiac sarcoplasmic reticulum in regard to specific phosphorylation of phospholamban we used a synthetic peptide (PLB-24) as *in vitro* model of the monomeric phospholamban. PLB-24 corresponds to the cytosolic part of the phospholamban monomer ($Met^1 - Asn^{30}$) with the amino acids Asp^2 to Arg^{25} and carries both identified phosphorylation sites (Ser^{16}, Thr^{17}). Our data demonstrate that SR vesicles isolated from rabbit myocardium possess activities of both PKA and CaMK which specifically phosphorylate PLB-24 at serine and threonine residues, respectively. Both phosphorylation sites of PLB-24 have been shown to remain accessible to their related protein kinase even when the adjacent site already is phosphorylated.

Methods

Preparation of cardiac sarcoplasmic reticulum fractions

Fractions of cardiac SR from about 10 g of frozen rabbit hearts powdered under liquid nitrogen were prepared by the method of Harigaya and Schwartz (5). The final membrane suspension was aliquoted and stored at −80 °C until use.

PLB-24 peptide synthesis

Synthesis of PLB-24 peptide (BioTez GmbH Berlin, FRG) was performed by the solid phase method and purified by reverse-phase HPLC on a Bischoft Polyencap 300 column (10 mm particle size). The identity of the purified peptide was verified by amino acid analysis.

PLB-24 peptide posphorylation

The phosphorylation reaction was carried out in a standard incubation mixture containing 25 mM PIPES pH 6.8, 10 mM $MgCl_2$, 100 μg bovine serum albumin, 5 μg PLB-24 and 20 μg SR protein. For assaying phosphorylation by endogenous PKA the incubation mixture was completed by 10 μM cAMP and 1 mM EGTA. For activating endogenous CaMK 100 μM $CaCl_2$ and 0.5 μM calmodulin (Calbiochem, USA) was added as well as 0.5 μg of PKI (inhibitor peptide of PKA, rabbit sequence, Sigma, USA). To specifically inhibit CaMK activity the calmodulin antagonist calmidazolium (Sigma, USA) and CaMKII (281–302) (Biomol, FRG), a peptide related to the autoinhibitory domain of the class II type enzyme, were used. Phosphorylation by endogenous PKG was measured in the presence of 10 μM cGMP and 0.5 μg PKI. For phosphorylation with exogenous protein kinase the purified enzyme was added to a final concentration of 100 nM and the standard incubation mixture was completed with 100 μM $CaCl_2$ and 0.5 μM calmodulin for CaMK and 10 μM cGMP in the case of PKG. The tubes were preincubated at 30 °C for 2 min. Then the phosphorylation reaction was initiated by the addition of $[\gamma\text{-}^{32}P]$ATP (Amersham, UK) to the final concentration of 50 μM (200 dpm/pmol). The total assay volume was 50 μl. The reaction was terminated by adding 10 μl of 15 % trichloroacetic acid. Denaturated protein was sedimented by centrifugation and 40 μl aliquots of the supernatant were spotted onto P 81 phosphocellulose filters (Whatmann, UK). The filters were immediately put into ice-cold 75 mM H_3PO_4 and subsequently washed three times for 5 min in 75 mM H_3PO_4. Filters were transferred into scintillation vials and 10 ml H_2O was added. Radioactivity bound to filters was quantitated by measuring the Cerenkov radiation in a liquid scintillation counter.

Phosphoamino acid analysis

Phosphorylation of PLB-24 was performed essentially as described above. Aliqouts of 40 μl of the acidified supernatant containing the phosphorylated PLB-24 were spotted onto 2×2 cm pieces of methanol-activated PVDF membrane (Immobilon, Serva, FRG) and left to dry for 15 to 30 min. Then the membranes were cut into small pieces, transferred to safe-lock reaction tubes and 500 μl of 6 M HCL was added to each sample. Before closing the tubes were gased with nitrogen. Hydrolysis was performed at 105 °C for the following time: 5 h for P-serine, 15 h for P-threonine and 8 h for both P-serine and P-threonine when PLB-24 had been phosphorylated by endogenous PKA and CaMK simultaneously. After hydrolysis supernatants were removed and lyophilized. The dried samples were dissolved in a small volume of thin-layer electrophoresis buffer containing P-serine and P-threonine (Sigma, USA) as standards and separated on cellulose thin-layer sheets (Merck, FRG) on a Pharmacia Phast electrophoresis system as described in (17). After separation thin-layer sheets were dried first with a hair-dryer and then for 30 min at 65 °C in an oven. Standards were visualized by spraying with ninhydrin solution followed by incubation at 65 °C. Radioactive labeled phosphoamino acids hydrolyzed from PLB-24 were detected by autoradiography on XBD-X-ray film (Fotochemische Werke GmbH Berlin, FRG).

Other methods

The catalytic subunit of cAMP-dependent protein kinase was prepared from bovine heart as described by Peters et al. (23). PKG from bovine lung was purified according to (29). CaMKII from rat brain was purified as in (1). Inhibition constants were calculated by nonlinear regression using the Inplot4 software (GraphPad Inc., USA).

Results

To confirm that the PLB-24 peptide possesses the same phosphorylation characteristics as described for native phospholamban purified exogenous protein kinases were used. Figure 1 shows the time-course of PLB-24 phosphorylation by equimolar concentrations of catalytic subunit of PKA, PKG and CaMKII. All three kinases were able to phosphorylate PLB-24 to about the same extent. The time-course for phosphorylation by CaMKII was slower, but finally reached the same plateau value for phosphate incorporation. The phosphoamino acid analysis of PLB-24 phosphorylated with catalytic subunit of PKA revealed entirely phosphoserine (Fig. 2). After phosphorylation with CaMKII there was phosphate incorporation detectable only as phosphothreonine. Thus, PLB-24 elicits phosphorylation properties as required and therefore was used as model substrate to study phospholamban phosphorylation specifically brought about by endogenous protein kinases of cardiac SR.

Figure 3 demonstrates the phosphorylation of PLB-24 by isolated fractions of cardiac SR under conditions established to specifically activate endogenous PKA, PKG and CaMK. Endogenous phosphatases were left unaffected in order to detect the potential of protein kinase activating conditions in native SR vesicles. There was no PLB-24 phosphorylation in the presence of cGMP, indicating that cardiac SR fractions used did not contain PKG activity. The phosphorylation of PLB-24 in the presence of cAMP was very similar to that obtained when Ca^{2+} and calmodulin was added with respect to time-course and maximal phosphate incorporation. In both cases the reaction reached the maximum within 5 min and remained at plateau levels up to 25 min. The average of maximal phosphate incorporation into PLB-24 (mean ± SEM of five separate experiments) was 0.60 ± 0.03 nmol ^{32}P/mg SR protein in the presence of cAMP and 0.61 ± 0.01 nmol ^{32}P/mg SR protein when Ca^{2+} and calmodu-

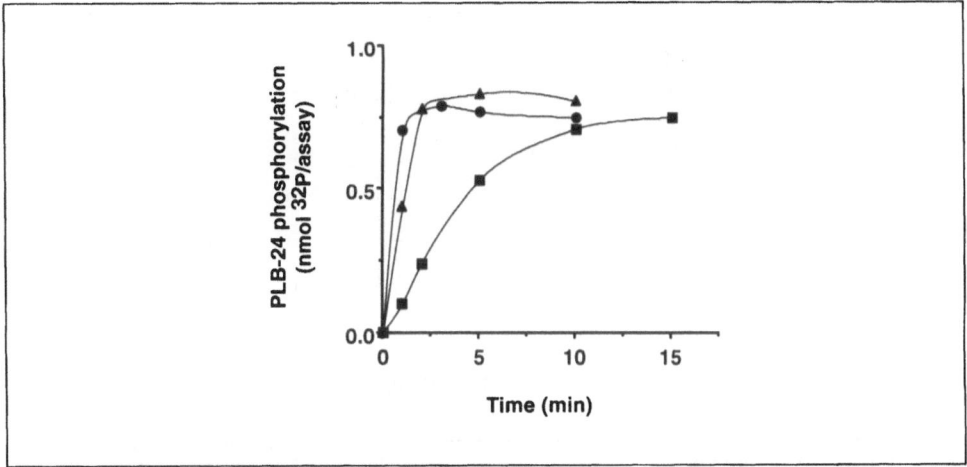

Fig. 1. Time-course of PLB-24 peptide phosphorylation by exogenous, purified protein kinases. Protein kinases were used in equimolar concentrations of 0.1 μM; (●) catalytic subunit of cAMP-dependent protein kinase, (▲) cGMP-dependent protein kinase, (■) Ca^{2+}/calmodulin-dependent protein kinase. For experimental details see the Methods section.

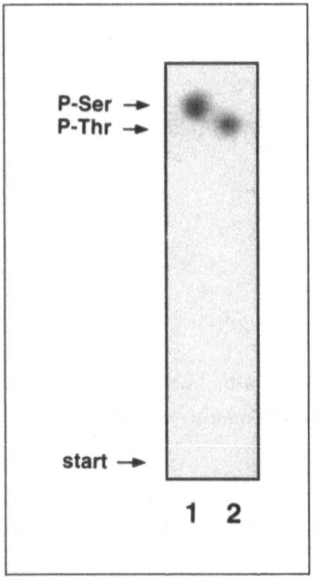

Fig. 2. Phosphoamino acid analysis of PLB-24 peptide phosphorylated by (1) catalytic subunit of cAMP-dependent protein kinase and (2) Ca^{2+}/calmodulin-dependent protein kinase. Details are given in the Methods section.

lin was added. To verify that these phosphorylation reactions were catalyzed by the respective endogenous kinases specific inhibitors were used (Fig. 4A and B). The highly specific inhibitor peptide for PKA completely blocked cAMP-induced PLB-24 phosphorylation with an IC_{50} of 0.2 μM. The phosphorylation of PLB-24 in the

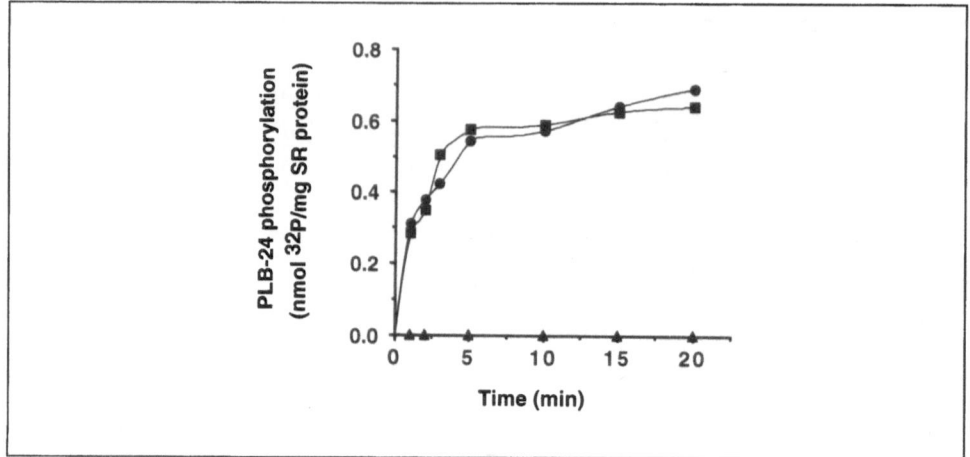

Fig. 3. PLB-24 peptide phosphorylation by endogenous protein kinases of cardiac sarcoplasmic reticulum. Conditions to activate specifically endogenous (●) cAMP-dependent protein kinase, (▲) cGMP-dependent protein kinase, (■) Ca^{2+}/calmodulin-dependent protein kinase are described in detail in the Methods section.

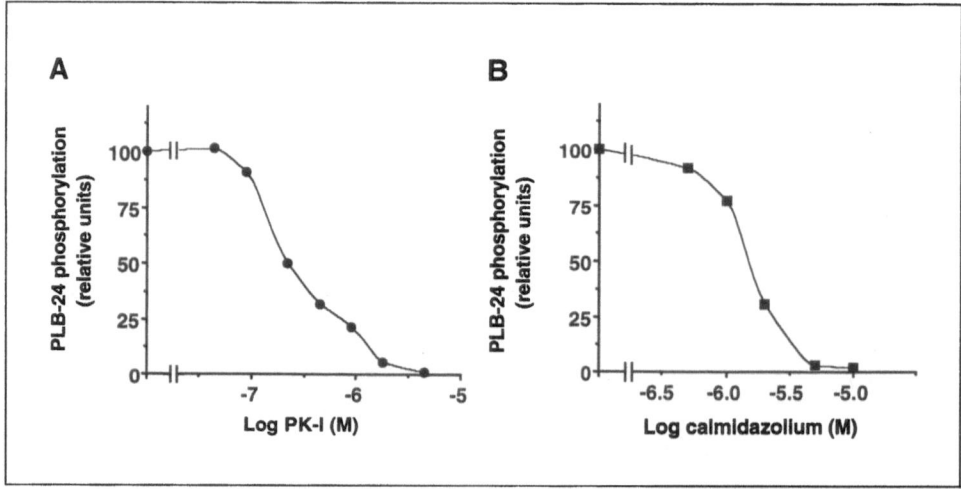

Fig. 4. Inhibition of PLB-24 peptide phosphorylation catalyzed by endogenous protein kinases of cardiac sarcoplasmic reticulum. **(A)** Inhibition of cAMP-dependent phosphorylation by the specific inhibitor peptide for cAMP-dependent protein kinase **(B)** Inhibition of Ca^{2+}/calmodulin-dependent phosphorylation by the calmodulin antagonist calmidazolium.

presence of Ca^{2+} and calmodulin was nearly abolished with increasing concentrations of the calmodulin antagonist calmidazolium. The IC_{50} was calculated to be 1.6 μM. Furthermore, the CaMKII (281–302) peptide, a specific inhibitor of the CaMK class II type enzyme, was found to be a sensitive blocker of protein kinase activity in the used SR preparations assayed with PLB-24 in the presence of Ca^{2+} and calmodulin. The obtained IC_{50} value of 2.5 μM is close to that obtained for endogenous δ-CaMKII in highly purified vesicles of cardiac SR (1). Phosphoamino acid analysis of PLB-24 phosphorylated under conditions as above showed phosphate incorporation specifically in serine residues in the presence of cAMP and in threonine residues when endogenous CaMK was activated by the addition of Ca^{2+} and calmodulin (Fig. 5). When both endogenous PKA and CaMK were activated simultaneously the phosphate incorporation was additive and occurred in serine as well as in threonine residues. Thus the assay conditions allow to specifically detect PLB-24 phosphorylation in sarcoplasmic reticulum vesicles catalyzed by endogenous PKA (SR-PKA) and the endogenous CaMK (SR-CaMK).

To answer the question whether possible interactions between the two phosphorylation sites in direct proximity (Ser^{16} and Thr^{17} in native phospholamban) may modulate their accessibility, phosphorylation experiments were performed with sequential activation of endogenous SR protein kinases (Fig. 6A and B). Without any additions to the reaction medium there was a significant unstimulated phosphorylation of PLB-24. This phosphorylation could be attributed to basal activities of SR-PKA and was abolished by the PKA-specific inhibitor peptide (data not shown). After activation of SR-PKA phosphate incorporation into PLB-24 reached the maximum within 5 min and remained at plateau levels up to 25 min (Fig. 6A). The activation of SR-CaMK after 10 min of SR-PKA reaction induced an additional rapid phosphorylation reaching maximum within the following 5 min. A similar pattern of additive phosphorylation was obtained when SR kinases were activated in the opposite sequence (Fig. 6B). Here the activation of SR-PKA, when PLB-24 phosphorylation by SR-CaMK already had reached plateau values, also led to an additional rapid phosphate

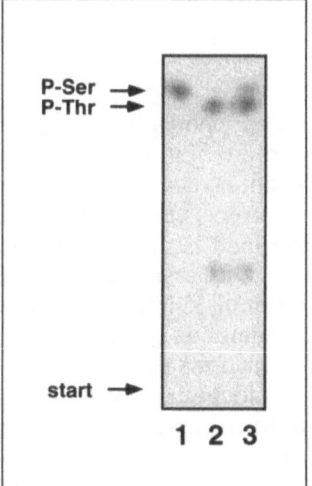

Fig. 5. Phosphoamino acid analysis of PLB-24 phosphorylated by endogenous protein kinases of cardiac sarcoplasmic reticulum. **(1)** Endogenous cAMP-dependent protein kinase and **(2)** endogenous Ca^{2+}/calmodulin-dependent protein kinase were activated as described in the Methods section. **(3)** Simultaneous activation of both endogenous protein kinases. In these experiments no EGTA or inhibitor peptide of cAMP-dependent protein kinase was present.

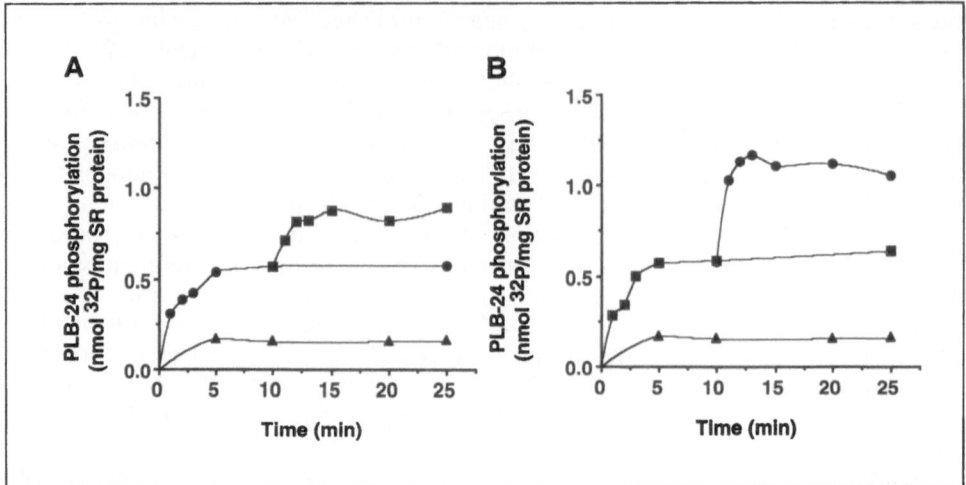

Fig. 6. Additive phosphorylation of PLB-24 by sequential activation of endogenous protein kinases of cardiac sarcoplasmic reticulum. **(A)** Initiation of cAMP-dependent phosphorylation followed 10 min later by activation of endogenous Ca^{2+}/calmodulin-dependent protein kinase. **(B)** Ca^{2+}/calmodulin-dependent phosphorylation followed after 10 min by activation of endogenous cAMP-dependent protein kinase. Conditions are as described in the Methods section except that no EGTA or inhibitor peptide of cAMP-dependent protein kinase was added to the assay mixture. (▲) unstimulated, (●) cAMP-stimulated, (■) Ca^{2+}/calmodulin-dependent phosphorylation of PLB-24.

incorporation. Thus endogenous protein kinases of cardiac SR can specifically phosphorylate PLB-24 completely independently from each other. The respective phosphorylation site remains accessible for the related kinase even when the proximal site is phosphorylated.

Discussion

Here we report on characteristics and dynamics of site-specific phosphorylation of the synthetic peptide PLB-24 by protein kinases intrinsic to membrane fractions of cardiac sarcoplasmic reticulum. PLB-24 corresponds to the amino acids 2 to 25 of the phospholamban monomer. This synthetic peptide has been used as model substrate to study properties of the adjacent phosphorylation sites Ser and Thr on the level of the hydrophilic entity of the monomeric phospholamban. Our experiments with exogenous as well as endogenous protein kinases revealed similar substrate properties for PLB-24 as described to be typical for native phospholamban (25).

   The synthetic peptide model system used is void of interactions due to the pentameric structure of native phospholamban in sarcoplasmic reticulum membranes as well as of the strong tendency of the complete monomer to form aggregates (18, 30). Recent studies have shown that in aqueous solution PLB-24 apparently does not keep a predominant secondary structure (7). Both the non-phosphorylated and the phosphorylated form of the peptide have been shown to adopt a primarily disordered conformation (21). Thus it is not likely that phosphorylation sites of a fraction of PLB-24 are masked or affected in their accessibility for protein kinases due to inter-molecular interactions. So the properties of phosphorylation sites of PLB-24 should be determined primarily by their surrounding amino acids.

Endogenous protein kinases in cardiac vesicle fractions, partially enriched in mem-branes of SR, phosphorylated PLB-24 with about the same potency in a cAMP-spe-cific as well as a Ca^{2+}/calmodulin-dependent fashion. Activating conditions for PKG failed to induce PLB-24 phosphorylation, although PLB-24 was an excellent sub-strate for exogenous, highly purified PKG. Apparently the membrane fractions used were devoid of PKG. Compared to PKA the concentration of PKG in cardiac myo-cytes has been estimated to be very low (20). Either cardiac SR membranes do not contain PKG or the enzyme is loosely associated with membrane structures and easily removed during the isolation procedure as it has been described for vascular smooth muscle (4).

It has been known for many years that cardiac SR contains a Ca^{2+}/calmodulin-dependent protein kinase that phosphorylates phospholamban (13, 15). But nature and properties of this SR-CaMK are only partially solved. SR-CaMK appears to be tightly bound to membranes of cardiac SR and only its partial purification has been described so far (10). Based on some of the known biochemical properties it has been proposed that SR-CaMK may belong to the family of the multifunctional Ca^{2+}/cal-modulin-dependent protein kinases, the CaMKII. Recently, we have characterized SR-CaMK in highly purified pig heart SR using the same PLB-24 peptide to be a dis-tinct form of the δ-CaMKII isozyme (1). Here we demonstrate that the SR-CaMK phosphorylates PLB-24 specifically at threonine residues and that time-course and extent of this phosphorylation is very similar to that obtained with SR-PKA. The inhibition of PLB-24 phosphorylation by the specific CaMKII inhibitor peptide indi-cates that it was catalyzed by a type II Ca^{2+}/calmodulin-dependent protein kinase intrinsic to the membrane preparations used.

Phosphorylation of phospholamban by PKA and CaMK *in vitro* was shown to be additive (26) and to occur specifically at Ser^{16} and Thr^{17}, respectively (31). Studies on intact heart preparations led to the hypothesis that cAMP-mediated phosphorylation is a prerequisite for Ca^{2+}/calmodulin-dependent phosphorylation of phospholamban (31). It remained unclear what is the base for this apparent priority of cAMP-mediated phosphorylation. One explanation, we were interested to study is that the phosphorylation sites situated in direct proximity interact in a way that determines the sequence of phosphorylation. In an early study the dynamics of sequential phos-phorylation was shown as phosphate incorporation into total cardiac SR membrane protein (15). But these data cannot be attributed directly to phosphorylation of phos-pholamban, because in cardiac SR there are substrates for CaMK others than phos-pholamban (6, 32). Using PLB-24 as model of the monomeric phospholamban we have demonstrated that endogenous SR-PKA and SR-CaMK are able to phosphory-late the adjacent phosphorylation sites in either sequence. Thus on the phospholam-ban monomer there is no priority of the PKA-specific Ser^{16} residue to become phos-phorylated. If there is a hierarchy in phosphorylation of Ser^{16} and Thr^{17} in the phos-pholamban molecule then it should be determined through interactions between the monomers or with the membrane environment. So in the intact heart most likely the site-specific phosphorylation of phospholamban and its sequence is defined by the mechanisms activating the related PKA and CaMK. Studies of physiological stimuli with intact cardiac preparations leading specifically to activation of CaMK and/or

PKA will contribute to further elucidate regulation and relevance of the multisite phosphorylation of phospholamban.

Acknowledgments   The authors thank Mrs. I. Ameln and Mrs. D. Vetter for excellent technical assistance. We also would like to thank Dr. U. Walter for his cooperation and support in the purification of cGMP-dependent protein kinase. Part of this work was supported by a grant from the Sonnenfeld-Stiftung Berlin, FRG. M. Kuschel is a recipient of a Sonnenfeld-Stiftung fellowship.

REFERENCES

1. Baltas L, Karczewski P, Krause E-G (1995) The cardiac sarcoplasmic reticulum phospholamban kinase is a distinct δ-CaM kinase isozyme. FEBS Lett 373: 71–75
2. Bilezikjian LM, Kranias EG, Potter JD, Schwartz A (1981) Studies on phosphorylation of canine cardiac sarcoplasmic reticulum by calmodulin-dependent protein kinase. Circ Res 49: 1356–1362
3. Colyer J, Wang JH (1991) Dependence of cardiac sarcoplasmic reticulum calcium pump activity on the phosphorylation status of phospholamban. J Biol Chem 266: 17486–17493
4. Cornwell TL, Pryzwanski KB, Wyatt TA, Lincoln TM (1991) Regulation of sarcoplasmic reticulum protein phosphorylation by localized cyclic GMP-dependent protein kinase in vascular smooth muscle cells. Mol Pharmacol 40: 923–931
5. Harigaya S, Schwartz A (1969) Rate of calcium binding and uptake in normal animal and failing human cardiac muscle. Circ Res 25: 781–794
6. Hohenegger M, Suko J (1993) Phosphorylation of the purified cardiac ryanodine receptor by exogenous and endogenous protein kinases. Biochem J 296: 303–308
7. Hubbard JA, MacLachlan LK, Meenan E, Salter CJ, Reid DG, Lahouratate P, Humphries J, Stevens N, Bell D, Neville WA, Murray KJ, Darker JG (1994) Confirmation of the cytosolic domain of phospholamban by NMR and CD. Mol Membr Biol 11: 263–269
8. Hughes G, East JM, Lee AG (1994) The hydrophilic domain of phospholamban inhibits the Ca^{2+} transport step of the Ca^{2+}-ATPase. Biochem J 303: 511–516
9. Inui JM, Kimura Y, Sasaki T, Tada M (1990) Molecular mechanisms of calcium uptake and release by sarcoplasmic reticulum. Japan Circ J 54: 1185–1191
10. Jett M-F, Schworer CM, Bass M, Soderling TR (1987) Identification of membrane-bound calcium, calmodulin-dependent protein kinase II in canine heart. Arch Biochem Biophys 255: 354–360
11. Karczewski P, Bartel S, Haase H, Krause E-G (1987) Isoproterenol induces both cAMP- and calcium-dependent phosphorylation of phospholamban in canine heart in vivo. Biomed Biochim Acta 46: 433–439
12. Kim HW, Steenart NAE, Ferguson DG, Kranias EG (1990) Functional reconstitution of the cardiac sarcoplasmic reticulum Ca^{2+}-ATPase with phospholamban in phospholipid vesicles. J Biol Chem 265: 1702–1709
13. Kranias EG, Bilezikjian LM, Potter JD, Piascik MT, Schwartz A (1980) The role of calmodulin in regulation of cardiac sarcoplasmic reticulum phosphorylation. Ann NY Acad Sci 356: 279–290
14. LePeuch CJ, Guilleaux J, DeMaille JG (1980) Phospholamban phosphorylation in the perfused rat heart is not solely dependent on β-adrenergic stimulation. FEBS Lett 114: 165–168
15. LePeuch CJ, Haiech J, Demaille JG (1979) Concerted regulation of cardiac sarcoplasmic reticulum calcium transport by cyclic adenosine monophosphate-dependent and calcium-calmodulin-dependent phosphorylations. Biochemistry 18: 5150–5157
16. Lindemann JP, Watanabe AM (1985) Phosphorylation of phospholamban in the intact myocardium. J Biol Chem 260: 4516–4525
17. Lippmann C, Lindschau C, Erdmann VA (1992) Thin-layer electrophoresis with PhastSystem facilitates analysis of phosphoamino acids from proteins bound to Immobilon. Electrophoresis 13: 666–668
18. Louis CF, Mafitt M, Jarvis B (1982) Factors that modify the molecular size of phospholamban, the 23,000-dalton cardiac sarcoplasmic reticulum phosphoprotein. J Biol Chem 257: 15182–15186
19. Luo W, Grupp I, Harrer J, Ponniah S, Grupp G, Duffy JJ, Doetschman T, Kranias EG (1994) Targeted ablation of the phospholamban gene is associated with markedly enhanced myocardial contractility and loss of β-adrenergic stimulation. Circ Res 75: 401–409

20. Mery P-F, Lohmann SM, Walter U, Fischmeister R (1991) Ca^{2+} current is regulated by cyclic GMP-dependent protein kinase in mammalian cardiac myocytes. Proc Natl Acad Sci USA 88: 1197–1201
21. Mortishiresmith RJ, Pitzenberger SM, Burke CJ, Middaugh CR, Garsky VM, Johnson RG (1995) Solution structure of the cytoplasmic domain of phospholamban – phosphorylation leads to a local perturbation in secondary structure. Biochemistry 34: 7603–7613
22. Raeymaekers L, Hofmann F, Casteels R (1988) Cyclic GMP-dependent protein kinase phosphorylates phospholamban in isolated sarcoplasmic reticulum from cardiac and smooth muscle. Biochem J 252: 269–273
23. Peters KA, Demaille JQ, Fischer EH (1977) Adenosine 3′:5′-monophosphate dependent protein kinase from bovine heart. Characterization of the catalytic subunit. Biochemistry 26: 5691–5697
24. Sasaki T, Inui M, Kimura Y, Kuzuya T, Tada M (1992) Molecular mechanisms of regulation of Ca^{2+} pump ATPase by phospholamban in cardiac sarcoplasmic reticulum. J Biol Chem 267: 1674–1679
25. Simmerman HKB, Collins JH, Theibert JL, Wegener AD, Jones LR (1986) Sequence analysis of phospholamban: identification of phosphorylation sites and two major structural domains. J Biol Chem 261: 13333:13341
26. Tada M, Inui M, Yamada M, Kadoma MA, Kuzuya T, Abe H, Kakiuchi S (1983) Effect of phospholamban phosphorylation catalyzed by adenosine 3′:5′-monophosphate- and calmodulin-dependent protein kinases on calcium transport ATPase of cardiac sarcoplasmic reticulum. J Mol Cell Cardiol 15: 335–346
27. Tada M, Katz A (1982) Phosphorylation of the sarcoplasmic reticulum and sarcolemma. Annu Rev Physiol 44: 401–423
28. Vorherr T, Chiesi M, Schwaller R, Carafoli E (1992) Regulation of the calcium ion pump of sarcoplasmic reticulum: Reversible inhibition by phospholamban and by the calmodulin binding domain of the plasma membrane calcium ion pump. Biochemistry 31: 371–376
29. Walter U, Miller P, Wilson F, Menkes D, Greengard P (1980) Immunological distinction between guanosine 3′:5′-monophosphate-dependent protein kinases. J Biol Chem 255: 3757–3762
30. Wegener AD, Simmerman HKB, Liepniekes J, Jones LR (1986) Proteolytic cleavage of phospholamban purified from canine sarcoplasmic reticulum vesicles: generation of a low resolution model of phospholamban structure. J Biol Chem 261: 5154–5159
31. Wegener AD, Simmerman HKB, Lindemann JP, Jones LR (1989) Phospholamban phosphorylation in intact ventricles. J Biol Chem 264: 11486–11474
32. Xu A, Hawkins C, Narayanan N (1993) Phosphorylation and activation of the Ca^{2+}-pumping ATPase of cardiac sarcoplasmic reticulum by Ca^{2+}/calmodulin-dependent protein kinase. J Biol Chem 268: 8394–8397

Authors' address:
Peter Karczewski, PhD
Max Delbrück Center for Molecular Medicine
Robert Rössle Straße 10
13125 Berlin-Buch, Germany

Sodium-calcium exchange: Recent advances

L. V. Hryshko, K. D. Philipson[1]

Division of Cardiovascular Sciences, St. Boniface General Hospital Research Centre, Winnipeg, Canada
[1] Cardiovascular Research Laboratories, UCLA School of Medicine, Los Angeles, USA

Abstract

Na-Ca exchange proteins are involved in Ca homeostasis in a wide variety of tissues. Unique Na-Ca exchangers have been identified by molecular biological approaches and it appears that these may represent a superfamily of ion transporters, similar to that identified for ion channels. Major advances in our understanding of these transporters have occurred in the past decade by combining molecular approaches with electrophysiological analyses. The regulatory and transport properties of Na-Ca exchangers are beginning to become understood in molecular detail. It also appears that the physiological roles of Na-Ca exchange may be quite complex. This brief review highlights some recent advances in Na-Ca exchange research obtained through the combination of molecular biological and electrophysiological approaches.

Key words Sodium-calcium exchange – regulation – exchanger isoforms

Introduction

Our ability to study Na-Ca exchange proteins has improved considerably in the past 6 years, in large part due to the application of molecular biological and electrophysiological techniques to investigate these transporters. The importance of the Na-Ca exchange system is well established in cardiac muscle. It is increasingly apparent that unique Na-Ca exchange proteins exist in other tissues and a more thorough understanding of their physiological roles is required. This review highlights some recent advances in Na-Ca exchange research with an emphasis on the cardiac Na-Ca exchanger, NCX1, as most studies have examined this prototypical exchanger.

Physiological function

In cardiac muscle, the Na-Ca exchanger plays a prominent role in contractile regulation. During regular patterns of cardiac stimulation, the same amount of Ca entering cells must be removed to maintain Ca homeostasis. The Na-Ca exchange system is the primary mechanism for this transsarcolemmal Ca efflux (3, 5, 15, 71). In general, the same amount of Ca entering through L-type Ca channels is removed by Na-Ca exchange (13). On a beat-to-beat basis, both sarcoplasmic reticular Ca uptake or Na-Ca exchange appear to be independently capable of mediating cardiac relaxation (4). In contrast, relaxation is markedly impaired if both of these systems are inhibited. Thus, the alternative Ca efflux or uptake pathways via sarcolemmal Ca-ATPases or mitochondria, do not appear to play substantial roles in physiological cardiac relaxation (4). Recently, antisense oligonucleotides directed against NCX1 have been used to verify the importance of this transporter in myocyte relaxation (6, 53). Treatment with antisense oligonucleotides completely inhibited the decay of Ca transients induced by caged Ca photorelease (53). Increases in intracellular Ca and Na-Ca exchange currents induced by extracellular Na removal were also abolished in this preparation. Antisense oligonucleotides have identified similar important roles for Na-Ca exchange in primary cultured neurons (6).

An increasing body of evidence supports the idea that reverse Na-Ca exchange may be involved in Ca entry during cardiac excitation and contribute to the Ca-induced Ca-release mechanism (42, 44–47). The majority of evidence for this role comes from voltage clamp experiments under conditions which eliminate Ca entry through L-type Ca channels. Under these conditions, Na entry through Na channels is thought to sufficiently elevate Na_i to activate reverse Na-Ca exchange (42). Even in the absence of sodium currents, reverse Na-Ca exchange may elevate Ca sufficiently to induce a sarcoplasmic reticulum Ca release (46). Inhibition of the exchanger by the inhibitory peptide, XIP, can partially prevent this reverse exchange-induced Ca release (41). Criticisms of this mechanism concern the use of elevated Na concentrations, loss of voltage control, and non-physiological sarcoplasmic reticular Ca loading (11, 83). This appears to be the case in guinea-pig coronary myocytes where reverse exchange can also induce a sarcoplasmic reticulum Ca release when intracellular sodium is elevated to very high levels (26). Recent studies in cardiac muscle have attempted to demonstrate this behaviour when physiological experimental conditions were employed (54, 55, 89, 90). Thus, while the physiological significance of this mechanism remains controversial, there is the interesting possibility that Na-Ca exchange may serve prominent roles in both contraction and relaxation of cardiac muscle.

The importance of Na-Ca exchange as a Ca efflux mechanism differs between species and within species during development. For example, Bers' group has demonstrated that in rat cardiac myocytes, only 7 % of the decline in intracellular Ca is attributable to Na-Ca exchange whereas this fraction is 28 % in rabbit myocytes (4). In general, it may be expected that species (eg. rat, mouse) which show a substantial dependence on sarcoplasmic reticular Ca cycling during excitation-contraction coupling will rely less so on Na-Ca exchange as a relaxation mechanism. Conversely, species (eg. rabbit, frog) with less robust sarcoplasmic reticular Ca cycling are likely to exhibit substantially greater fluxes through Na-Ca exchange. This reciprocal relationship between the importance of the sarcoplasmic reticulum and the Na-Ca exchange system appears to be maintained during development (65, 87). In general, the Na-Ca exchange system appears to play a prominent role in Ca fluxes in immature hearts prior to the development of the T tubular system and sarcoplasmic reticulum. Fetal and newborn rabbit hearts exhibit 2.5 fold more exchanger protein than adult hearts based on immunoreactivity studies (1). Similar developmental disparities were observed for Na-dependent Ca uptake into sarcolemmal vesicles in rabbit (1) although no difference was observed in a study using canine hearts (28). Exchanger transcript levels peak near birth in rabbit and rat myocytes and then exhibit a postnatal decline (10). Immunocytochemical localization studies have shown intense labeling in the T tubular system of adult guinea-pig myocytes (23). Developmentally, labeling is confined to the peripheral sarcolemma in immature rabbit myocytes. As the T tubular system and the sarcoplasmic reticulum develop, labeling of the exchanger becomes evident in these regions (16). Interestingly, a T tubular localization might situate the exchanger in proximity to the sarcoplasmic reticulum Ca release channel, a requisite for reverse Na-Ca exchange to be effective in contributing to SR Ca release.

The existence and operation of Na-Ca exchange systems have been documented in a wide variety of tissue types. A partial list includes cardiac, smooth, and skeletal muscle, neural, pancreatic and renal tissue, paracrine and amacrine cells, myometrium, blood, bone, and chromaffin cells (2, 7–9, 20, 24, 27, 30, 38–40, 43, 57, 62, 64, 66, 67, 76, 79, 84, 85, 88). A related protein, the Na-Ca, K exchanger is expressed primarily in the retina. This protein, Retx, differs both functionally and structurally from the cardiac exchanger (68, 78, 81). The majority of functional studies have focused on cardiac and neural tissues for which Na-Ca exchange was originally described. As discussed below, it is now evident that distinct Na-Ca exchange proteins are expressed in a tissue specific manner. These unique exchangers are a consequence of tissue-specific alternative splicing (40, 43). However, Na-Ca exchanger isoforms have also been identified which are the products of different genes (50, 67, 69). At present, detailed functional distinctions between these various exchanger proteins have not yet been described. This multiplicity of exchangers might have been anticipated given the considerable differences in Ca handling in different tissue types.

Na-Ca exchange proteins

The NCX1 cDNA encodes a protein composed of 970 amino acids with an approximate molecular weight of 120 kD (67). During biosynthesis and processing, a signal sequence of 32 amino acids is cleaved and N-linked glycosylation occurs at a single residue, Asn-9 (21, 35). Cleavage of the signal peptide has been verified by amino acid sequencing of the purified exchanger (21). Recent studies have demonstrated that functional expression of NCX1-type exchange proteins still occurs in constructs lacking the signal sequence, indicating the presence of internal topogenic signals for correct membrane insertion (25, 56, 80). A variety of expression systems have been used successfully for heterologous expression of exchange proteins including Xenopus oocytes (67), HeLa (24, 57), cos and 293 (39), CHO (17), BHK (69) and insect cells (49). In addition, Na-Ca exchange function is being examined in transgenic mice (51) which should provide new opportunities to investigate the physiology of this transport system.

Hydropathy analysis of the primary sequence for NCX1 predicts 11 transmembrane spanning regions with a large intervening hydrophilic region between transmembrane segments 5 and 6 (67, 73). The cytoplasmic orientation of this large intervening loop has been established using monoclonal antibodies (75). Identification of a cleaved signal sequence and glycosylation at position Asn-9 constrains the N-terminus to the extracellular surface (21, 35). However, few other details of the topology predicted by hydropathy analysis are established. Schwarz and Benzer (82) have identified an intramolecular homology for Na-Ca exchangers suggestive of a gene duplication event during the evolution of these proteins. Transmembrane segments 2 and 3 exhibit similarity to transmembrane segments 8 and 9. This intramolecular homology is conserved among all identified exchangers (74).

The above description provides the defining criteria for identifying members of the exchanger superfamily (74). That is, members possess similar secondary structure to NCX1 and inter- and intramolecular homology for transmembrane segments 2,3 and 8,9. Included in this family are NCX1 and its various splice variants. Splicing is observed near the C-terminus of the large cytoplasmic loop (40). NCX2 and NCX3 represent the products of different genes and are expressed primarily in brain and skeletal muscle based on Northern analysis (50, 69). The retinal Na-Ca,K exchanger exhibits these characteristics despite virtually no additional homology (78). Finally, large scale genome sequencing projects have led to the identification of putative exchangers including ones from yeast, *C.elegans,* and *E.coli* (74). The sequences of these latter exchangers are so divergent that a Na-Ca exchange function remains speculative (74).

Regulatory properties

A variety of regulatory influences have been described for the cardiac Na-Ca exchanger. NCX1 exhibits altered transport properties as a consequence of both intrinsic and extrinsic (environmental) factors. Extrinsic factors which have been studied in detail include voltage, ATP, pH, redox state, and the membrane environment (12, 17, 19, 29, 32, 34, 72, 77, 86). Activation of the Na-Ca exchanger by phosphorylation has been identified in the squid axon (18) and more recently in smooth muscle cells (37). Stimulation of β-adrenergic receptors appears to alter exchange function in frog cardiac muscle (22).

Intrinsically, NCX1 is regulated by both Na and Ca, in addition to transporting these ions (31). The giant excised patch technique has been particularly useful for the characterization of many of these properties. Na regulation leads to a partial inactivation of exchange currents in response to the application of cytoplasmic Na (31, 33). The Kd for this effect is similar to the Kd for transport, suggesting that the fully Na loaded exchanger can partition between active and inactive states. A physiological role for this inactivation mechanism is not immediately apparent. The operation of this mechanism has been demonstrated in intact cardiac myocytes, albeit under non-physiological conditions (60).

As first recognized in the squid giant axon, the cardiac Na-Ca exchanger is regulated by cytoplasmic Ca (63). From giant excised patch experiments, it has been possible to characterize this mechanism in detail (31, 34). Using conditions to measure reverse Na-Ca exchange, transported and regulatory Ca can be separated to the opposite membrane surfaces. Under these conditions, the application of micromolar

Ca to the cytoplasmic surface of the patch leads to a marked augmentation of outward exchange current for both NCX1 and NCX2 (31, 34, 50, 59, 61). In the absence of regulatory Ca, the exchange current is almost completely eliminated. This is striking given the fact that the electrochemical gradient is barely altered by this intervention. Thus, analogous to gating in ion channels, the exchanger can be "gated" by cytoplasmic Ca.

While a physiological role for Ca regulation is not completely established, this may serve as a means of coupling Ca influx to efflux. The Kd for regulation of 0.3 μM seems reasonable for this possibility (31, 34, 61). Ca regulation occurs slowly over a time-course of seconds under many experimental conditions (61). Consequently, the regulatory mechanism may sense the time averaged Ca over the course of several contraction-relaxation cycles. Increases in Ca entry or stimulation rates would increase time-averaged Ca levels and consequently up-regulate exchange function. Conversely, lower heart rates or levels of contractility would require less Ca efflux and this would be sensed by a reduction in time-averaged Ca levels at the regulatory Ca binding site. This possibility remains to be established.

The regulatory Ca binding site has been identified for NCX1 and comprises a segment of 137 amino acids within the large cytoplasmic loop of the exchanger (48, 61). Within this segment, there are two highly acidic regions thought to be involved in regulatory Ca binding. Mutation of specific amino acids within these acidic regions decreased ^{45}Ca binding affinity for fusion proteins expressing portions of the cytoplasmic loop (48). Similarly, a decrease in Ca affinity for functional regulation was observed for these mutants as assessed by the giant excised patch technique (61). The mechanism by which Ca binding is transduced to the transport machinery is unknown.

The regulatory Ca binding site is highly conserved among different exchangers. The acidic amino acid segments thought to be involved in Ca binding for NCX1, NCX2, and the Na-Ca exchanger from Drosophila exhibit greater than 75 % amino acid identity (36, 50, 61). This high degree of homology is perhaps surprising given the fact that all of these three exchangers show differences in their patterns of Ca_i regulation (36, 50, 61). In particular, Ca_i regulation is completely opposite for the Drosophila Na-Ca exchanger compared to NCX1 and NCX2 (36). That is, in response to cytoplasmic Ca application, the Drosophila Na-Ca exchanger is inhibited, in contrast to the observed stimulation in NCX1 and NCX2. Recently, we have studied mutations in the putative regulatory Ca binding region of the Drosophila exchanger and have confirmed that analogous mutations to those in NCX1 alter Ca_i regulation (14). Studies are currently underway investigating the transduction mechanism.

Physiological implications

Advances in our understanding of the diversity and functional properties of Na-Ca exchange proteins have occurred rapidly. However, more questions have been raised than answered. For example, cardiac muscle operates over a wide functional range, in large part, due to variations in Ca entry. Obviously then, Ca efflux must adjust to maintain Ca homeostasis. Given that Na-Ca exchange is the predominant mechanism for Ca efflux, it is surprising that so little is known regarding how this is accomplished. Does Ca_i regulation of the exchanger account entirely for this variable gain or do other physiological mechanisms operate? Is the exchanger simply present in such a large excess that Ca efflux is assured over a wide physiological range? Transgenic animal experiments may help provide answers to these questions. Na regulation of the exchanger has been documented in intact myocytes but a physiological role has not been established. Does ATP-dependent regulation of the exchanger contribute to Ca overload under such conditions as ischemia-reperfusion injury? Several studies have shown that Na-Ca exchange currents contribute to the transient inward currents during oscillatory afterpotentials (52, 70). However, the role of Na-Ca exchange in cardiac arrhythmogenesis still requires further investigation. Would bypassing the Na pump and directly modulating Na-Ca exchange produce a better inotropic agent than digitalis? It seems likely that a more comprehensive picture of Na-Ca exchange function will emerge within the next few years.

REFERENCES

1. Artman M (1992) Sarcolemmal Na^+-Ca^{2+} exchange activity and exchanger immunoreactivity in developing rabbit hearts. Amer J Physiol 263: H1506–H1513
2. Balasubramanyam M, Rohowsky-Kochan C, Reeves JP, Gardner JP (1994) Na^+/Ca^{2+} exchange-mediated calcium entry in human lymphocytes. J Clin Invest 94: 2002–2008
3. Barry WH, Bridge JHB (1993) Intracellular calcium homeostasis in cardiac myocytes. Circulation 87: 1806–1815
4. Bassani JWM, Bassani RA, Bers DM (1994) Relaxation in rabbit and rat cardiac cells: species-dependent differences in cellular mechanisms. J Physiol 476: 279–293
5. Bers DM (1991) Excitation-Contraction Coupling and Cardiac Contractile Force. Kluwer Academic Publications, Dordrecht Boston London
6. Bland KS, Takahashi K, Islam S, Michaelis ML (1996) Effects of NCX-1 antisense oligodeoxynucleotides on cardiac myocytes and primary neurons in culture. In: Hilgemann DW, Philipson KD, Vassort G (eds) Sodium-Calcium Exchange: Proceedings of the Third International Conference. New York Academy of Sciences, New York
7. Blaustein MP (1988) Sodium/calcium exchange and the control of contractility in cardiac muscle and vascular smooth muscle. J Cardiovasc Pharmacol 12: S56–S68
8. Blaustein MP (1989) Sodium-calcium exchange in cardiac, smooth, and skeletal muscles: key to control of contractility. In: Hoffman JF, Glebisch G (Eds) Current Topics in Membranes and Transport. Academic Press, Inc, San Diego, V34: 289–330
9. Blaustein MP, DiPolo R, Reeves JP, Eds (1991) Sodium-Calcium Exchange: Proceedings of the Second International Conference. New York Academy of Sciences, New York
10. Boerth SR, Zimmer DB, Artman M (1994) Steady-state mRNA levels of the sarcolemmal Na^+-Ca^{2+} exchanger peak near birth in the developing rabbit and rat hearts. Circ Res 74: 354–359
11. Bouchard RA, Clarke RB, Giles WR (1993) Regulation of unloaded cell shortening by sarcolemmal sodium-calcium exchange in isolated rat ventricular myocytes. J Physiol 469: 583–599
12. Bridge JHB, Spitzer KW, Ershler PR (1988) Relaxation of isolated ventricular cardiomyocytes by a voltage-dependent process. Science 241: 823–825
13. Bridge JHB, Smolley JR, Spitzer KW (1990) The relationship between charge movements associated with I_{Ca} and I_{Na-Ca} in cardiac myocytes. Science 248: 376–378
14. Buchko J, Hnatowich M, Hryshko LV (1996) The same regulatory Ca^{2+} binding site is employed by NCX1 and Calx for opposite Ca_i^{2+} regulation phenotypes. Biophys J (submitted)
15. Cannell MB (1991) Contribution of sodium-calcium exchange to calcium regulation in cardiac muscle. Ann N Y Acad Sci 639: 428–443
16. Chen F, Mottino G, Klitzner TS, Philipson KD, Frank JS (1995) Distribution of the Na^+/Ca^{2+} exchange protein in developing rabbit myocytes. Am J Physiol 268: C1126–C1132

17. Condrescu M, Gardner JP, Chernaya G, Aceto JF, Kroupis C, Reeves JP (1995) ATP-dependent regulation of sodium-calcium exchange in chinese hamster ovary cell transfected with the bovine cardiac sodium-calcium exchanger. J Biol Chem 270: 9137–9146
18. DiPolo R, Beauge L (1987) In squid axons, ATP modulates Na^+-Ca^{2+} exchange by a Ca_i^{2+}-dependent phosphorylation. Biochim Biophys Acta 897: 347–354
19. Doering AE, Lederer WJ (1993) The mechanism by which cytoplasmic protons inhibit the sodium-calcium exchanger in guinea-pig heart cells. J Physiol 466: 481–499
20. Dominguez JH, Mann C, Rothrock JK, Bhati V (1991) Na^+-Ca^{2+} exchange and Ca^{2+} depletion in rat proximal tubules. Amer J Physiol 261: F328–F335
21. Durkin JT, Ahrens DC, Pan YCE, Reeves JP (1991) Purification and amino-terminal sequence of the bovine cardiac sodium-calcium exchanger. Arch Biochim Biophys 290: 369–375
22. Fan J, Shuba Y, Morad M (1995) Modulation of sodium-calcium exchanger by beta-adrenergic agonists in frog ventricular myocytes. Biophys J 68: 136a
23. Frank JS, Mottino G, Reid D, Molday RS, Philipson KD (1992) Distribution of the Na^+-Ca^{2+} exchange protein in mammalian cardiac myocytes: an immunoflourescence and immunocolloidal gold-labeling study. J Cell Biol 117: 337–345
24. Furman I, Cook O, Kasir J, Rahamimoff H (1993) Cloning of two isoforms of the rat brain Na^+-Ca^{2+} exchanger gene and their functional expression in HeLa cells. Fed Eur Biochem Soc 319: 105–109
25. Furman I, Cook O, Kasir J, Low W, Rahamimoff (1995) The putative amino-terminal signal peptide of the cloned rat brain Na^+-Ca^{2+} exchanger gene (Rbe-1) is not mandatory for functional expression. J Biol Chem 270: 19120–19127
26. Ganitkevich VY, Isenberg G (1993) Ca^{2+} entry through Na^+-Ca^{2+} exchange can trigger Ca^{2+} release from Ca^{2+} stores in Na^+-loaded guinea-pig coronary myocytes. J Physiol 468: 225–243
27. Gleason E, Borges S, Wilson M (1994) Control of transmitter release from retinal amacrine cells by Ca^{2+} influx and efflux. Neuron 13: 1109–1117
28. Hanson GL, Schilling WP, Michael LH (1993) Sodium-potassium pump and sodium-calcium exchange in adult and neonatal canine cardiac sarcolemma. Amer J Physiol 264: H320–H326
29. Haworth RA, Goknur AB (1992) ATP dependence of calcium uptake by the Na-Ca exchanger of adult heart cells. Circ Res 71: 210–217
30. Herchuelz A, Lebrun P (1993) A role for Na/Ca exchange in the pancreatic B cell: studies with thapsigargin and caffeine. Biochem Pharmacol 45: 7–11
31. Hilgemann DW (1990) Regulation and deregulation of cardiac Na^+-Ca^{2+} exchange in giant excised sarcolemmal membrane patches. Nature 344: 242–245
32. Hilgemann DW, Collins A (1992) Mechanism of cardiac Na^+-Ca^{2+} exchange current stimulation by MgATP: possible involvement of amiophospholipid translocase. J Physiol 454: 59–82
33. Hilgemann DW, Matsuoka S, Nagel GA, Collins A (1992) Steady-state and dynamic properties of cardiac sodium-calcium exchange: sodium-dependent inactivation. J Gen Physiol 100: 905–932
34. Hilgemann DW, Collins A, Matsuoka S (1992) Steady-state and dynamic properties of cardiac sodium-calcium exchange: secondary modulation by cytoplasmic calcium and ATP. J Gen Physiol 100: 933–961
35. Hryshko LV, Nicoll DA, Weiss JN, Philipson KD (1993) Biosynthesis and initial processing of the cardiac sarcolemmal Na^+-Ca^{2+} exchanger. Biochim Biophys Acta 1151: 35–42
36. Hryshko LV, Nicoll DA, Matsuoka S, Weiss JN, Schwarz E, Benzer S, Philipson KD (1995) Anomolous regulation of the Na^+-Ca^{2+} exchanger from Drosophila. Biophys J 68: 410a
37. Iwamoto T, Wakabayashi S, Shigekawa M (1995) Growth factor-induced phosphorylation and activation of aortic smooth muscle Na^+/Ca^{2+} exchanger. J Biol Chem 270: 8996–9001
38. Kaplan JH, Kennedy BG, Somlyo AP (1987) Calcium-stimulated sodium efflux from rabbit vascular smooth muscle. J Physiol 388: 245–260
39. Kofuji P, Hadley RW, Kieval RS, Lederer WJ, Schulze DH (1992) Expression of the Na-Ca exchanger in diverse tissues: a study using the cloned human cardiac Na-Ca exchanger. Am J Physiol 263: C1241–C1249
40. Kofuji P, Lederer WJ, Shulze DH (1994) Mutually exclusive and cassette exons underlie alternatively spliced isoforms of the Na/Ca exchanger. J Biol Chem 269: 5145–5149
41. Kohmoto O, Levi AJ, Bridge JHB (1994) Relation between reverse sodium-calcium exchange and sarcoplasmic reticulum calcium release in guinea pig ventricular cells. Circ Res 74: 550–554
42. Leblanc N, Hume JR (1990) Sodium current-induced release of calcium from cardiac sarcoplasmic reticulum. Science 248: 372–376
43. Lee SL, Yu ASL, Lytton J (1994) Tissue-specific expression of Na^+-Ca^{2+} exchanger isoforms. J Bio Chem 269: 14849–14852
44. Levesque PC, Leblanc N, Hume JR (1994) Release of calcium from guinea pig cardiac sarcoplasmic reticulum induced by sodium-calcium exchange. Cardiovasc Res 28: 370–378

45. Levi AJ, Brooksby P, Hancox JC (1993) One hump or two? The triggering of calcium release from the sarcoplasmic reticulum and the voltage dependence of contraction in mammalian cardiac muscle. Cardiovasc Res 27: 1743–1757
46. Levi AJ, Brooksby P, Hancox JC (1993) A role for depolarisation induced calcium entry on the Na-Ca exchange in triggering intracellular calcium release and contraction in rat ventricular myocytes. Cardiovasc Res 27: 1677–1690
47. Levi AJ, Spitzer KW, Kohmoto O, Bridge JHB (1994) Depolarization-induced Ca entry via Na-Ca exchange triggers SR release in guinea pig cardiac myocytes. Amer J Physiol 266: H1422–H1433
48. Levitsky DO, Nicoll DA, Philipson KD (1994) Identification of the high affinity Ca^{2+}-binding domain of the cardiac Na^+-Ca^{2+} exchanger. J Biol Chem 269: 22847–22852
49. Li Z, Smolley CD, Bridge JHB, Frank JS, Philipson KD (1992) Expression of the cardiac Na^+-Ca^{2+} exchanger in insect cells using a baculovirus vector. J Biol Chem 267: 7828–7833
50. Li Z, Matsuoka S, Hryshko LV, Nicoll DA, Bersohn MM, Burke EP, Lifton RP, Philipson KD (1994) Cloning of the NCX2 isoform of the plasma membrane Na^+-Ca^{2+} exchanger. J Biol Chem 269: 17434–17439
51. Li Z, Wu RY, Nicoll DA, Philipson KD (1994) Expression of the canine Na/Ca exchanger in transgenic mouse hearts. Biophys J 66: A331
52. Lipp P, Pott L (1988) Transient inward current in guinea-pig atrial myocytes reflects a change of sodium-calcium exchange current. J Physiol 397: 601–630
53. Lipp P, Schwaller B, Niggli E (1995) Specific inhibition of Na-Ca exchange function by antisense oligodeoxynucleotides. FEBS Lett 364: 198–202
54. Litwin SE, Webster GS, Bridge JHB (1995) Further evidence that reverse Na-Ca exchange can trigger SR calcium release. Biophys J 68: 135a
55. Litwin SE, Bridge JHB (1996) Evidence that reverse Na-Ca exchange can trigger SR Ca release. In: Hilgemann DW, Philipson KD, Vassort G (eds) Sodium-Calcium Exchange: Proceedings of the Third International Conference. New York Academy of Sciences, New York
56. Loo TW, Ho C, Clarke DM (1995) Expression of a functionally active human renal sodium-calcium exchanger lacking a signal sequence. J Biol Chem 270: 19345–19350
57. Low W, Kasir J, Rahaminoff H (1993) Cloning of the rat heart Na^+-Ca^{2+} exchanger and its functional expression in HeLa cells. FEBS 316: 63–67
58. Matsuoka S, Hilgemann DW (1992) Steady-state and dynamic properties of cardiac sodium-calcium exchange: ion and voltage dependencies of the transport cycle. J Gen Physiol 100: 963–1001
59. Matsuoka S, Nicoll DA, Reilly RF, Hilgemann DW, Philipson KD (1993) Initial localization of regulatory regions of the cardiac sarcolemmal Na^+-Ca^{2+} exchanger. Proc Natl Acad Sci 90: 3870–3874
60. Matsuoka S, Hilgemann DW (1994) Inactivation of outward Na^+-Ca^{2+} exchange current in guinea-pig ventricular myocytes. J Physiol 476: 443–458
61. Matsuoka S, Nicoll DA, Hryshko LV, Levitsky DO, Weiss JN, Philipson KD (1995) Regulation of the cardiac Na^+-Ca^{2+} exchanger by Ca^{2+}: mutational analysis of the Ca^{2+}-binding domain. J Gen Physiol 105: 403–420
62. Milanick MA (1989) Na-Ca exchange in ferret red blood cells. Amer J Physiol 256: C390–C398
63. Miura Y, Kimura J (1989) Sodium-calcium exchange current: dependence on internal Ca and Na and competitive binding of external Na and Ca. J Gen Physiol 93: 1129–1145
64. Morishita F, Kawarabayashi T, Sakamoto Y, Shirakawa (1995) Role of the sodium-calcium exchange mechanism and the effect of magnesium on sodium-free and high-potassium contractures in pregnant human myometrium. Amer J Obstet Gynecol 172: 186–195
65. Nakanishi T, Jarmakani JM (1981) Effect of extracellular sodium on mechanical function in the newborn rabbit. Dev Pharmacol Ther 2: 188–200
66. Nakasaki Y, Iwamoto T, Hanada H, Imagawa T, Shigekawa M (1993) Cloning of the rat aortic smooth muscle Na^+/Ca^{2+} exchanger and tissue-specific expression of isoforms. J Biochem 114: 528–534
67. Nicoll DA, Longoni S, Philipson KD (1990) Molecular cloning and functional expression of the cardiac sarcolemmal Na^+-Ca^{2+} exchanger. Science 250: 562–565
68. Nicoll DA, Barrios BR, Philipson KD (1991) Na^+-Ca^{2+} exchangers from rod outer segments and cardiac sarcolemma: comparison of properties. Amer J Physiol 260: C1212–C1216
69. Nicoll DA, Quednau B, Qui Z, Xia YR, Lusis AJ, Philipson KD (1996) Cloning of a third mammalian Na^+-Ca^{2+} exchanger: NCX3. Biophys J (in press)
70. Nilius B, Albitz R, Linde T (1988) Mechanisms involved in generation of oscillatory afterpotentials in myocardium. Biomed Biochim Acta 47: 163–171
71. O'Neill SC, Valdeolmillos M, Lamont C, Donoso P, Eisner DA (1991) The contribution of Na-Ca exchange to relaxation in mammalian cardiac muscle. Ann NY Acad Sci 639: 444–452
72. Philipson KD (1990) The cardiac Na^+-Ca^{2+} exchanger: dependence on membrane evironment. Cell Biol Intl Rep 14: 305–309
73. Philipson KD, Nicoll DA (1992) Na^+-Ca^{2+} exchange. Curr Op Cell Biol 4: 678–683

74. Philipson KD, Nicoll DA, Matsuoka S, Hryshko LV, Levitsky DO, Weiss JN (1996) Molecular regulation of the Na$^+$-Ca^{2+} exchanger. Proceedings of the Third International Conference on Sodium-Calcium Exchange. New York Academy of Sciences, New York

75. Porzig H, Li Z, Nicoll DA, Philipson KD (1993) Mapping of the cardiac sodium-calcium exchanger with monoclonal antibodies. Amer J Physiol 265: C748–C758

76. Powis DA, Clark CL, O'Brien KJ (1994) Lanthanum can be transported by the sodium-calcium exchange pathway and directly triggers catecholamine release from bovine chromaffin cells. Cell Calcium 16: 377–390

77. Reeves JP, Bailey CA, Hale CC (1986) Redox modification of sodium-calcium exchange activity in cardiac sarcolemmal vesicles. J Biol Chem 261: 4948–4955

78. Reilander H, Achilles A, Friedel U, Maul G, Lottspeich F, Cook NJ (1992) Primary structure and functional expression of the Na/Ca,K exchanger from bovine rod photoreceptors. EMBO J 11: 1689–1695

79. Reilly RF, Shugrue CA (1992) cDNA cloning of a renal Na$^+$-Ca^{2+} exchanger. Amer J Physiol 262: F1105–F1109

80. Sahin-Toth M, Nicoll DA, Frank JS, Philipson KD, Friedlander M (1995) The cleaved N-terminal signal sequence of the cardiac Na$^+$-Ca^{2+} exchanger is not required for functional membrane integration. Biochem Biophys Res Comm 212: 968–974

81. Schnetkamp PPM, Basu DK, Szerencsei RT (1989) Na$^+$-Ca^{2+} exchange in bovine rod outer segments requires and transports K$^+$. Amer J Physiol 257: C153–C157

82. Schwarz E, Benzer S (1996) Expression and evolution of Calx, a sodium-calcium exchanger of Drosophila melanogaster. (submitted)

83. Sham JSK, Cleeman L, Morad M (1992) Gating of the cardiac Ca^{2+} release channel: the role of Na$^+$ current and Na$^+$-Ca^{2+} exchange. Science 255: 850–853

84. Short CL, Monk RD, Bushinsky DA, Krieger NS (1994) Hormonal regulation of Na$^+$-Ca^{2+} exchange in osteoblast-like cells. J Bone Mineral Res 9: 1159–1166

85. Simchowitz L, Cragoe EJ (1988) Na$^+$-Ca^{2+} exchange in human neutrophils. Amer J Physiol 254: C150–C164

86. Vemuri R, Philipson KD (1987) Phospholipid composition modulates the Na$^+$-Ca^{2+} exchange activity of cardiac sarcolemma in reconstituted vesicles. Biochim Biophys Acta 937: 258–268

87. Vetter R, Kemsies C, Schulze W (1987) Sarcolemmal Na$^+$-Ca^{2+} exchange and sarcoplasmic reticulum Ca^{2+} uptake in several cardiac preparations. Biomed Biochim Acta 46: S375–S381

88. Vigne P, Breittmayer JP, Duval D, Frelin C, Lazdunski M (1988) The Na$^+$/Ca^{2+} antiporter in aortic smooth muscle cells. J Biol Chem 263: 8078–8083

89. Vites AM, Wasserstrom JA (1995) Calcium influx via Na/Ca exchange and calcium current can both trigger transient contractions in cat ventricular myocytes. Biophys J 68: 135a

90. Wasserstrom JA, Vites AM (1995) Na-Ca exchange triggers contraction in rat ventricular myocytes. Biophys J 68: 135a

Authors' address:
Kenneth D. Philipson, PhD
Cardiovascular Research Laboratories
UCLA School of Medicine
Los Angeles, California, 90095-1760 USA

Expression and function of the cardiac Na^+/Ca^{2+} exchanger in postnatal development of the rat, in experimental-induced cardiac hypertrophy, and in the failing human heart

R. Studer, H. Reinecke, R. Vetter[1], J. Holtz[2], H. Drexler

Universitätsklinik, Innere Medizin III, Kardiologie und Angiologie, Freiburg, Germany
[1] Max-Delbrück-Centrum, Berlin-Buch, Germany
[2] Institut für Pathophysiologie, Universität Halle, Germany

Abstract

The diastolic and systolic dysfunction in the failing heart appear to be related to the altered Ca^{2+} handling of the cardiac myocyte. Disturbed Ca^{2+} handling might also affect influx and efflux of other ions, including Na^+. In this context, the cardiac sarcolemmal Na^+/Ca^{2+} exchanger represents an important exchange mechanism of Ca^{2+} versus Na^+ transport across the sarcolemma. Expression and function of cardiac Na^+/Ca^{2+} exchanger is highest in newborn rats and declines gradually in postnatal development. In pressure overload-induced hypertrophy, expression of cardiac Na^+/Ca^{2+} exchanger is increased and translated into increased Na^+/Ca^{2+} exchanger activity similar to the early phase of postnatal development in the rat. This suggests a common underlying mechanism in the control of Na^+/Ca^{2+} exchanger expression in the immature and the hypertrophied myocardium. Similar to experimental-induced hypertrophy, mRNA, protein and activity of Na^+/Ca^{2+} exchanger is increased in the failing human heart suggesting an increase in the number of functional exchanger molecules rather than an enhanced exchange rate by preexisting exchanger molecules. The potential functional implications of an increased cardiac Na^+/Ca^{2+} exchanger activity in human heart failure may be limitation of diastolic intracellular Ca^{2+} overload. However, this may increase the arrhythmogenic potential of the failing heart, since additional Na^+ influx via Na^+/Ca^{2+} exchanger may affect the membrane potential.

Key words Cardiac Na^+/Ca^{2+} exchanger – expression and function – postnatal development – cardiac hypertrophy and failure – Ca^{2+} overload – arrhythmogenic potential – reversed mode

Introduction

Sarcoplasmic reticulum (SR) Ca^{2+} pumping and sarcolemmal (SL) Na^+/Ca^{2+} exchange are two major processes responsible for reducing cytosolic Ca^{2+} from a high systolic level to a low resting level during cardiac relaxation. The SR Ca^{2+}-ATPase extrudes Ca^{2+} from the cytosol into the lumen of the SR and the Na^+/Ca^{2+} exchanger mediates the movement of cytosolic Ca^{2+} across the sarcolemma to the extracellular space (5). In rodent cardiomyocytes, the SR Ca^{2+}-ATPase is thought to handle approximately 80 % of cellular Ca^{2+} during a contraction-relaxation cycle, whereas up to 20 % of Ca^{2+} movement can be attributed to the Na^+/Ca^{2+} exchanger (3, 4). However, this relationship may vary among species (5, 26), during development of species (17, 29) and in pathological states (24). The predominant role of the Na^+/Ca^{2+} exchanger appears to be removal of cytosolic Ca^{2+} out of the cardiomyocyte in exchange for extracellular Na^+ (exchanger's forward mode). As three Na^+ ions are exchanged for one Ca^{2+} an inwardly directed current results. However, in the initial phase of excitation-contraction coupling. Na^+/Ca^{2+} exchange may occur in the opposite direction (exchanger's reversed mode). In this respect, recent studies have implicated a putative role for the Na^+/Ca^{2+} exchanger in the activation of contraction by providing a source of Ca^{2+} to trigger the release of additional Ca^{2+} from cardiac SR (19). To elucidate the putative role of the Na^+/Ca^{2+} exchanger in excitation-contraction coupling in the failing heart, we investigated expression and function of cardiac Na^+/Ca^{2+} exchanger in experimental-induced hypertrophy of the rat and in patients with end-stage heart failure in comparison to normal early postnatal and mature myocardium.

Results and discussion

Developmental changes in mRNA steady state levels of Na^+/Ca^{2+} exchanger and SR Ca^{2+}-ATPase were measured in rat heart by Northern blot analysis (Fig. 1). Northern blot analysis revealed transcripts of 7.2 kb for the Na^+/Ca^{2+} exchanger and 4.3 kb for the SR Ca^{2+}-ATPase which were both detectable at all developmental stages studied (Fig. 1). As shown in Fig. 1, Na^+/Ca^{2+} exchanger gene expression was highest at the very late fetal stage and at day 1 post partum and declined with increased postnatal age. This decline was accompanied by a corresponding increase in the gene expression of SR Ca^{2+}-ATPase. Interestingly, Na^+/Ca^{2+} exchanger mRNA levels correlated to the relative levels of immunoreactive Na^+/Ca^{2+} exchanger protein suggesting that mRNA levels are translated into corresponding Na^+/Ca^{2+} exchanger protein levels (data not shown). Figure 2 demonstrates Na^+/Ca^{2+} exchanger and SR Ca^{2+}-ATPase transport activities in crude membrane preparations from developing rat hearts. Similar to the gene expression, the Na^+/Ca^{2+} exchanger activity – measured as Na^+-dependent Ca^{2+} uptake – declines and the SR Ca^{2+}-ATPase activity – measured as oxalate-supported Ca^{2+} uptake – increases during postnatal development of the rat. Thus, in postnatal development of the rat the expression and function of the Na^+/Ca^{2+} exchanger is inversely related to the expression and function of the SR Ca^{2+}-ATPase. These results together with previous findings, either on the cardiac Na^+/Ca^{2+} exchanger (2, 7) or the SR Ca^{2+}-ATPase expression (10, 18, 21) in fetal, neonatal and adult rat myocardium, suggest a coordinated control at the pretranslational level in the developmental regulation of both the Na^+/Ca^{2+} exchanger and the SR Ca^{2+}-ATPase. This is consistent with previous findings which demonstrated that transsarcolemmal Ca^{2+} movements play a greater role in the control of the contraction and relaxation in newborn compared to mature myocardium of adult animals (17, 27, 32), while SR Ca^{2+} release and reuptake function is depressed (9, 27, 32, 33).

Knowledge of the molecular mechanisms determining the developmental differences in cardiac Ca^{2+} handling may be of particular interest with respect to the molecular mechanisms responsible for a defective Ca^{2+} homeostasis in hypertrophied and failing hearts (6, 24). Embryonic development, postnatal growth, and

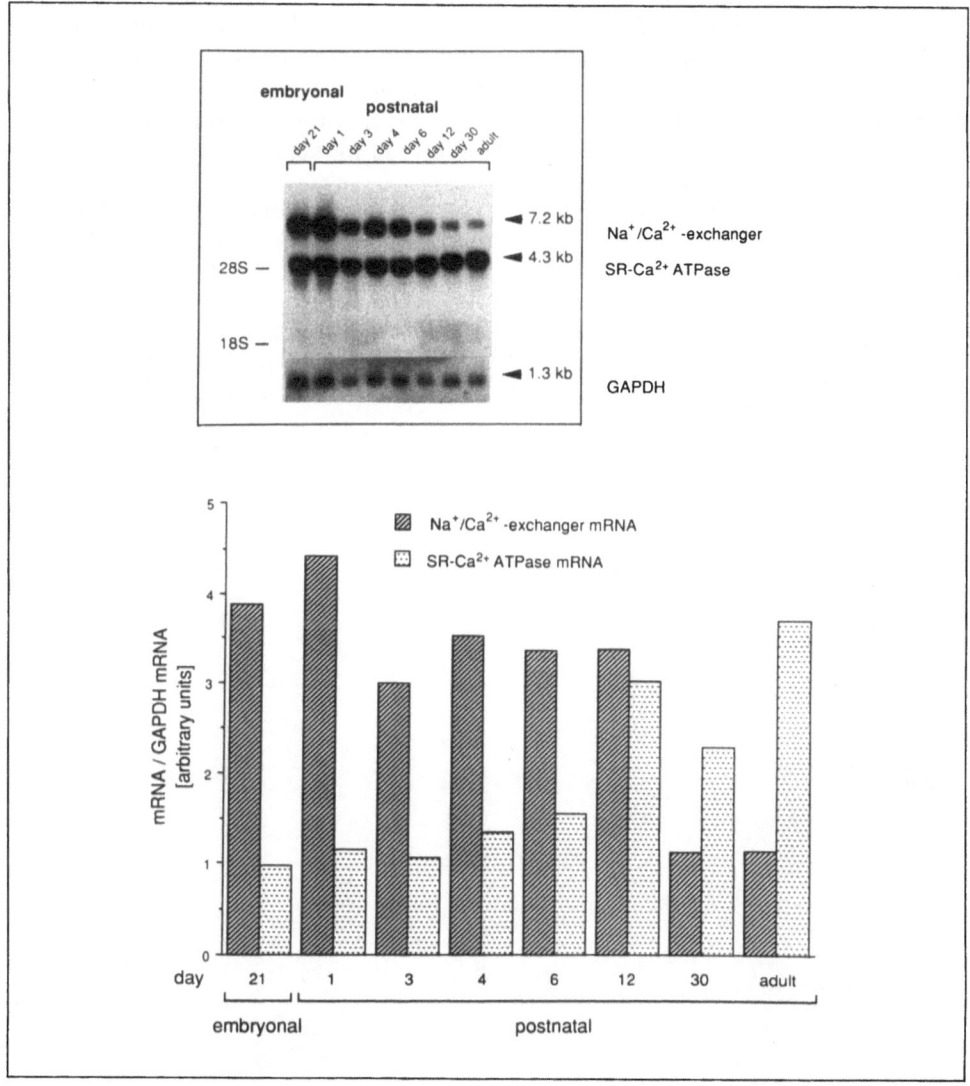

Fig. 1. Developmental gene expression of Na$^+$/Ca^{2+} exchanger and SR Ca^{2+}-ATPase in rat myocardium (34). Left-hand side, Northern blot analysis of the Na$^+$/Ca^{2+} exchanger (7.2 kb), SR Ca^{2+}-ATPase (4.3 kb) and Glyceraldehyde-3-phosphate dehydrogenase (GAPDH; 1.3 kb). The positions of 18S and 28S rRNA are indicated. Right-hand side, bar graphs showing steady-state mRNA levels of Na$^+$/Ca^{2+} exchanger and SR Ca^{2+}-ATPase normalized to the respective GAPDH mRNA signal in rat heart during development: fetal day 21 (21 G) and postnatal days 1, 3, 4, 6, 12, 30, and 150 (adult).

adaptation of the adult heart to increased workload are controlled by the coordinated temporal and spacial expression of cardiac muscle genes (8). Both qualitative and quantitative changes in gene expression appear to be involved, including those in the immediate early gene program and other more long-term changes in gene expression (8). There is now strong evidence that the decrease in SR Ca^{2+}-ATPase expression can contribute to defective Ca^{2+} handling in different experimental models of overload-induced hypertrophy and in end-stage human heart failure (for review see 1; 14; 31). However, the role of the Na^+/Ca^{2+} exchanger in cardiac hypertrophy and failure remains controversial. While recent studies demonstrated an early up-regulation of the expression of the Na^+/Ca^{2+} exchanger along with an enhanced Na^+/Ca^{2+} exchanger activity in response to pressure overload-induced hypertrophy (16, 25) and cardiomyopathy (15), an earlier report by Hanf and co-workers (12) described a reduced Na^+/Ca^{2+} exchanger activity in vesicular membrane preparations of hypertrophied rat hearts. To address this controversy, we investigated expression and function of the Na^+/Ca^{2+} exchanger in pressure overload-induced hypertrophy of the rat and in end-stage human heart failure.

As shown in Fig. 3, cardiac Na^+/Ca^{2+} exchanger protein level is increased in pressure overload-induced hypertrophy in comparison to sham-operated rats and is translated into increased Na^+/Ca^{2+} exchanger activity. Therefore, we believe that in pressure overload-induced hypertrophy of the rat, expression and activity of Na^+/Ca^{2+} exchanger is, indeed, increased, similar to the expression and activity of the Na^+/Ca^{2+} exchanger in early postnatal development of the rat. This may suggest a common underlying mechanism in the control of Na^+/Ca^{2+} exchanger gene expression in

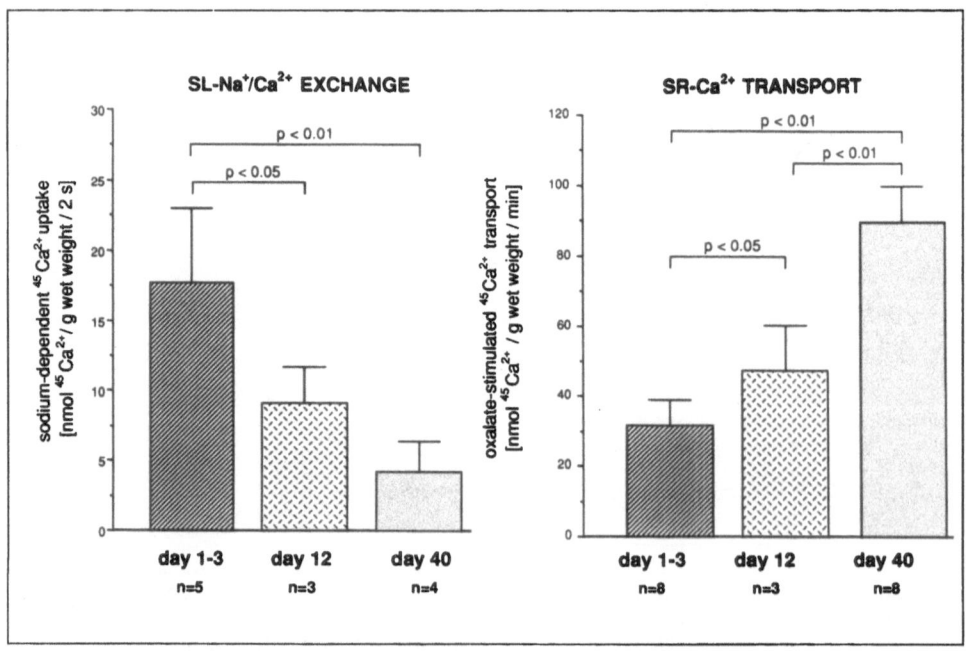

Fig. 2. Reciprocal changes of SL-Na^+/Ca^{2+} exchange and SR-Ca^{2+} transport activities in crude membrane preparations from postnatal developing rat hearts (34).

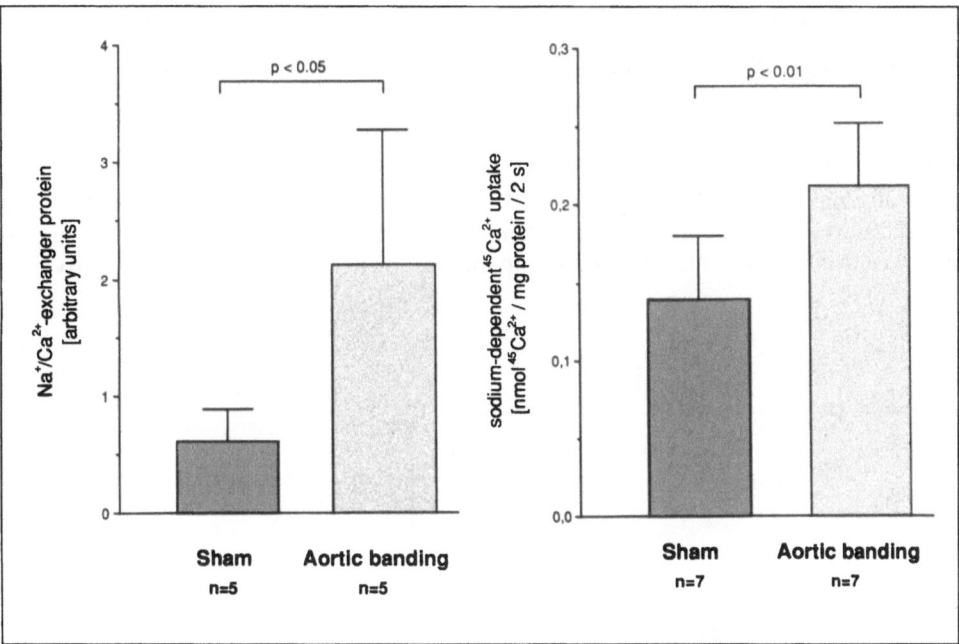

Fig. 3. Protein level and activity of the cardiac Na^+/Ca^{2+} exchanger in pressure overload-induced hypertrophy due to abdominal aortic banding compared to sham-operated rats (30).

the immature and the hypertrophied/failing myocardium. Figure 4 shows expression and activity of the Na^+/Ca^{2+} exchanger in nonfailing hearts (NF) obtained from organ donors and in failing hearts obtained from patients undergoing heart transplantation because of coronary artery disease (CAD) or because of dilated cardiomyopathy (DCM). Similar to our observations in experimental-induced hypertrophy, there was an increase of Na^+/Ca^{2+} exchanger expression (mRNA as well as protein level) and activity in CAD and DCM as compared to nonfailing hearts. This suggests that the enhanced Na^+/Ca^{2+} exchanger activity is due to an increase in the number of functional Na^+/Ca^{2+} exchanger molecules rather than to an enhanced Na^+/Ca^{2+} exchanger rate by preexisting Na^+/Ca^{2+} exchanger molecules indicating a regulation at the pretranslational level.

What might be the potential functional implications of an increased Na^+/Ca^{2+} exchanger activity in human heart failure? Several studies have described alterations of SR function in human heart failure. Intracellular Ca^{2+} measurements using aequorin showed that Ca^{2+} transients in muscles from failing human hearts were markedly prolonged in both Ca^{2+} release and uptake phases (11, 23). Ca^{2+} uptake rates were reported to be diminished in right ventricular biopsy samples from failing hearts (20), and mRNA and protein levels of the SR Ca^{2+}-ATPase were shown to be decreased in left ventricular specimens from patients with heart failure (22, 31). Therefore, an attractive hypothesis is that the decrease in the density of SR Ca^{2+} pumps, which leads to a slower rate of Ca^{2+} uptake into the SR, may account for prolongation of Ca^{2+} transients (11, 23) and impaired isometric relaxation in the failing human heart (13). In the face of a decreased SR Ca^{2+}-ATPase gene expression and impaired LV function in the failing human heart (11, 13, 14, 20, 22, 23), the increase in Na^+/Ca^{2+} exchanger activity may represent an important compensatory mechanism, which may limit diastolic intracellular Ca^{2+} overload and therefore, support diastolic relaxation by extruding Ca^{2+} from the cardiomyocyte along with an influx of Na^+ reflecting a net inward current (3 Na^+ versus 1 Ca^{2+}). However, the benefit of enhanced Na^+/Ca^{2+} exchanger activity for diastolic Ca^{2+} removal is compromised by an additional influx of Na^+ which, in turn, may contribute to delayed afterdepolarizations and, therefore be associated with an increased risk of arrhythmias. In the initial phase of excitation-contraction coupling increased Na^+/Ca^{2+} exchanger activity may

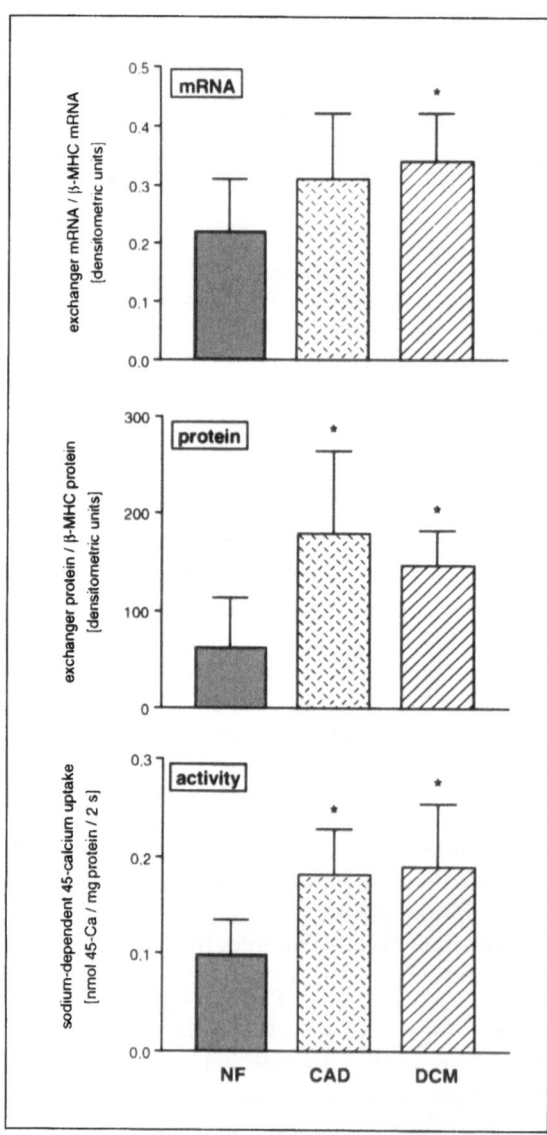

Fig. 4. Bar graphs showing mRNA level, protein level and activity of the Na^+/Ca^{2+} exchanger in patients with coronary artery disease (CAD) and dilated cardiomyopathy (DCM) compared to nonfailing controls (NF).
* = p < 0.05, ANOVA followed by Student-Newman-Keuls test; β-MHC, β-myosin heavy chain (28, 31).

trigger additional Ca^{2+} from the SR by working in reversed mode that might have a positive intropic effect.

Acknowledgments This work was supported by grants from the Deutsche Forschungsgemeinschaft (Dr 148/6-1, Ve 136/1–3).

REFERENCES

1. Arai M, Matsui H, Periasamy M (1994) Sarcoplasmic reticulum gene expression in cardiac hypertrophy and heart failure. Circ Res 74: 555–564
2. Artman M (1992) Sarcolemmal Na$^+$-Ca^{2+} exchange activity and exchanger immunoreactivity in developing rabbit hearts. Am J Physiol 263: H1506–H1513
3. Bers DM, Bridge JHB (1989) Relaxation of rabbit ventricular muscle by Na-Ca exchange and sarcoplasmic reticulum calcium pump. Circ Res 65: 334–342
4. Bers DM, Lederer WJ, Berlin JR (1990) Intracellular Ca transients in rat cardiac myocytes: role of Na-Ca exchange in excitation-contraction coupling. Am J Physiol 258: C944–C954
5. Bers DM, Bassani JW, Bassani RA (1993) Competition and redistribution among calcium transport systems in rabbit cardiac myocytes. Cardiovasc Res 27: 1772–1777
6. Bing OHL, Brooks WW, Conrad CH, Sen S, Perreault CL, Morgan JP (1991) Intracellular calcium transients in myocardium from spontaneously hypertensive rats during the transition to heart failure. Circ Res 68: 1390–1400
7. Boerth SR, Zimmer DB, Artman M (1994) Steady-state mRNA levels of the sarcolemmal Na$^+$-Ca^{2+} exchanger peak near birth in developing rabbit and rat hearts. Circ Res 74: 354–359
8. Chien KR, Zhu H, Knowlton KU, Miller Hance W, Van Bilsen M, O'Brien TX, Evans SM (1993) Transcriptional regulation during cardiac growth and development. Annu Rev Physiol 55: 77–95
9. Fabiato A (1982) Calcium release in skinned cardiac cells: variation with species, tissues, and development. Fed Proc 41: 2238–2244
10. Fisher DJ, Tate CA, Philips S (1992) Developmental regulation of the sarcoplasmic reticulum calcium pump in the rabbit heart. Pediatr Res 31: 474–479
11. Gwathmey JK, Copelas L, MacKinnon R, Schoen FJ, Feldman MD, Grossman W, Morgan JP (1987) Abnormal intracellular calcium handling in myocardium from patients with end-stage heart failure. Circ Res 61: 70–76
12. Hanf R, Dubraix I, Marotte F, Lelievre LG (1988) Rat cardiac hypertrophy. Altered sodium-calcium exchange activity in sarcolemmal vesicles. FEBS Letters 236: 145–149
13. Hasenfuss G, Mulieri LA, Leavitt BJ, Allen PD, Haeberle JR, Alpert NR (1992) Alteration of contractile function and excitation-contraction coupling in dilated cardiomyopathy. Circ Res 70: 1225–1232
14. Hasenfuss G, Reinecke H, Studer R, Meyer M, Pieske B, Holtz J, Holubarsch C, Posival H, Just H, Drexler H (1994) Relation between myocardial function and expression of sarcoplasmic reticulum Ca^{2+}-ATPase in failing and nonfailing human myocardium. Circ Res 75: 434–442
15. Hatem SN, Sham JSK, Morad M (1994) Enhanced Na$^+$-Ca^{2+} exchange activity in cardiomyopathic syrian hamster. Circ Res 74: 253–261
16. Kent RL, Rozich JD, McCollam PL, McDermott DE, Thacker UF, Menick DR, McDermott PJ, Cooper IV G (1993) Rapid expression of the Na$^+$-Ca^{2+} exchanger in response to cardiac pressure overload. Am J Physiol 265: H1024–H1029
17. Klitzner TS (1991) Maturational changes in excitation-contraction coupling in mammalian myocardium. J Am Coll Cardiol 17: 218–225
18. Komuro I, Kurabayashi M, Shibazaki Y, Takaku F, Yazaki Y (1989) Molecular cloning and characterization of a Ca^{2+} + Mg^{2+}-dependent adenosine triphosphatase from rat cardiac sarcoplasmic reticulum. Regulation of its expression by pressure overload and developmental stage. J Clin Invest 83: 1102–1108
19. Leblanc N, Hume JR (1990) Sodium current-induced release of calcium from cardiac sarcoplasmatic reticulum. Science 248: 372–376
20. Limas CJ, Olivari M, Goldenberg IF, Levine TB, Benditt DG, Simon A (1987) Calcium uptake by cardiac sarcoplasmic reticulum in human dilated cardiomyopathy. Cardiovasc Res 21: 601–605

21. Lompré A-M, Lambert F, Lakatta EG, Schwartz K (1991) Expression of sarcoplasmic reticulum Ca^{2+}-ATPase and calsequestrin genes in rat heart during ontogenic development and aging. Circ Res 69: 1380–1388
22. Mercadier J-J, Lompré A-M, Duc P, Boheler KR, Fraysse JB, Wisnewsky C, Allen PD, Komajda M, Schwartz K (1990) Altered sarcoplasmic reticulum Ca^{2+}-ATPase gene expression in human ventricle during end-stage heart failure. J Clin Invest 85: 305–309
23. Morgan JP, Erny RE, Allen PD, Grossman W, Gwathmey JK (1990) Abnormal intracellular calcium handling: a major cause of systolic and diastolic dysfunction in ventricular myocardium from patients with heart failure. Circulation 61 Suppl III: III21–32
24. Morgan JP (1991) Mechanisms of disease – abnormal intracellular modulation of calcium as a major cause of cardiac contractile dysfunction. New Engl J Med 325: 625–632
25. Nakanishi H, Makino N, Hata T, Matsui H, Yano K, Yanaga T (1989) Sarcolemmal Ca^{2+} transport activities in cardiac hypertrophy caused by pressure overload. Am J Physiol 257: H349–H356
26. Negretti N, O'Neill SC, Eisner DA (1993) The relative contributions of different intracellular and sarcolemmal systems to relaxation in rat ventricular myocytes. Cardiovasc Res 27: 1826–1830
27. Ostádalová I, Kolár F, Ostádal B, Rohlicek V, Rohlicek J, Prochazka J (1993) Early postnatal development of contractile performance and responsiveness to Ca^{2+}, verapamil and ryanodine in the isolated rat heart. J Mol Cell Cardiol 25: 733–740
28. Reinecke H, Studer R, Vetter R, Holtz J, Drexler H (1995) Cardiac Na^+/Ca^{2+} exchange activity in patients with end-stage heart failure. Cardiovasc Res, in press
29. Seguchi M, Harding JA, Jarmakani JM (1986) Developmental change in the function of sarcoplasmic reticulum. J Mol Cell Cardiol 18: 189–195
30. Studer R, Reinecke H, Vetter R, Holtz J, Drexler H (1993) Enhanced expression and function of the Na^+/Ca^{2+} exchanger in rat ventricular hypertrophy and in myocardium of neonatal rats. (Abstract) Circulation 88 Suppl I: 86
31. Studer R, Reinecke H, Bilger J, Eschenhagen T, Böhm M, Hasenfuß G, Just H, Holtz J, Drexler H (1994) Gene expression of the cardiac Na^+-Ca^{2+} exchanger in end-stage human heart failure. Circ Res 75: 443–453
32. Tanaka H, Shigenobu K (1989) Effect of ryanodine on neonatal and adult rat heart: developmental increase in sarcoplasmic reticulum function. J Mol Cell Cardiol 21: 1305–1313
33. Vetter R, Kemsies C, Schulze W (1987) Sarcolemmal Na^+-Ca^{2+} exchange and sarcoplasmic reticulum Ca^{2+} uptake in several cardiac preparations. Biomed Biochim Acta 46: S375–S381
34. Vetter R, Studer R, Reinecke H, Kolár F, Ostádalová I, Drexler H (1995) Reciprocal changes in the post-natal expression of the sarcolemmal Na^+-Ca^{2+} exchanger and SERCA2 in rat heart. J Mol Cell Cardiol 27: 1689–1701

Authors' address:
Roland Studer PhD
Universitätsklinik
Innere Medizin III
Kardiologie und Angiologie
Breisacher Str. 33
79106 Freiburg, Germany

Plasma membrane calcium pump: structure, function, and relationships

E. Carafoli

Laboratory of Biochemistry III, Swiss Federal Institute of Technology (ETH), Zürich, Switzerland

Abstract

The plasma membrane Ca-pump (134 kDa) is stimulated by calmodulin and by other treatments (exposure to acidic phospholipids, treatments with proteases, phosphorylation by protein kinases A or C, self-association to form oligomers). It is the product of four genes (in humans), but additional isoforms originate through alternative mRNA spicing. Most of the pump mass protrudes into the cytoplasm with three main units. The calmodulin binding domain is located in the C-terminal protruding unit. The domain is a positively charged segment of about 25 residues. The calcium-activated protease calpain activates the pump by removing its calmodulin binding domain and the portion C-terminal to it. The-resulting 124 KDa fragment has been used to test the suggestion of an autoinhibitory function of the calmodulin binding domain. The latter interacts with two domains of the pump, one located close to the active site in the mid-cytoplasmic protruding unit, the other in the first (N-terminal) protruding unit. The isoforms of the pump show variations in the regulatory domains, e.g., alternative mRNA splicing can eliminate the domain phosphorylated by protein kinase A, or alter the sensitivity of the pump to calmodulin. This occurs by inserting sequences rich in His between calmodulin binding subdomains A and B. The inserted domain(s) confer pH sensitivity to the binding of calmodulin. Calcium binding sites have been found in acidic regions preceding and following the calmodulin binding domain.

Key words   Calcium pump – calmodulin – calpain

The plasma membrane Ca-pump (PMCA) is the largest of all P-type ion pumps, i.e., pumps which form a phosphorylated intermediate in the catalytic cycle (an aspartyl-phosphate) and are inhibited by vanadate. The PMCA pump interacts with Ca with high affinity, but has a low total Ca transporting capacity. This property makes it inadequate to rapidly eject large amounts of Ca, as required, for exampie, by the functional cycle of heart cells. Thus, in these cells, the pump is quantitatively over-shadowed by a larger system, the NaCa exchanger. First discovered in erythrocytes, the PMCA pump has been subsequently found in many other cells, and is now assumed to be an obligatory component of eucaryotic plasma membranes. It is stimulated by calmodulin and, in its absence, by a number of alternative treatments like the exposure to acidic phospholipids (including the phosphorylated derivatives of phosphatidyl-inositol), a controlled treatment with proteases, e.g., trypsin or calpain, phosphorylation reactions by protein kinases A or C and self-association to form dimers or, more likely, oligomers.

Cloning work (4, 8) in the late 1980s has shown that the pump is a single polypeptide chain of molecular mass about 134 KDa. It is the product of a multigene family: four genes have been recognized in humans, and they have been assigned to chromosomes 1, 3, 12 and x. Numerous additional isoforms then originate through alternative mRNA spicing. The general architecture of the pump (Fig. 1) follows the general pattern of the P-type pump family, i.e., most of the pump mass protrudes into the cytoplasmic medium, very short loops connecting the putative transmembrane domain on the external side. Ten putative transmembrane domains have been identified, four concentrated in the N-terminal portion of the pump and six in the C-terminal portion. The transmembrane organization of the pump has been, to a large part, directly validated by work with monoclonal antibodies and with other chemical labelling techniques. Three main units protrude into the cytosol, the first between transmembrane domains 2 and 3, the second between transmembrane domains 4 and 5, and the third from transmembrane domain 10. The first protruding unit has been proposed, based on the analogy with other P-type pumps, to permit the coupling of ATP hydrolysis to the transport of Ca and is thus sometimes called the transducing unit. The protruding portions of the pump (Fig. 1) consist of antiparallel β-sheets, a-helices and parallel β-sheets. The domain protruding between transmembrane segments 4 and 5 contains the active site(s) of the pump (i.e., the site of aspartyl-phos-

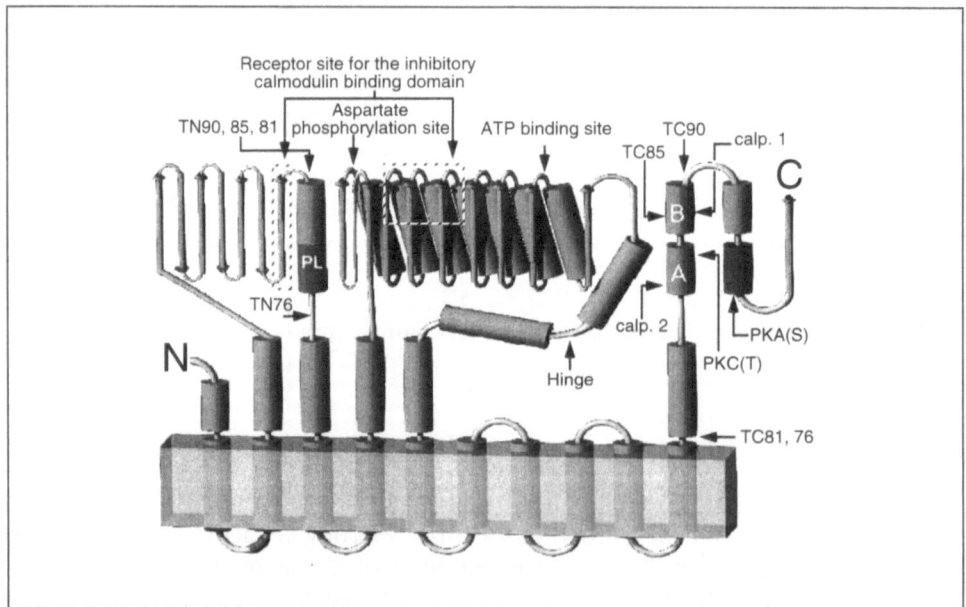

Fig. 1. Membrane architecture and domain definition of the PMCA pump. Cylinders indicate predicted α-helices, arrows β-sheets. The two calmodulin binding sub-domains are indicated by A and B. Calp 1 and calp 2 are the two sequential sites of calpain cleavage. PKA (S) and PKC (T) are sites of serine and threonine kinase phosphorylation: PKA only phosphorylates one of the isoforms of the pump. TC is the notation for the C-terminal cleavage by trypsin, TN that of the N-terminal cleavage. PL is the main domain responsive to acidic phospholipids.

phate formation and the binding site for ATP), and is assumed to be connected to the membrane by a flexible "hinge" in its C-terminal portion which permits the catalytic aspartic acid to approach the bound ATP during the reaction cycle.

The calmodulin binding domain of the pump has been identified with the help of bifunctional crosslinkers coupled to calmodulin (James et al., 1988), and located in the last protruding unit of the pump. The domain is a positively charged segment of about 25 residues, which has a strong α-helix propensity in its N- and C-terminal portions (sub-domains A and B). Work with trypsin has shown that the pump is sequentially degraded to fragments of electrophoretic molecular masses 90, 85, 81, 76 KDa. The 90 KDa fragment has low basal activity and is stimulated by both calmodulin and acidic phospholipids. During the formation of the 85 and 81 KDa fragments, the pump gradually loses its sensitivity to calmodulin, but retains that to acidic phospholipids, whereas the formation of the 76 KDa fragment is accompanied by the loss of phospholipid sensitivity as well. The removal of the calmodulin binding domain and of the pump portion C-terminal to it during the formation of these fragments leads to the stimulation of the basal activity of the pump, suggesting that the domain acts as an autoinhibitor of the pump. In the formation of the 90 to 76 KDa fragments, trypsin also cuts the pump between putative transmembrane domains 2 and 3, but it is doubtful whether the portion of the pump N-terminal to the cut is actually removed. The Ca-dependent protease calpain also activates the pump, and does so by removing in two steps its calmodulin binding domain and the portion C-terminal to it. The resulting 124 KDa fragment has been used to test the suggestion of the autoinhibitory function of the calmodulin binding domain. The latter, suitably derivatized with a photoactivatable crosslinker (2) has been found to label two domains of the pump, one located between the sites of aspartyl-phosphate formation and of ATP-binding, the other in the first protruding unit of the pump. The finding that the "receptor" sites for the calmodulin binding domain are located in close proximity to the active site(s) of the pump conveniently rationalizes the "inhibitory" action of the domain. The calmodulin binding domain can be phosphorylated by protein kinase C, leading to some activation of the basal activity of the pump (9). The calmodulin-binding domain has been prepared synthetically with a phosphate on the threonine that is the substrate for protein kinase C (6): the phosphorylated domain is unable to inhibit the fully active 124 kDa calpain product. This establishes a striking parallel with the Ca-pump of sarcoplasmic reticulum which is kept inhibited by the association of the accessory protein, phospholamban, and which is reactivated by the removal of phospholamban from its binding site by kinase-directed phosphorylations.

On the N-terminal side, trypsin cleaves the pump between transmembrane domains two and three. The N-termini of the fragments of 90, 85, 81 KDa differ from that of the 76 KDa fragment by a heavily charged stretch of about 40 residues. Work with the synthetic C-terminal portion of the stretch, which is very rich in basic amino acids (labelled PL in Fig. 1), has shown (1) it to be one of the sites of the pump responsible for the response to acidic phospholipids (the other site appears to be the calmodulin binding domain itself).

None of the isoforms of the pump show variations in the domains which are preserved throughout the family of P-type ion motive ATPases, e.g., the domains surrounding the active site(s). Most of the diversity concerns the regulatory domains and leads to differences in regulatory properties, e.g., alternative mRNA splicing can eliminate the domain phosphorylated by protein kinase A (PKA(S) in Fig. 1). A particularly interesting mRNA splicing process leads to inserts of increasing length between calmodulin binding subdomains A and B. The newly inserted domain(s) duplicate somewhat the original calmodulin binding domain, except that the positively charged amino acids are histidines instead of arginines and lysines. This confers to the newly inserted domain(s) pH sensitivity in the binding of calmodulin, and may thus endow the pump with additional modulation possibilities.

One domain of the pump which is still unknown is that containing the catalytic Ca binding site. By analogy with suggestions on the Ca pump of sarcoplasmic reticulum, this Ca binding site could be located within some of the transmembrane domains. Mutagenesis work on selected residues in some of the transmembrane domains are in line with the prediction. Other Ca binding sites, possibly regulatory, have recently been found immediately C- and N-terminal to the calmodulin binding domain (6).

Despite the similarity of the plasma membrane and the endoplasmic reticulum Ca pumps, the two enzymes are targeted to two different membranes. Chimeric constructs of the two proteins have shown that the region encompassing the first two transmembrane domains of the SERCA pump contains a strong endoplasmic reticulum retention signal. Chimeric constructs in which the first two transmembrane domains of the PMCA pump are followed by the remainder of the SERCA pump are still largely retained in the reticulum: i.e., the SERCA pump contains additional endoplasmic reticulum retention signals elsewhere in the molecule that outweigh those present in the first two PMCA transmembrane domains (3).

REFERENCES

1. Brodin P, Falchetto R, Vorherr T, Carafoli E (1992) Identification of two domains which mediate the binding of activating phospholipids to the plasma membrane Ca^{2+} pump. Eur J Biochem 204: 939–946
2. Falchetto R, Vorherr T, Brunner J, Carafoli E (1991) The plasma membrane Ca^{2+} pump contains a site that interacts with its calmodulin binding domain. J Biol Chem 266: 2930–2936
3. Foletti D, Guerini D, Carafoli E (1995) Subcellular targeting of the endoplasmic reticulum and plasma membrane Ca^{2+} pumps: a study using recombinant chimeras. FASEB J 9: 670–680
4. Greeb J, Shull GE (1989) Molecular cloning of a third isoform of the calmodulin-sensitive plasma membrane Ca^{2+}-transporting ATPase that is expressed predominantly in brain and skeletal muscle. J Biol Chem 264: 18569–18576
5. Hofmann F, Anagli J, Carafoli E, Vorherr T (1994) Phosphorylation of the calmodulin binding domain of the plasma membrane Ca^{2+} pump by protein kinase C reduces its interaction with calmodulin and with its pump receptor site. J Biol Chem 269: 24298–24303
6. Hofmann F, James P, Vorherr T, Carafoli E (1993) The C-terminal domain of the plasma membrane Ca^{2+} pump contains three high affinity binding sites. J Biol Chem 268: 10252–10259
7. James P, Maeda M, Fischer R, Verma AK, Krebs J, Penniston JT, Carafoli E (1988) Identification and primary structure of a calmodulin-binding domain of the Ca^{2+} pump of human erythrocytes. J Biol Chem 263: 2905–2910
8. Verma AK, Filoteo AG, Stanford RD, Wieben ED, Penniston JT, Strehler EE, Fischer R, Heim R, Vogel G, Mathews S, Strehler-Page, M-A, James P, Vorherr T, Krebs J, Carafoli E (1988) Complete primary structure of a human plasma membrane Ca^{2+} pump. J Biol Chem 263: 14152–14159
9. Wang KKW, Wright LC, Machan CL, Allen BC, Conigrave AD, Roufogalis BD (1991) Protein kinase C phosphorylates the carboxyl terminus of the plasma membrane Ca^{2+}-ATPase from human erythrocytes. J Biol Chem 266: 9078–9085

Authors' address:
Ernesto Carafoli
Laboratory of Biochemistry III
Swiss Federal Institute of
Technology (ETH),
Universitätsstr. 16
8092 Zürich, Switzerland

Regulation of mRNA-expression of the sarcolemmal calmodulin-dependent calcium pump in cardiac hypertrophy

B. Krain,[1] A. Hammes, L. Neyses

Department of Medicine, University of Würzburg, Würzburg, Germany
[1] Present address: Institute for Molecular Biology, Hannover Medical School, Germany

Abstract

While the sarcolemmal calmodulin-dependent calcium pump (PMCA) is thought to play a minor role in beat-to-beat sarcolemmal Ca^{2+}-movements in the myocardium compared to the Na^+/Ca^{2+}-exchanger, its role in long-term processes such as growth and differentiation has not been explored. In a first step to address this question we, therefore, asked whether mRNA expression of the four PMCA isoforms and/or splicing variants was altered during normal and hypertrophic growth of the myocardium and during differentiation of skeletal myoblasts. Differentiation of L6 rat myoblasts to myotubes was paralleled by novel expression of PMCA 3f (i.e., isoform 3, splice variant f). In myocardial cells, transition from the neonatal to the adult phenotype was accompanied by novel expression of PMCA 3e while all other isoforms and splice variants remained stable. This splicing of PMCA 3 was dramatically accelerated by hypertrophic stimuli. In the adult SHR model of hypertrophy no qualitative changes in PMCA expression pattern occurred. We conclude: (1) isoform 3 is the most plastic isoform in the myocardium; (2) PMCA 3e may either determine functions of the adult myocardium or be involved in the transition from the neonatal to the adult phenotype; (3) together with the experiments in myogenic model systems, these results suggest a role of the sarcolemmal calcium pump in long-term processes such as myocardial growth and hypertrophy.

Key words Sarcolemmal Ca^{2+} pump – hypertrophy – myocardial growth – myogenic differentiation – alternative splicing

Introduction

In mammalian cells the calmodulin-dependent plasma membrane Ca^{2+}-ATPase (PMCA) is a ubiquitous Ca^{2+}-transporting system which extrudes Ca^{2+} from the cytoplasm (for a review see ref. 10). While the function of the sarcoendoplasmic Ca^{2+}-ATPase (SERCA) has been well characterized, the exact role of the PMCA for calcium homeostasis remains less clear. Open questions include: What is the function of the striking isoform diversity of the pump with at least 4 (for a review see ref. 11), possibly five (6) genes (isoforms) on different chromosomes and numerous splice variants? Does the PMCA take part in calcium sparks in the cytosol? How is the pump regulated on a short – and long term basis? Is it involved in growth and differentiation?

In myocardium, skeletal muscle, neurones, and perhaps smooth muscle, the regulation of Ca^{2+}-export is further compounded by the presence of an active sodium/calcium exchanger (25). In the heart this system, together with SERCA, is believed to sustain most of the calcium homeostasis on a beat-to-beat basis and the PMCA has been assigned a minor role (3; reviewed in 19).

We have recently shown that the PMCA may have a role in more long-term processes, because differentiation of myogenic cells directs alternative splicing of the constitutive PMCA isoforms 1 and 4 (17). Alternative splicing occurs in region C, the major known regulatory region which confers calmodulin sensitivity. The more N-terminal splice region A presumably participates in regulation of the pump by acidic phospholipids. For nomenclature of the splice variants in splice region C see Fig. 1.

In the present work we investigated whether alternative splicing in these pivotal regions also accompanied maturation of the myocardium from the neonatal to the adult phenotype and whether this pattern was altered in hypertrophic heart growth. Myogenic in vitro differentiation was used as a model system. We here demonstrate that myogenic differentiation does not only direct alternative splicing of the PMCA isoforms 1 and 4 but also transcription of an isoform not previously demonstrated in myogenic cells (PMCA 3). Conversion of rat skin fibroblasts to myotubes by overexpression of the myogenic determination genes myogenin, myf5, and myf6 also dictated alternative splicing of the PMCA. The transition from the neonatal to the adult phenotype is accompanied by new expression of PMCA 3e. In striking contrast with other genes [e.g., cardiac α-actin (31), α-myosin-heavy-chain (20), Na^+/K^+-ATPase (33), reviewed in refs. (24) and (27)], expression of PMCA 3e was markedly accelerated by hypertrophic stimuli while the other isoforms showed no qualitative alteration and may, therefore, resemble the unaltered isoform expression of SERCA in cardiac hypertrophy (13). Therefore, in the myocardium the PMCA may play a role in long-term growth processes rather than in beat-to-beat calcium regulation.

Materials and methods

Preparation of isolated neonatal cardiomyocytes

Cardiomyocytes from 1-day-old Wistar Kyoto rats (WKY) were prepared according to the method described by Simpson and Savion (32).

Cells were enzymatically treated and preplated for 75 min in Ham's F-10/10 %, FCS (fetal calfserum)/10 % HS (horseserum) at 37 °C and 5 % CO_2 to reduce the number of nonmyocardial cells (NMCs). The enriched fraction was counted and 75,000 viable cells (trypan blue exclusion test) were plated per cm^2 in gelatine-coated culture dishes (0.5 % porcine gelatine, Sigma). 15–18 h later the medium was replaced by Ham's F-10 medium containing insulin 10 μg/ml (Serva, Heidelberg, Ger-

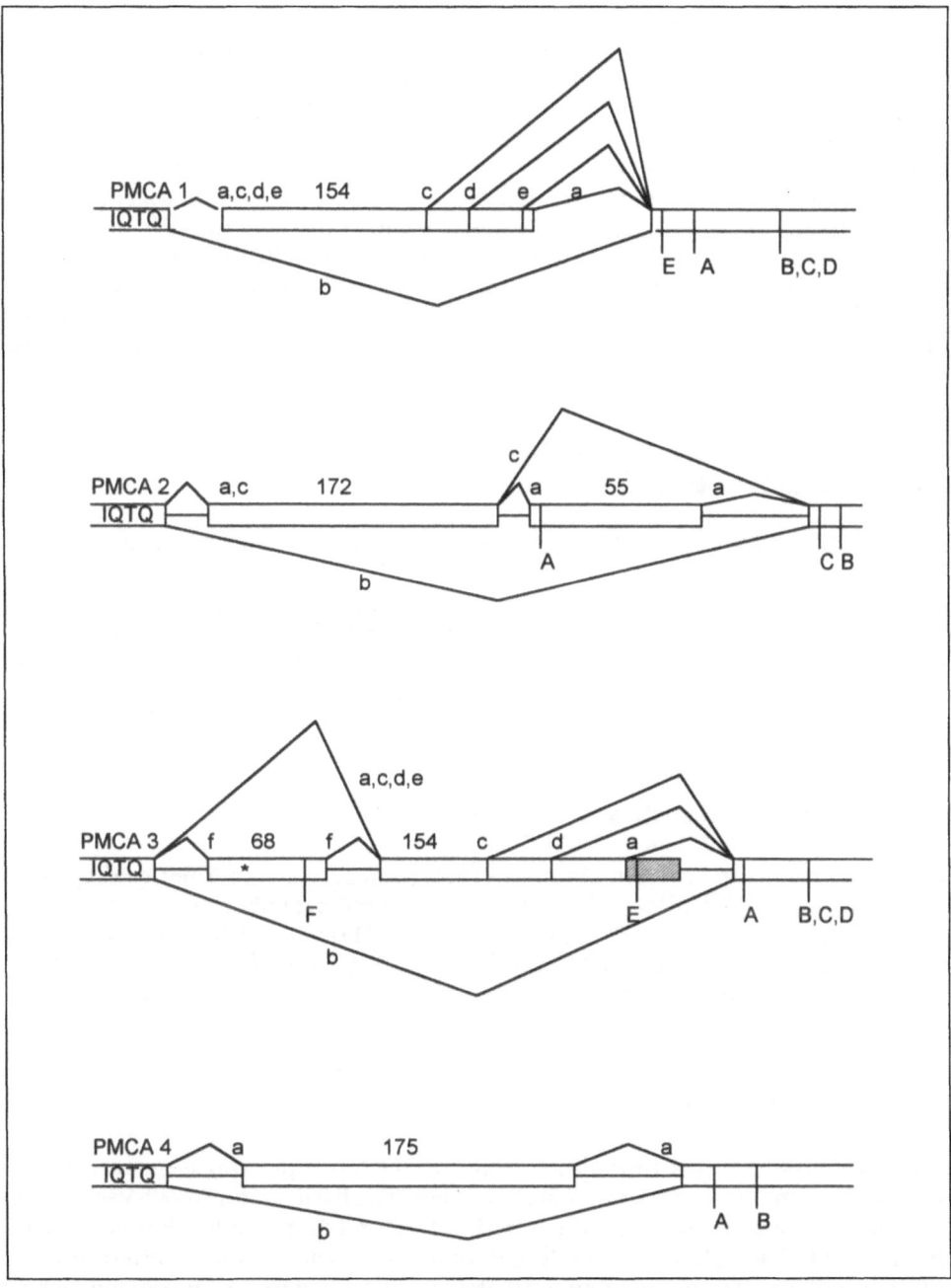

Fig. 1 Scheme of the alternative splicing variants of plasma membrane Ca^{2+}-ATPase (PMCA) isoforms 1, 2, 3, and 4 at the calmodulin binding site (region C). Exons are represented by boxes and introns are represented by horizontal lines. The numbers indicate the sizes (in bp) of the alternatively spliced exons. The diagram of each gene starts with the last four amino acids of the exon encoding the constant region of the calmodulin-binding domain. Lowercase letters indicate the splicing patterns, and uppercase letters indicate the position of stop codons in the mRNAs encoding the corresponding PMCA splice variants. In PMCA 3, *represents the potential phosphorylation site for the cGMP-dependent protein kinase. The hatched box represents an extension of 154bp exon and is followed by an alternative polyadenylation site that is used by PMCA 3c and 3f mRNAs.

many); vitamin C 0.1 mmol/L (Sigma); vitamin B_{12} 1.5 μmol/L (Serva); transferrin 10 μg/ml (Sigma); NaSe 20 nmol/L (Sigma); bromodeoxyuridine 0.1 mmol/L (Sigma). This procedure yielded about 97 % beating cardiomyocytes as assessed by light microscopy and troponin T immunofluorescent staining.

Hypertrophic stimuli were added to the cells after 15–18 h in culture. This time was termed 0 hours (h). Angiotensin II (Sigma) was added at a concentration of 10^{-7} M every 24 h for 48 h, while isoproterenol (Sigma) and phenylephrine (Serva, Heidelberg, Germany) were added once at a concentration of 10^{-5} M for 48 h.

To assess the degree of hypertrophy the number of cells in culture dishes was counted (20 random fields) and the protein content determined. Cells were lysed with 10 % trichloracetic acid (TCA) at 4 °C for 1 h, rinsed two times with TCA, and dissolved in 1 ml of 1 % SDS at 37 °C. The cell protein fraction was quantified by the Lowry method (21).

Isolation of adult cardiomyocytes

Adult cardiomyocytes from Wistar Kyoto rats (WKY) and spontaneously hypertensive rats (SHR) (10 and 20 weeks old; Charles River Wega, Bad Sulzfeld, Germany) were isolated by the collagenase method. Collagenase/hyaluronidase perfusion of the isolated hearts was performed according to Powell (28) with modifications of Rose and Kammermeier (29). After the final 2 % bovine serum gradient, more than 99 % of all cells were cardiomyocytes as assessed by troponin T staining.

Cell culture and differentiation

L6 myoblasts (35) and rat skin fibroblasts (FR) (purchased from American Type Culture Collection, ATCC, Rockville, MD) were cultured in Dulbecco's modified Eagle medium (DMEM; GIBCO BRL, Gaithersburg, MD) with 10 % FCS. Differentiation of L6 myoblasts was induced by substituting 2 % HS (v/v) for 10 % FCS. Addition of 10^{-6} M insulin (Serva) induced complete differentiation within 5–7 days.

Transfection of fibroblasts

Rat skin fibroblasts (FR-fibroblasts) were transfected with expression vectors containing different myogenin determination genes. The basic vector pEMSVscribe (18) contains the constitutive viral promoter MSV LTR and the polyadenylation sequence from SV 40. The following muscle determination factors were inserted into the pEMSVscribe vector by the unique EcoRI site: 1.5 kb cDNA of myogenin lacking only the first 22 nucleotides of the 5' untranslated region (34), 1.8 kb cDNA of myoD (12), 1.4 kb cDNA of myf5 (8), 1.3 kb cDNA of myf6 (7).

Myogenin and myoD cDNA were kind gifts from Dr. Woodring Wright (Southwestern Medical Center, Dallas, USA). Myf5 and myf6 cDNA were provided by H. H. Arnold (Institut für Biochemie und Biotechnologie, Technische Universität Braunschweig, Germany). Transfection was performed by electroporation at 340 mV and 960 μF (Gene Pulser, BIORAD, Munich, Germany). After transfection the cells were plated at 5×10^6 cells/24 cm^2 dish. Twelve hours later, the cells were rinsed and fed with differentiation medium (DMEM plus 2 % HS and 10^{-6} M insulin). Myotube formation started after about 3 days and continued over the next 10 days. Muscle-specific differentiation was confirmed by demonstration of myotubes and by measurement of the muscle-specific creatine phosphokinase activity using the hexo-kinase/glucose-6-phosphate dehydrogenase coupled enzyme assay (Sigma, St. Louis, MO). Control cells were transfected with the pEMSVscribe vector without the muscle-specific determination factors.

Detection of the different plasma membrane calcium-ATPase isoform-specific mRNAs and their splicing variants by reverse transcription PCR (RT-PCR)

The procedure of RNA preparation, reverse transcription, amplification by RT-PCR, and analysis of the PCR products by Southern blotting has been described elsewhere (17). Splicing variants 3f and 3e were detected by the following primer pair. Forward primer: 5'-GTCCAATTTGGAGGGAAGCC-3'; reverse primer: 5'-CCAGGTGCCATTTATGAG AG-3'. Primer pairs used for the PMCA 1, 3, and 4 specific mRNA in the splice region A are presented in Table 1.

Semiquantitative analysis of PCR products

Semiquantitative analysis (sometimes also called quantitative PCR) was carried out for the splicing variants of the PMCA 1, 2, and 4 in the splicing region C.

To avoid artifactual results in quantitative PCR, the kinetics of the reaction was determined for each primer pair used in semiquantitative analysis. The RT-PCR reaction was identical to that described in ref. 17 except that 0.8 μCi [α-^{32}P] dCTP was

Table 1 Primer sequences for the various rat plasma membrane Ca^{2+}-ATPase isoforms for the alternative splicing region A

Rat PMCA isoform	Primer pair sequence	PMCA splice variants	Length of the cDNA	Length of PCR product
PMCA 1	997: 5'-GGCGAGTCTG ACCATGTTAAG-3' 1308: 5'-GTCTTTCTCA TCACCATCTCC-3'	1	4084 bp	312 bp
PMCA 3	1467: 5'-GATCCTATGC TGCTCTCAGGC-3' 1849: 5-CCATCCACAA CGAAGGTCTC-3'	3H 3F	4441 bp 4399 bp	425 bp 383 bp
PMCA 4	1059*: 5'-CTGCTGCCT GCAGATGGAATC-3' 1399*: 5'-TTGTCGATT CCCTCTGGCTG-3'	4H 4F	4463 bp 4421 bp	341 bp 299 bp

Numbers specify the 5'-position of the primer sequence on the cDNA. Splice variants in the region A are designated by capital letters; * primer sequences from human PMCA 4, as only the C-terminus is known for the rat PMCA.

added to the reaction mix. After 25, 30, 35, 40, and 45 cycles, reaction tubes were removed and 20 μl of the reaction mix loaded on an agarose gel. The PCR products were cut out under UV-light, melted in 500 μl H$_2$O at 95 °C and the radioactivity measured by Cerenkov counting. After 40 cycles the PCR reactions were still in the exponential phase for all three primer pairs examined. Semiquantitative analysis was, therefore, performed at 40 cycles.

Results

To be able to create hypotheses about a possible function of the plasma membrane calcium pump (PMCA) in long term processes such as growth and differentiation, we examined mRNA-expression of PMCA splice variants in regions C and A in L6 cells (Figs. 2 and 3). The PMCA mRNA splice variants in region C showed a more complex expression pattern in L6 myotubes than in L6 myoblasts (Figs. 2a and 2b). In addition to the results by Hammes et al. (17), which showed the expression of PMCA splicing variants 1c, 1d, and 4a in L6 myotubes in addition to PMCA 1b and 4b in L6 myoblasts, a novel splicing variant could be detected for the PMCA 3 using suitable primer pairs. Myoblast differentiation was accompanied by novel expression of PMCA 3f (Fig. 2b); the PMCA 3e specific PCR fragment in myoblasts showed extremely low abundance and could only be detected on radioactive Southern blots after 40 PCR cycles. Therefore, this PMCA 3e expression is probably of little significance.

PMCA 2 and splice variants of PMCA 3 other than 3e and 3f were not detected in L6 cells. The mRNA splicing pattern of the PMCA in region A did not change upon myogenic differentiation (Fig. 3). Only the PMCA 1-specific 312 bp-fragment as well as PMCA 3H (very faint band in L6 myoblasts) and PMCA 4H and 4F were found in L6 myoblasts and myotubes.

These experiments identified PMCA 3 as the most plastic isoform in muscle differentiation and in myocardial cells. We, therefore, concentrated on this isoform.

Regulation of PMCA 3 expression by myogenic determination factors

The isoform variant switch of PMCA 3 upon myogenic differentiation raised the question whether the observed switches in PMCA 3 mRNA-expression were induced by muscle-specific factors and whether different myogenic determination factors directed different isoform splicing patterns. We, therefore, transfected fetal rat skin fibroblasts (FR-fibroblasts) with the pEMSVscribe vector containing the cDNA of either of the myogenic determination factors myogenin, myoD, myf5, or myf6 under the control of a constitutive viral promotor (see methods). FR-fibroblasts could be successfully transformed into myotubes with pEMSVscribe+myogenin, pEMSVscribe+myf5, pEMSVscribe+myf6, but for unknown reasons not with pEMSVscribe+myoD, as examined by the formation of multinucleated myotubes and creatine kinase assay (results not shown). PMCA 3 mRNA-expression is depicted in Fig. 4. FR-fibroblasts cultured in 10 % FCS (v/v) expressed PMCA 3f. FR-fibroblasts which were transfected with the pEMSVscribe vector without the myogenic deter-

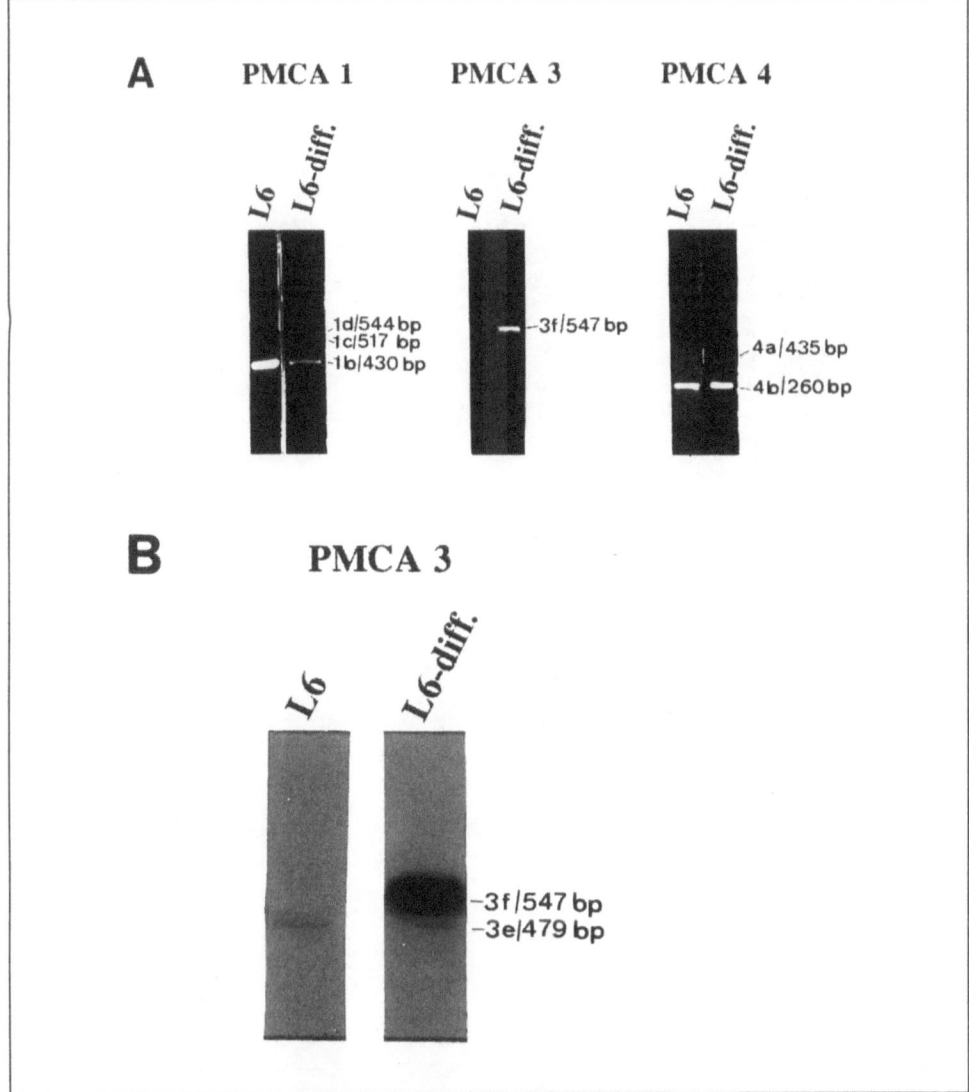

Fig. 2 Plasma membrane Ca^{2+}-ATPase (PMCA) isoform-specific mRNA pattern in splice region C in L6 myoblasts and myotubes (L6-diff.). **A)** PMCA isoform-specific mRNA pattern in splicing region C. PMCA 1 products were separated on a 2.5 % Meta Phor-agarose gel, the other fragments on 2 % agarose gels. A PCR product of about 390 bp (middle band in PMCA 4) was probably due to amplification of an unrelated mRNA. It yielded no signal on Southern blots. Differentiation medium was present for 5–7 days. PMCA 2 expression was not detected. Results for PMCA 1 and PMCA 4 have been published elsewhere (17) and are shown here for comparison. **B)** Southern blot analysis of PMCA 3 specific PCR products of L6 myoblasts and myotubes. L6 myoblasts expressed very low amounts of PMCA 3e (only detectable on radioactive Southern blots, not in the original agarose gel), L6 myotubes expressed PMCA 3f mRNA only.

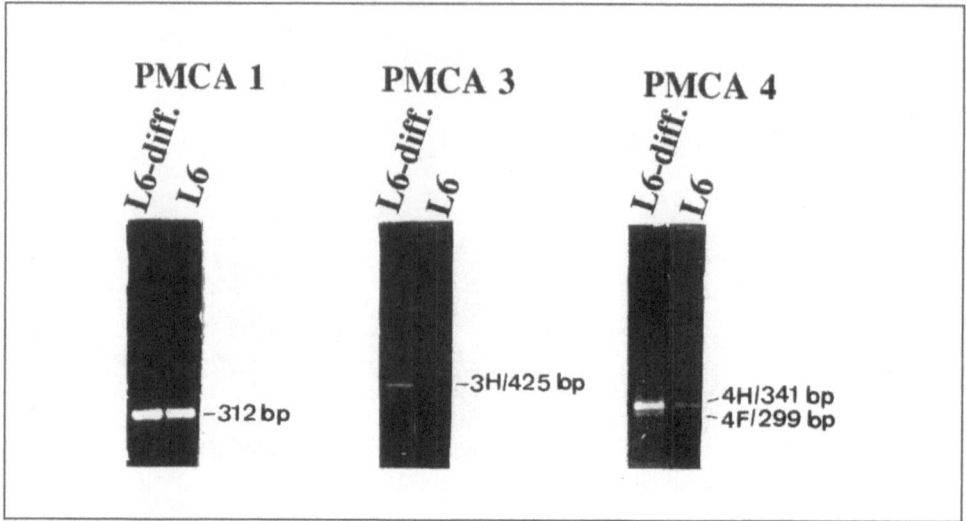

Fig. 3   PMCA isoform-specific mRNA pattern in splicing region A. No differentiation-specific differences in PMCA 1 and 4 mRNA-expression could be found. PMCA 3 was almost undetectable in myoblasts (see Fig. 2B).

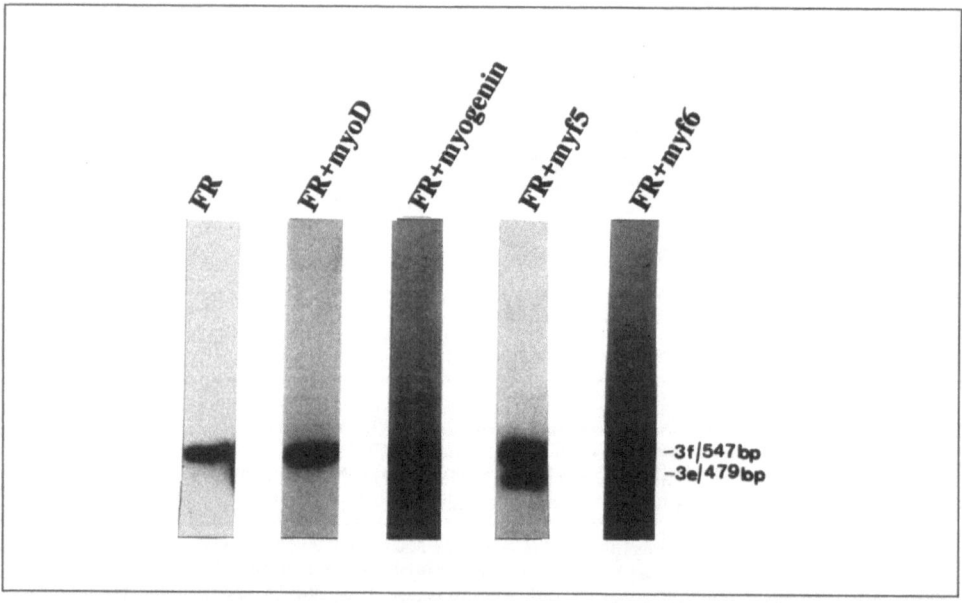

Fig. 4   Isoform variant switch of the plasma membrane Ca^{2+}-ATPase in FR-fibroblasts expressing different myogenic determination factors. Southern blot analysis of the PCR products are shown.
FR = control with FR-fibroblasts transfected with empty pEMSVscribe vector. FR + myoD, FR + myogenin, FR + myf5, FR + myf6: FR cells expressing the respective cDNA under the control of a constitutive viral promoter. Myotube formation started about 3 days after transfection with myogenin cDNA, myf5, or myf6 cDNA. RT-PCR was performed after 14 days. Transfection of FR-fibroblasts with myoD cDNA did not result in the formation of multinucleated myotubes suggesting that the transcription factor environment of FR cells was not permissive for differentiation with myoD.

mination factors expressed PMCA 3f, as well as FR-fibroblasts transfected with pEMSVscribe+myoD cDNA. FR-fibroblasts transfected with pEMSVscribe+ myogenin cDNA, pEMSVscribe+myf5 cDNA, and pEMSVscribe+myf6 cDNA expressed PMCA 3e in addition to PMCA 3f. This PMCA 3 mRNA-expression pattern varied from that found in L6 myotubes. Because of the endogenous expression of PMCA 3f mRNA in FR-fibroblasts, a qualitatively new induction of PMCA 3f upon differentiation could not be demonstrated but there might be quantitative differences. These results demonstrate that PMCA 3 splicing is specifically activated by muscle-specific determination genes. Different myogenic factors induce no differences in alternative splicing, possibly due to cross-induction of the myogenic determination factors (14). This also suggested that splicing of PMCA 3 may be essential either for the differentiation process or for the differentiated muscle phenotype.

Growth-dependent PMCA 3 mRNA-expression in cardiac myocytes

The results presented above strongly indicated a possible role of PMCA isoform variants for the function of differentiated myogenic cells and/or for the differentiation process itself. We then examined whether a similar process could be demonstrated in the myocardium. Comparison of PMCA mRNA-expression in the splicing region C showed that PMCA 3e mRNA-expression was growth-specific (Fig. 5). Analogous to fibroblasts transfected with the myogenic determination genes, PMCA 3e was increasingly expressed in cardiomyocytes from 7 day, 10, and 20 week old animals (for PMCA 3e expression in 20 week old cardiomyocytes see Fig. 6 third lane). One day old rat cardiomyocytes expressed PMCA 3f but not PMCA 3e. PMCA 1, 2, and 4 showed no qualitative changes in PMCA mRNA-expression when neonatal PMCA

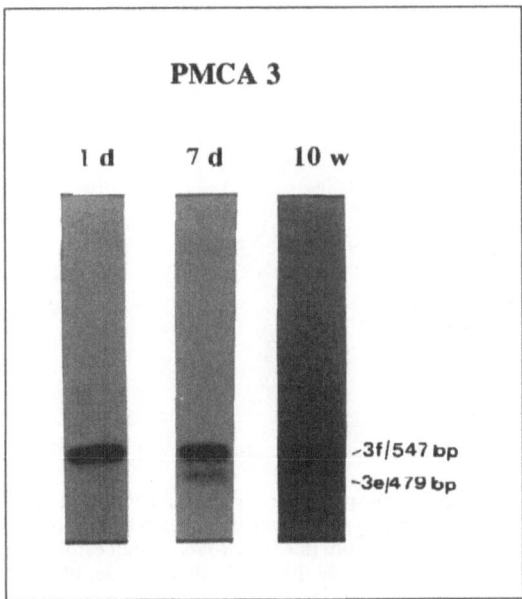

Fig. 5 Growth-specific PMCA 3e mRNA-expression in WKY rat cardiomyocytes at different ages. PMCA 3f mRNA was expressed in cardiomyocytes of all ages examined. PMCA 3e mRNA was not expressed in one day old (1 d) cardiomyocytes, but was expressed in seven day old (7 d) and ten week old (10w) cardiomyocytes. PMCA 3e expression in 20 week old cardiomyocytes is shown in Fig. 6, third lane. Note the increasing expression of PMCA 3e compared with 3f.

mRNA-expression was compared to PMCA mRNA-expression in adult (10 and 20 weeks) rat cardiomyocytes. A typical pattern of PMCA splice variants in adult cardiomyocytes is shown in Fig. 6.

PMCA mRNA-expression in cardiac hypertrophy

We then asked: if PMCA 3e expression is characteristic of normal cell growth, will PMCA 3e expression also change in hypertrophic growth and will there be a tendency towards expression of an antecedent phenotype as described for many contractile proteins in cardiac hypertrophy?

Two models of hypertrophy were investigated: First neonatal rat cardiomyocytes treated with three hypertrophic stimuli, for example, angiotensin II (30), isoproterenol and phenylephrine (4) and second adult isolated cardiomyocytes from spontaneously hypertensive rats (SHR).

The neonatal hypertrophy model showed no qualitative differences of PMCA splicing form expression for PMCA 1, 2, and 4 between normal and hypertrophic cardiomyocytes treated with either of the three stimuli. All cells expressed PMCA 1b, 1c, 1d, PMCA 2b, 2c, 2a, PMCA 4b, and 4a (data not shown). Furthermore, the PMCA mRNA-expression pattern of these isoforms was qualitatively identical to the PMCA mRNA-expression pattern of adult cardiomyocytes. The expression of PMCA 3e in hypertrophied neonatal cardiomyocytes was, however, altered when compared with controls (Fig. 7). PMCA 3e mRNA was not expressed in the 0 h con-

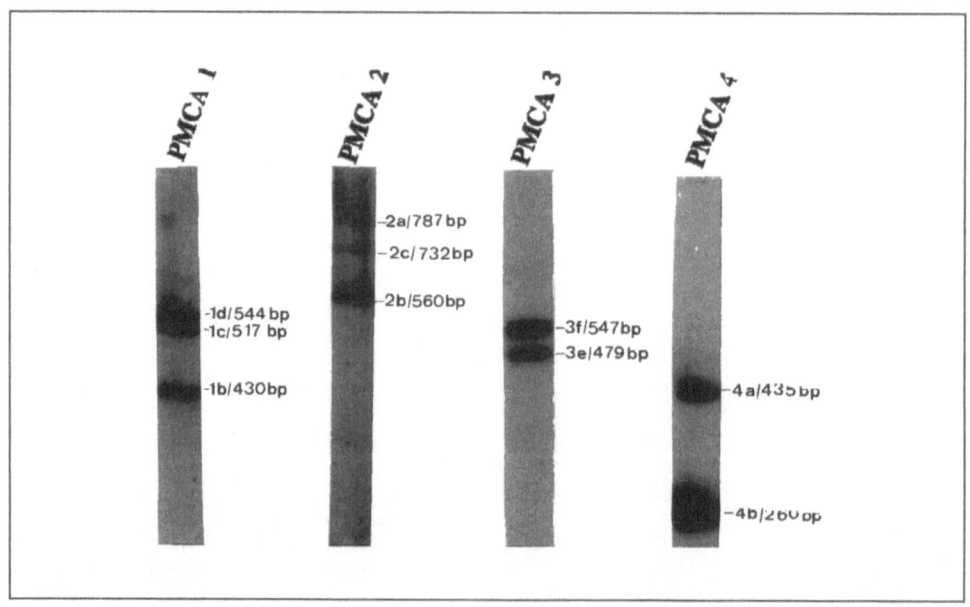

Fig. 6 Plasma membrane Ca^{2+}-ATPase (PMCA) mRNA splicing pattern in region C in adult cardiomyocytes from 20 week old Wistar Kyoto rats (WKY). This expression pattern was detected in both 10 and 20 week old spontaneously hypertensive rats (SH-rats) and Wistar Kyoto rats (WKY-rats). Adult cardiomyocytes expressed PMCA mRNA 1b, 1c, 1d, PMCA 2 mRNA 2a, 2b, 2c, PMCA 3 mRNA 3f, 3e, PMCA 4 mRNA 4b, and 4a.

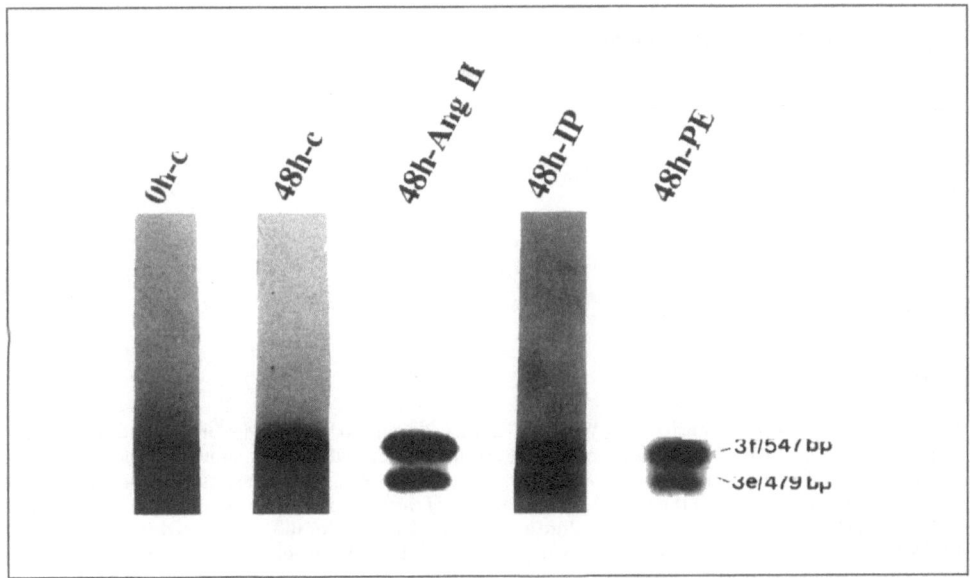

Fig. 7 PMCA 3e/3f mRNA-expression in neonatal cardiomyocytes and in myocytes that were treated with various hypertrophic stimuli. Southern blot analysis of the specific PCR-products. Neonatal cardiomyocytes (0 h–c, c for control) were treated with various hypertrophic stimuli for 48 h. Angiotensin II was added every 24 h (10^{-7} M; 48 h-Ang II), isoproterenol (48 h-IP) and phenylephrine (48 h-PE) were added to a final concentration of 10^{-5} M. Control: untreated neonatal cardiomyocytes (48 h-c). The relative degree of hypertrophy as assessed by protein content was: 0 h-c: 1; 48 h-c: 1.2; 48 h-Ang II: 1.3; 48 h-IP: 1.6; 48 h-PE: 1.7 (n = 3).

trols and only weakly expressed in the 48 h controls (only detected on radioactive Southern blots, not in agarose gels). PMCA 3e mRNA-expression was greatly accelerated by all three hypertrophic stimuli. Therefore, no reversion of the expression pattern towards the neonatal (antecendent) phenotype but rather acceleration towards the adult phenotype was conferred by these stimuli.

As a further model of hypertrophy PMCA mRNA-expression pattern was examined in 10 and 20 week old cardiomyocytes from spontaneously hypertensive rats SHR and in age-matched controls. Ten week old SHR cardiomyocytes had 25 % and 20 week old cells 27 % hypertrophy by cell volume compared to controls. The PMCA mRNA-expression pattern for PMCA 1, 2, 3, and 4 in splicing region C was identical to the one in Fig. 6. Also the expression pattern showed no qualitative differences between 10 and 20 week old SHR cardiomyocytes and age-matched controls. All cardiomyocytes, examined expressed PMCA 1b, 1c, 1d, PMCA 2b, 2c, 2a, PMCA 3f, 3e, PMCA 4b and 4a.

Furthermore, we performed quantification of the mRNA of the various splicing variants. Even after rigorous standardization of the PCR protocol, this resulted in a high variability, well described for other systems. Therefore, an internal standardization was performed for the splicing variants of each isoform (Table 2); this permitted the assessment of the relative abundance of the splice variants within each isoform, but obviously precludes comparison between isoforms. The relative amounts of PMCA splicing variants within each isoform remained relatively stable in SHR and WKY.

Table 2 Semiquantitative PCR-analysis of the relative amounts of the PMCA mRNA splicing variants within one isoform in adult rat cardiomyocytes

	WKY-10W	SHR-10W	WKY-20W	SHR-20W
PMCA 2				
1 c + d	0.64 ± 0.24	0.68 ± 0.21	0.38 ± 0.17	0.73 ± 0.16
1 b	1	1	1	1
PMCA 2				
2 a	0.88 ± 0.19	0.92 ± 0.27	0.83 ± 0.11	0.90 ± 0.35
2 c	0.74 ± 0.12	0.73 ± 0.25	0.74 ± 0.20	0.74 ± 0.19
2 b	1	1	1	1
PMCA 4				
4 a	0.12 ± 0.03	0.14 ± 0.03	0.16 ± 0.07	0.10 ± 0.02
4 b	1	1	1	1

SHR: spontaneously hypertensive rats. WKY: Wistar Kyoto rats: 10 W: isolated cardiomyocytes from ten week old animals. 20 W: isolated cardiomyocytes from 20 week old animals. Note that the ratio of the amount of the splicing variants refers to one isoform only. The amount of the shortest PCR product was set equal to 1, and the amount of the other splicing variants of the same isoform were expressed as a fraction of 1. No conclusions can be drawn for absolute abundance of mRNA for the splicing variants and between the isoforms. The standard deviation is given in parentheses. The 10 week old groups consisted of 4 animals each; the 20 week old groups consisted of 6 animals each. One PCR reaction was performed for each animal for PMCA 1. PMCA 1c and 1d were counted together because of the close proximity of the bands. PCR-reactions in double were performed for each animal for PMCA 2 and PMCA 4. The differences between the groups found were not significant (Wilcoxon's rank sum test).

Discussion

While first, though still incomplete, insights into the function of the PMCA and its isoform diversity begin to emerge (for review see 10), very little is known about its expression and potential role in heart muscle and myogenic cell lines widely used for the investigation of terminal differentiation.

As a first step toward the goal of defining the role of the PMCA in this context our results show that (1) differentiation of L6 cells dictates expression of a new splice variant of the pump (PMCA 3f), (2) all myogenic factors (except for myoD which does not induce muscle differentiation in FR rat skin fibroblasts) dictate an identical splicing pattern of PMCA 3, (3) in analogy to FR-fibroblasts transfected with myogenic determination factors, in the myocardium, transition from the neonatal to the adult phenotype is accompanied by novel expression of PMCA 3e mRNA, and (4) in the neonatal cardiac hypertrophy model PMCA 3e mRNA-expression is accelerated compared to normal growth. In cardiomyocytes from 10 and 20 week old SHR PMCA expression is qualitatively unaltered compared to WKY controls. PMCA 1, 2, and 4 are examples of genes that display no reversion to a developmentally antecedent phenotype in cardiac hypertrophy.

For PMCA isoforms 1, 2, and 4 this finding is analogous to the SERCA isoform expression where no isoform switches have been found in models of cardiac hypertrophy. In contrast to the stable expression pattern of PMCA 1, 2, and 4 (this paper), SERCA (13), and skeletal α-actin in humans (5), isoform changes in hypertrophy have been reported for (among other genes) rat α-actin genes (31), myosin-heavy-chain genes (20), and the α-subunit of the Na$^+$/K$^+$-ATPase (33). The genes for contractile proteins showed an enhanced expression of isoforms typical of the fetal/neonatal phenotype, whereas expression of isoforms characteristic of the adult phenotype was depressed (for review see ref. 27). In contrast to these results, PMCA 3e expression was accelerated by the hypertrophic process.

While the question concerning the mechanisms governing developmental regulation of PMCA 3 is difficult to address because the promoter region of the PMCA 3 is unknown, our data allow one to derive testable hypotheses about the potential function of this pump.

In a somewhat simplified view, calcium regulation in the heart and other tissues can be divided into short- and long-term processes. In the shortest temporal unit of cardiac action, i.e., one contraction/relaxation cycle, the PMCA does not appear to play a major role. When all other calcium-transporting systems of isolated rat or guinea-pig cardiomyocytes were inhibited, outward calcium transport by the PMCA only accounted for a small fraction of the calcium flux (3; review: 19). Direct inhibition of the pump in this kind of experiment is currently not possible due to the lack of a specific inhibitor. Although most of these experiments were carried out at 20–23 °C and the PMCA may contribute more to the outward calcium transport at physiological temperature, our results do not conflict with this view because they primarily address cardiac functions other than contraction.

In this context, it has been recently demonstrated that in the myocardium and various other cells the PMCA is highly spatially restricted to structures known as caveolae (15). Although long known, the function of these structures is only beginning to be unraveled (1). Caveolae are the preferred location of glycosylphosphatidylinositol (GPI)-anchored membrane proteins, some of which mediate potocytosis, i.e., concentration of small molecules such as calcium, cAMP, or adenosine and subsequent release into the cytosol. Caveolae may not be preformed structures of the cell membrane but rather form upon multimerization signals bringing together molecules which then travel to caveolae (22). A form of the inositol 1,4,5-trisphosphate-receptor like Ca^{2+}-channel has been shown to be colocalized in caveolae (16), and it is, therefore, conceivable that the PMCA may function to regulate calcium fluxes in these storage sites. A further speculation could be that ANP released from hypertrophied ventricular myocardium (2) or angiotensin II released from hypertrophied myocardium as an autocrine agent in stretch-mediated hypertrophy (30) is exocytosed via the caveolar route and hence the PMCA could be regulating this process. It is an obvious hypothesis from our results that PMCA 3e may be related to this process. This view is supported by the accelerated expression of PMCA 3e in hypertrophied neonatal cardiomyocytes. It is also possible that the PMCA may dictate translational efficiency in cardiac growth (23).

To study long-term regulation of the pump we chose the model of myogenic differentiation. This allowed us to create hypotheses about changes that may occur in normal and hypertrophic heart growth. We identified here novel expression of PMCA 3 in the process of myogenic differentiation. All myogenic factors which were able to induce the muscle phenotype in rat skin fibroblasts, i.e., myogenin, myf5 and myf6, but for unknown reasons not myoD, were able to direct alternative splicing of PMCA 3 and novel expression of PMCA 3e. This shows that PMCA 3e expression occurs downstream of myf/myogenin expression and PMCA 3e expression is not induced by some unknown factor in the medium used for differentiation (e.g., insulin and/or horse serum).

In the heart we were able to demonstrate that PMCA 3 (not previously identified in the myocardium) occurred in neonatal cardiac myocytes and that maturation to the adult phenotype was accompanied by alternative splicing of this isoform.

Interestingly, the PMCA 3 isoform is the only isoform containing a 68nt-exon which is spliced in in PMCA 3f but spliced out in PMCA 3e. The 68nt-exon contains a potential phosphorylation site for the cGMP-dependent protein kinase (9). Hence, alternative splicing of PMCA 3 in (normal and hypertrophic) growth could regulate sensitivity toward regulation by cGMP.

Another obvious hypothesis about the function of PMCA 3e is that it may be related to the cessation of spontaneous beating which occurs in the same time range, e.g., by increasing calcium efflux in a spatially restricted compartment in addition to changes in the calcium channel (26). It is also possible that adult, but not neonatal, cardiomyocytes respond to endo-paracrine stimuli which require the presence of the novel splice variant, perhaps in membrane caveolae (see discussion above).

If PMCA isoform expression is related to normal cardiac growth, could variations in PMCA expression pattern also be typical of cardiac hypertrophy? Our original hypothesis was that reversion to a more undifferentiated phenotype would take place in a manner similar to the "fetal isoform theory" for contractile proteins (24, 27). Surprisingly, not only did we find no change in PMCA isoform composition in cardiac hypertrophy, but there was an acceleration of PMCA 3e expression in neonatal cells when hypertrophic stimuli were applied. In cardiac myocytes from SHR, the PMCA expression pattern remained stable compared to WKY. A quantitative difference in mRNA accumulation could still be present, but exploratory analysis using quantitative PCR showed that these changes, if present, would be below the detection limits of this method. Clearly, for a definitive answer to this question the production of isoform-specific antibodies will have to be awaited. With this caveat in mind, our results suggest the hypothesis that PMCA 3e may have a role in the development of cardiac hypertrophy, e.g., by influencing secretion of autocrine stimuli such as angiotensin II from caveolae (see above).

The overall conclusion from the results presented here is that it is reasonable to put forward the hypothesis that the sarcolemmal calmodulin-dependent calcium pump may be involved in growth and differentiation in myogenic, myocardial, and possibly other cells.

Acknowledgments We thank W. Wright (Southwestern Medical Center, Dallas, Texas) for providing the pEMSVscribe+myogenin and pEMSVscribe+myoD plasmids and H. H. Arnold and T. Braun (Technische Universität, Braunschweig, Germany) for providing pEMSVscribe+myf5 and pEMSVscribe+myf6. We thank G. Shull (University of Cincinnati, Cincinnati, Ohio) for sending us the full length cDNA for rat PMCA isoforms 1 and 2 and special thanks to E. Carafoli and T. Stauffer (University of Zuerich, Switzerland) for many helpful discussions and technical suggestions. The technical assistance of Silke Oberdorf is gratefully acknowledged. This work was supported by Deutsche Forschungsgemeinschaft, TP B6, SFB 355.

REFERENCES

1. Anderson RGW (1993) Caveolae: where incoming and outgoing messengers meet. Proc Natl Acad Sci USA 90: 10909–10913
2. Argentin S, Ardati A, Tremblay S, Lihrmann I, Robitaille L, Drouin J, Nemer M (1994) Developmental stage-specific regulation of atrial natriuretic factor gene transcription in cardiac cells. Mol Cell Biol 14: 777–790
3. Bers DM, Bassani JWM, Bassani RA (1993) Competition and redistribution among calcium transport systems in rabbit cardiac myocytes. Cardiovasc Res 27: 1772–1777
4. Bishopric NH, Kedes L (1991) Adrenergic regulation of the skeletal α-actin gene promoter during myocardial cell hypertrophy. Proc Natl Acad Sci 88: 2132–2136
5. Boheler KR, Carrier L, de la Bastie D, Allen PD, Komajada M, Mercadier JJ, Schwartz K (1991) Skeletal actin mRNA increases in the human heart during ontogenic development and is the major isoform of control and failing human hearts. J Clin Invest 88: 323–330
6. Brand P, Neve RL, Kammerscheidt R, Rhodas RE, Vanaman TC (1992) Analysis of the tissue-specific distribution of mRNAs encoding the plasma membrane calcium-pumping ATPases and characterization of an alternatively spliced form of PMCA 4 at the cDNA and genomic level. J Biol Chem 267: 4376–4385
7. Braun T, Bober E, Winter B, Rosenthal N, Arnold HH (1990) Myf-6, a novel member of the human gene family of myogenic determination factors/ evidence for a gene cluster on chromosome 12. EMBO J 9: 821–831
8. Braun T, Buschhausen-Denker, Bober E, Tannich E, Arnold HH (1989) A novel human factor related to but distinct from MyoD1 induces myogenic conversion in 10T1/2 fibroblasts. EMBO J 8: 701–709
9. Burk SE, Shull GE (1992) Structure of the rat plasma membrane Ca^{2+}-ATPase isoform 3 gene and characterization of alternative splicing and transcription products. J Biol Chem 267: 19683–19690
10. Carafoli E, Guerini D (1993) Molecular and cellular biology of plasma membrane calcium ATPase. Trends in Cardiovasc Med 3: 177–184
11. Carafoli E, Stauffer T (1993) The plasma membrane calcium pump: functional domains, regulation of the activity, and tissue specificity of isoform expression. J Neurobiol 3: 312–324
12. Davis RL, Weintraub H, Lassar AB (1987) Expression of single transfected cDNA converts fibroblasts to myoblasts. Cell 51: 987–1000
13. de la Bastie D, Levitsky D, Rappaport L, Mercadier J-J, Marotte F, Wisnewsky C, Brovkovich V, Schwarz K, Lompré A-M (1990) Function of the sarcoplasmic reticulum and expression of its Ca^{2+}-ATPase gene in pressure overload-induced cardiac hypertrophy in the rat. Circ Res 66: 554–564
14. Emerson CP (1990) Myogenesis and developmental control genes. Curr Opinion Cell Biol 2: 1065–1075
15. Fujimoto T (1993) Calcium pump of the plasma membrane is localized in caveolae. J Cell Biol 120: 1147–1157
16. Fujimoto T, Nakade S, Miyawaki A, Mikoshiba K, Ogawa K (1992) Localization of inositol 1,4,5-trisphosphate receptor-like protein in plasmalemmal caveolae. J Cell Biol 119: 1507–1513
17. Hammes A, Oberdorf S, Strehler EE, Stauffer T, Carafoli E, Vetter H, Neyses L (1994) Differentiation-specific isoform mRNA expression of the calmodulin-dependent plasma membrane Ca^{2+}-ATPase. FASEB J 8: 428–435
18. Harland R, Weintraub H (1985) Translation of mRNA injected into Xenopus oocytes is specifically inhibited by antisense RNA. J Cell Biol 101: 1094–1099
19. Langer GA (1994) Myocardial Calcium Compartmentation. Trends Cardiovasc Med 4: 103–109
20. Lompré A-M, Schwartz K, d'Abis A, Lacombe G, Van Thiem N, Swynghedauw B (1979) Myosin isoenzyme redistribution in chronic heart overload. Nature 282: 105–107
21. Lowry OH, Rosebrough NJ, Farr AL, Randall RJ (1951) Protein measurement with the Folin phenol reagent. J Biol Chem 193: 265–275
22. Mayor S, Rothberg KG, Maxfield FR (1994) Sequestration of GPI-anchored proteins in caveolae triggered by cross-linking. Science 264: 1948–1951
23. Morgan HE, Gordon EE, Kira Y, Chua BHL, Russo LA, Peterson CJ, McDermott PJ, Watson PA (1987) Biochemical mechanisms of cardiac hypertrophy. Ann Rev Physiol 49: 533–543
24. Nadal-Ginard B, Mahdavi V (1990) Molecular basis of cardiac performance. J Clin Invest 84: 1693–1700
25. Nicoll DA, Longoni S, Philipson KD (1990) Molecular cloning and functional expression of the cardiac sarcolemmal Na^+/Ca^{2+} exchanger. Science 250: 562–565
26. Nuss HB, Houser SR (1993) T-type Ca^{2+} current is expressed in hypertrophied adult feline left ventricular myocytes. Circ Res 73: 777–782
27. Parker TG, Schneider MD (1991) Growth factors, proto-oncogenes, and plasticity of the cardiac phenotype. Annu Rev Physiol 53: 179–200

28. Powell T (1988) Methods for isolation and preparation of single adult myocytes. In: Clark WA, Decker RS, Borg TK (eds) Biology of Adult Myocytes. Elsevier, Amsterdam: 9–13

29. Rose H, Kammermeier H (1986) Contraction and metabolic activity of electrically stimulated cardiac myocytes from adult rats. Pfluegers Archiv 407: 116–118

30. Sadoshima J, Xu Y, Slayter HS, Izumo S (1993) Autocrine release of angiotensin II mediates stretch-induced hypertrophy of cardiac myocytes in vitro. Cell 75: 977–984

31. Schwartz K, de la Bastie D, Bouveret P, Oliviero P, Alonso S, Buckingham M (1986) α-skeletal actin mRNA accumulates in hypertrophied adult rat hearts. Circ Res 12: 551–555

32. Simpson P, Savion S (1982) Differentiation of rat cardiomyocytes in single cell cultures with and without proliferating nonmyocardial cells. Circ Res 50: 101–116

33. Sweadner KJ, Herrera VLM, Amato S, Moellmann A, Gibbons DK, Repke KRH (1994) Immunologic identification of Na^+, K^+-ATPase isoforms in myocardium. Isoform change in deoxycorticosterone acetate-salt hypertension. Circ Res 74: 669–678

34. Wright WE, Sassoon DA, Lin VK (1989) Myogenin, a factor regulating myogenesis, has a domain homologous to myoD. Cell 56: 607–617

35. Yaffe D (1968) Retention of differentiation potentialities during prolonged cultivation of myogenic cells. Proc Natl Acad Sci USA 61: 477–483

Authors' address:
L. Neyses MD
Department of Medicine
University of Würzburg
Josef-Schneider-Str. 2
97080 Würzburg, Germany

Molecular mechanisms regulating the myofilament response to Ca^{2+}: Implications of mutations causal for familial hypertrophic cardiomyopathy

K. A. Palmiter, R. J. Solaro

University of Illinois at Chicago, Department of Physiology and Biophysics, Chicago, USA

Abstract

In this chapter we consider a current perception of the molecular mechanisms controlling myofilament activation with emphasis on alterations that may occur in familial hypertrophic cardiomyopathy (FHC). FHC is a sarcomeric disease (100) with an autosomal dominant pattern of heritability (27, 51). There is a substantial body of evidence implicating missense mutations in the β-MHC gene as causal for the development of this disease. Recently, mutations in genes of two thin filament regulatory proteins, cardiac troponin T(cTnT) and α-tropomyosin (α-Tm), have also been linked to FHC. The commonality among the functional consequences of these mutations remains an important question. This review discusses how these pathological mutations may impact the activation process by disrupting critical structure function relations in both the thick and thin filaments.

Key words Cardiomyopathy – myofilament activation – β-myosin heavy chain – troponin T – tropomyosin

In striated muscle, highly ordered protein structures impose the functional interactions that govern myofilament activation. Any changes which disrupt these structures have the potential to perturb functional interactions among the myofilament proteins. An understanding of the functional consequences of altered protein structure has taken on new significance with the identification of mutations in the β-myosin heavy chain (β-MHC), cardiac troponin T (cTnT), and α-tropomyosin (α-Tm) genes as causal for the same disease, familial hypertrophic cardiomyopathy (FHC).

Familial hypertrophic cardiomyopathy

FHC is a genetically heterogeneous disease with a familial (27), autosomal dominant pattern of inheritance (19, 27, 91). The disease is distinguished from other primary hypertrophic cardiomyopathies by the significant sarcomeric disarray (for review see (15)). Patients with FHC have massive asymmetric ventricular hypertrophy. Their hearts hypercontract and are less compliant. This leads to reduced left ventricular (LV) volume capacity and rapid emptying of a small stroke volume resulting in little or no volume reserve. In some patients the mitral valve comes into contact with the thickened LV septum which produces an outflow obstruction. The disease can be clinically asymptomatic and often leads to sudden death usually at the onset of strenuous exercise (6, 15, 50, 52). As of this writing, single, missense, point mutations in four distinct genetic loci, including those on chromosome 1q3 (105) (TnT mutations, 15q2 (99) (α-Tm mutations), 14q1 (32, 38) (β-MHC mutations), and 11q11 (7), have been implicated as causal for this disease. How is it that single point mutations in functionally related, yet distinct proteins can be causal for the same disease? It is likely that the answer lies in an understanding of how these point mutations influence the process of myofilament activation.

Myofilament activation

In relaxed myofilaments, the thin filament is in an inhibited "off" state in which interactions between thick filament cross-bridges and actin are weak or blocked. Release from the inhibited state involves steric, allosteric and cooperative interactions among the proteins in a thin filament functional unit (seven actins, one tropomyosin, one troponin complex) and the myosin head. Activation also spreads along the length of the thin filament from functional unit to functional unit, in part, via tropomyosin end-to-end overlap regions. The troponin regulatory complex is made up of three proteins, troponin C (TnC) which binds Ca^{2+}, troponin I (TnI) the inhibitory protein, and troponin T (TnT) the tropomyosin binding protein. In cardiac muscle, the transition from the relaxed to the activated state is triggered by Ca^{2+} binding to a single regulatory site at the N-terminus of TnC. Figure 1 illustrates how protein-protein interactions may change when the myofilaments undergo this transition. Under relaxing conditions (panel A) the C-terminal domain of TnC containing two high affinity Ca^{2+}/Mg^{2+} binding sites is anchored to the thin filament by a structural interaction with the N-terminal domain of TnI). The N-terminal, or regulatory domain of TnC interacts weakly with TnI, which is strongly bound to actin under these conditions, and troponin T (TnT) is strongly bound to Tm. Ca^{2+} binding to TnC initiates a cascade of changes in these protein-protein interactions such that TnI-actin affinity is decreased and TnI-TnC affinity is increased. Furthermore, conformational changes transmitted through TnT to Tm are thought to promote the actin-cross-bridge reaction. The switching on of the activated state by TnC-Ca^{2+} is therefore allosteric-acting at some distance from the cross-bridge binding site on actin. Steric mechanisms involving movements of TnI (98) (and possibly TnT) and Tm (41, 69) are also apparent. The movement of both TnI and Tm may be important in removing a steric block of the actin-cross-bridge reaction. This is an important aspect of the activation process in that it involves cooperative activation of a near neighbor functional unit by force generating cross-bridges communicated through contiguous Tm molecules. Thus' activation may spread along the thin filament as functional units are engaged in the contraction cycle (42, 56, 58). The exact nature of the activation

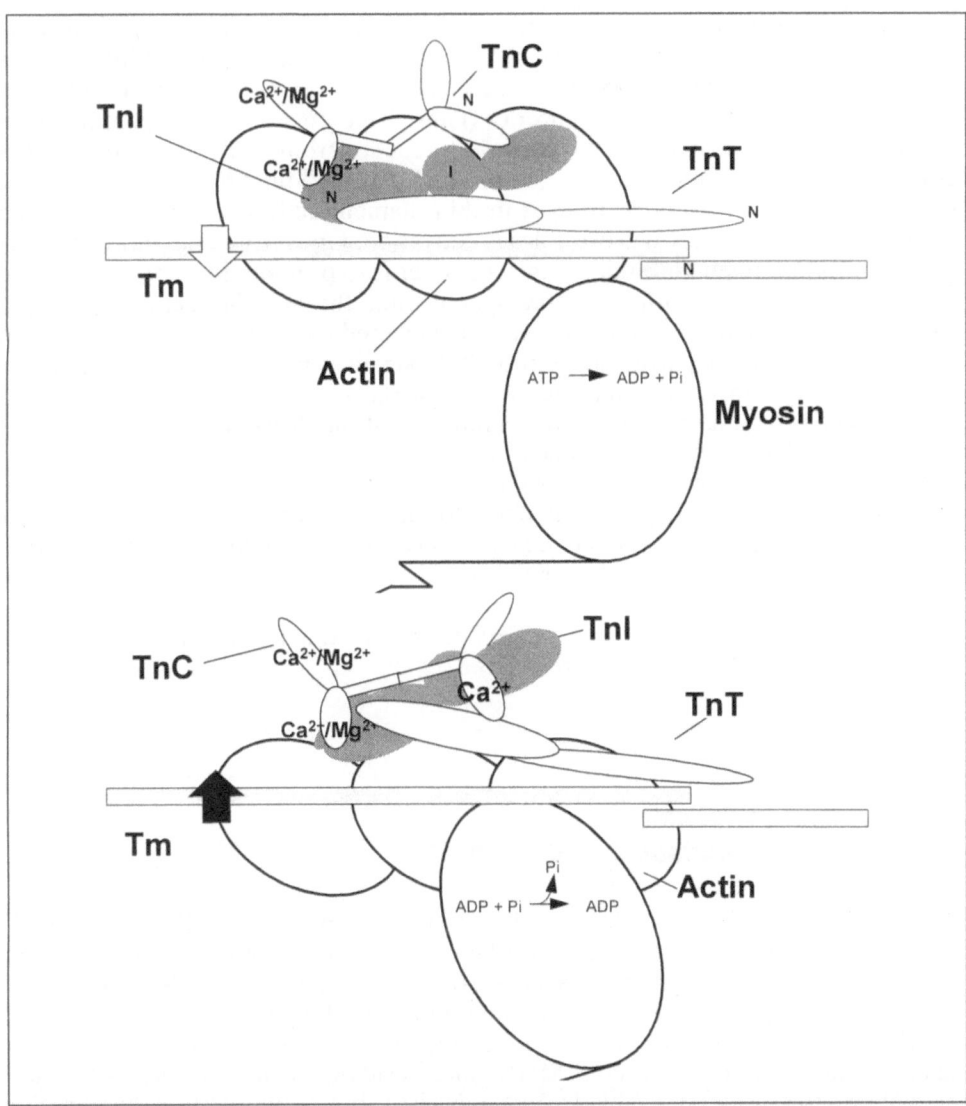

Fig. 1. Schematic representation of the two states of myofilament activation which indicates the various roles that each of the thin filament proteins and the myosin S1 head play in the two states of activation: panel A, relaxed, and panel B, activated. The amino terminal domains of the thin filament proteins are denoted with an N. Proteins are not drawn to scale and represent only approximate interaction sites. Panel A, Under relaxed conditions the actin-cross-bridge reaction is in a blocked or weak binding state due to the steric blocking position of tropomyosin (denoted by the arrow). Either ATP or ADP-Pi is bound at the S1 head. The C-terminal region of TnT is tightly bound to tropomyosin (around amino acid Cys 190 of that protein) and TnI (the inhibitory region, I) is tightly bound to actin. TnC and TnI maintain a structural interaction involving their C- and N-terminal regions, respectively. There is no Ca^{2+} bound to the N-terminal, regulatory site of TnC and only weak interaction of this TnC domain with TnI. Panel B, activation occurs when Ca^{2+} binds to the N-terminal regulatory site of TnC. This promotes a cascade of changes in protein interactions that result in: i) strong N-terminal TnC-TnI (inhibitory region) interaction, ii) weakened TnI-actin interaction iii) weakened C-terminal TnT-Tm interaction, quite possibly prompted by this region of TnT lifting off of the thin filament, iv) a movement of Tm, (denoted by the arrow) induced by the changes in the troponin proteins (and later by the cross-bridge reaction) that promotes strong actin-cross-bridge interaction, v) isomerization of the myosin S1 head and release of Pi to form strong actin-crossbridge interaction and production of force.

process remains controversial. Two modes of activation have been proposed. One involves "all or none" recruitment of cross-bridges, whereas the other involves graded activation of cross-bridges through changes in the rate of transition from a weak to a strong binding state. Lehrer (42) has proposed a compelling model incorporating both release of the actin-cross-bridge reaction from a blocked state as well as cross-bridge isomerization from a "weak" to a "strong" binding state. The model incorporates the role of cross-bridges in thin filament activation. Importantly, the model indicates that Ca^{2+} has two roles in activation. One is to recruit blocked cross-bridges into thin filament binding, and the other is to promote isomerization to the force-generating state. With myofilament activation, the cross-bridges react strongly with the thin filament in an interaction cycle powered by the hydrolysis of ATP (42, 56, 58, 113). Thus, a particular contractile state may be perceived as a balance between the allosteric and steric activation of the myofilaments by bound cross-bridges. The force that is generated is a function of the distribution of cross-bridge states and the force generated by each state.

According to this concept of myofilament activation, cross-bridges are not only the molecular motors impelling thin filaments toward the center of the sarcomere, but they are also involved in cooperative activation of the myofilaments. In human ventricular muscle, the cross-bridges participating in these reactions contain the β-myosin heavy chain which accounts for 95 % of the myosin isoform population (94). Of the mutations which are causal for FHC those affecting the heavy chain region of the β-myosin isoform are best characterized.

β-myosin isoform mutations and role in FHC

The β-myosin protein can be divided, by enzymatic cleavage, into a S1 (head) and S2 (tail) region (43). The S2-tail region is filamentous and assembles with neighboring myosins to make up the backbone structure of the thick filament. The S1 region of the protein is where actin and light chain binding, as well as the enzymatic (ATPase) activity of the myosin molecule occurs (43, 87). As of this writing, more than 40 distinct missence mutations in the β-MHC gene, residing on chromosome 14q1, have been shown to cause FHC (Table 1). Virtually all the mutations occur in the S1 region of the molecule or close to the S1/S2 junction and result in a change in the charge of an amino acid that was otherwise very strongly conserved (for reviews see (17, 49)), a hybrid α-MHC/β-MHC molecule (95), or a deletion/truncation of the β-MHC amino acid sequence (17). Interestingly, none of the mutations map to regions of known functional significance such as the ATP, actin, or light chain binding domains (87).

Patients with β-MHC mutations present with a wide spectrum of clinical symptoms (extent of hypertrophy, angina, dyspnea, syncope) none of which can be absolutely correlated with one particular mutation(s) (18, 20, 22, 107). However, studies correlating the clinical prognostic implications of specific β-MHC mutations show promising predictive value (2, 17, 107).

It is generally thought that the distinguishing phenotypic characteristic of FHC was the result of incorporation of mutant myosin molecules that ultimately disrupt thick filament or sarcomere formation (47, 92). When transfected into COS cells, at least seven β-MHC mutants, including two of the most lethal mutations, Arg403Gln and Arg453Cys, induce the expression of a diffuse nonfilamentous myosin phenotype 30–50 % of the time (47, 92). In muscle cells this would be expected to result in sarcomeric disarray. Even so, a substantial population of transfected cells did form filamentous structures with the same phenotype as wild-type myosin. This suggests that sarcomeric disarray in vivo may be the result of hypertrophy, secondary, to changes in the function of myosin with respect to myofilament activation. This idea is substantiated by data that show the Arg403Gln mutation significantly decreases the

Table 1. Mutations in the human β-MHC gene causal for familial hypertrophic cardiomyopathy

Mutation	Exon affected	Charge change	Prognosis
Ala26Val (17)	3	no	*
Arg54stop (17)	3	N/A	*
Val59Ile (17)	3	no	*
Thr124Ile (17)	5	no	*
Arg143Gln (17)	5	yes, (+) to (O)	*
Try162Cys (17)	5	*	*
Asn187Lys (17)	7	yes, (O) to (+)	*
Asn232Ser (17)	8	no	*
Arg249Gln (107)	9	yes, (+) to (O)	56 % disease penetrance (22)
Gly256Glu (21)	9	yes, (O) to (−)	*
Arg403Gln (26, 107, 108)	13	yes, (+) to (O)	high sudden death, high disease penetrance (22, 107)
Arg403Trp (2)	13	yes, (+) to (O)	*
Arg403Cys (2)	13	yes, (+) to (−)	*
Arg453Cys (107)	14	yes, (+) to (−)	poor pronosis (17, 107)
Phe513Cys (2)	15	no	little effect on patient survival (2)
Gly584Arg (107, 108)	16	yes, (O) to (+)	no conclusive data (107)
Asp587Val (17)	16	yes, (−) to (O)	*
Val606Met (107, 108)	16	no	excellent prognosis (17, 107)
Lys615Asn (20)	16	yes, (+) to (O)	*
Gly716Arg (2)	19	yes, (0) to (+)	*
Arg719Trp (2, 14)	19	yes, (+) to (O)	significant reduction in life expectancy (17, 107)
Arg723Cys (107)	20	yes, (+) to (O)	*
Pro731Leu (17)	20	no	*
Ile736Met (17)	20	no	*
Gly741Arg (22)	20	yes, (O) to (+)	*
Gly741Trp (17)	20	no	*
Arg741Gln (22)	20	yes, (+) to (O)	*
Asp778Gly (17)	21	yes, (−) to (O)	*
Arg870His (17)	22	*	*
Leu908Val (1, 22)	23	no	low disease penetrance (17, 107)
Glu924Lys (107)	23	yes, (−) to (+)	no conclusive data (107)
Glu917Lys (17)	23	yes, (−) to (+)	low incidence of sudden death (17)
Glu935Lys (17)	23	yes, (−) to (+)	*
Glu949Lys (107)	23	yes, (−) to (+)	no conclusive data (107)
Gly1931–1935 (17, 48)	40	deletion mutant	*
α/β-MHC hybrid (95)	recombination exon 27		*

* information is currently not available   (O) = neutral,   (+) = basic,   (−) = acidic

actin activated ATPase activity of the β-MHC molecule (93). Moreover, using an in vitro motility assay, Cuda et al. (16) reported that the rate of actin filament sliding is decreased (also seen in the Leu908Val mutation) because the affinity of the mutant myosin for actin is increased. It is possible, therefore, that mutant myosin heads impose a drag on filament shortening, thereby increasing the work load of the heart during contraction.

Thin filament protein mutations and FHC

β-MHC mutations, however, are not the only mutations implicated as causal for FHC. Single, missense, point mutations and/or deletion/truncation mutants of, both cardiac troponin T (cTnT) and α-tropomyosin (α-Tm) have also been described as causal for this disease. Thus, it is important to examine how these mutations may affect the structural integrity of the proteins, and thereby lead to a disruption of the activation process.

Troponin T

TnT, the tropomyosin binding unit of the troponin complex, has been fully characterized in fast skeletal muscle as an elongated molecule (24, 62) which upon treatment with chymotrypsin, splits into two functional domains, TnT1 and TnT2 (97) (Fig. 2). TnT1 makes up the N-terminal 3/5ths of the TnT protein. This region has been shown to interact, in a Ca^{2+}-independent manner, with the C-terminal region of Tm extending over the end-to-end overlap regions of adjacent Tm molecules (45, 57, 70). TnT2 makes up the C-terminal 2/5ths of the protein and is involved in the major Ca^{2+}-sensitive conformational changes in TnT (37).

TnT1/CB3

The TnT1 region can be further divided, by cyanogen bromide (CB) digestion, into a CB3 (residues 1–70) and CB2 domain (residues 71–151) (79). There is controversy concerning the function of the CB3 region of TnT1. Deletion of the first 45 N-terminal amino acids of rabbit skeletal TnT (2/3 of CB3) strengthens Tm-TnT binding (65) suggesting a negative influence of the CB3 region on TnT-Tm interactions. Additionally, CB3 fragments do not bind to α-Tm (72). This region of TnT is highly variable in amino acid sequence and length. Tissue-specific, and developmental regulation of exons 4–8 by alternative mRNA splicing in rat skeletal muscle results in at least 10, and potentially 64 different N-terminal isoforms (3, 4). The same process occurs in rat and human cardiac muscle (39, 103). In bovine cardiac muscle there are two N-terminal isoforms (28, 88) which have been shown to confer subtle differences on TnC-Ca^{2+} affinity (101) and on the Ca^{2+}-senstivity of the actin-activated myosin ATPase of reconstituted myofilament preparations (102). Given that crystallization studies

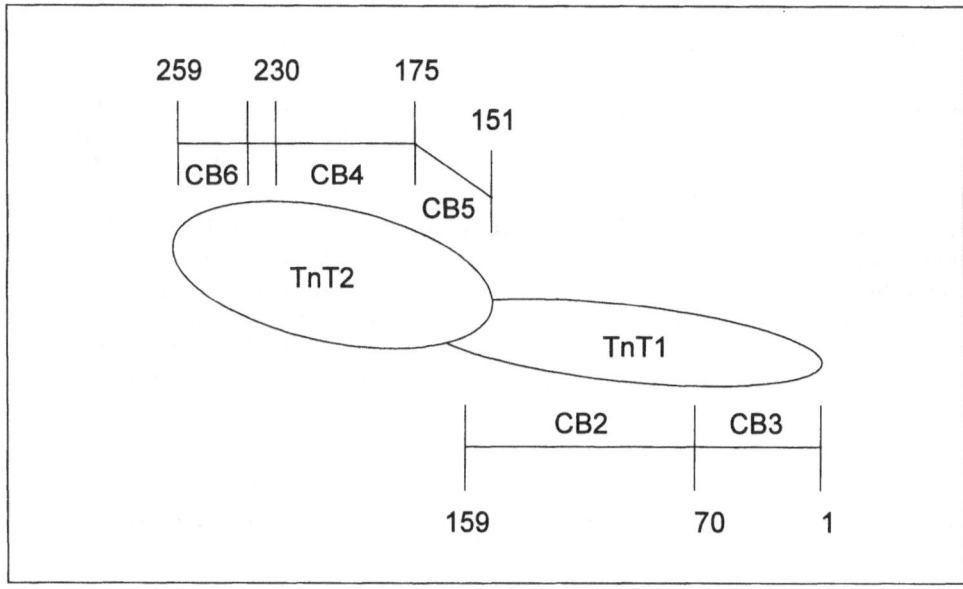

Fig. 2. Schematic representation of rabbit fast skeletal TnT. Treatment of TnT with chymotrypsin splits the protein into two major fragments, TnT1 and TnT2. Treatment of these fragments with cyanogen bromide yields five major functional fragments denoted CB2-6 each of which have been characterized with respect to their binding interactions. Functional characterization of the fragments awaits further experimentation but the relative contribution of some of the regions is known, as explained in the text.

show CB3-Tm binding (109), it is likely that the highly variable, yet regulated, generation of N-terminal isoforms has a functional role in modulating myofilament activation.

TnT1/CB2

The CB2 domain of TnT is a highly α-helical (75), expansive region of TnT defined as residues 71–151. The importance of this region with respect to thin filament activation is becoming clear. CB2 has been previously shown to bind to Tm (75) supporting the idea that the function of TnT was to anchor the Tn complex onto the thin filament (33, 84). Binding studies isolating the CB2 domain reinforced this idea. Deletion mutants of TnT have defined the CB2 region as critical for anchoring Tn-Tm to actin (111). Additionally, lysine reactivity studies show a perturbation in the CB2 region of TnT with TnI and TnC binding, supporting TnT's structural role (34). What is apparent, with respect to the TnT mutations causal for FHC, is the importance of the CB2 region in linking the TnT2 domain and the extreme N-terminal region of TnT (CB3) involved in Tm end-to-end interactions. Four of the eight mutations discovered in TnT which are causal for FHC are point mutations which affect amino acids in, or near, the CB2 domain of the protein (Table 2), (illustrated in Fig. 3). CB2 is a region of significant amino acid periodicity which spans approximately 7–8 residues (about 13Å stretches) and which is linear in the disposition of its acidic and basic residues (67). While the Ile79Asn mutation does not induce a charge change, it does result in a polar amino acid substitution at a position where normally a nonpolar residue would exist. In the Phe110Ile mutation there is also no charge change however isoleucine is less hydrophobic than phenylalanine, which could affect stacking interactions. The other two point mutations both result in a charge change; the Arg92Gln replaces a basic amino acid with a neutral amino acid, and the Glu163Lys is a negative to positive charge replacement. Another mutation, the ΔGlu160 results in a deletion of a glutamic acid from within the TnT amino acid sequence. Either of these mutations may result in structural modifications that locally destabilize the highly α-helical CB2 domain. If destabilization occurs transmission of the activating signal may be disrupted in several ways. First, structural destabilizing of the CB2 region of TnT could change the Ca^{2+}-insensitive TnT1-Tm interactions. This would be of some significance since the TnT1 domain (including the CB2 region) may be the invariant link tethering the troponin complex to Tm in the presence of Ca^{2+} (109).

Table 2. Mutations in the human cardiac TnT gene causal for familial hypertrophic cardiomyopathy

Mutation	Exon affected	Charge change	Prognosis
Ile7100Asn (100)	8	no	*
Arg1002Gln (100)	100	yes, (+) to (O)	*
Phe110Ile (106)	100	no	*
ΔGlu160 (106)	11	N/A	*
Glu163Lys (106)	14	yes, (−) to (+)	*
Glu244Asp (49)	15	no	*
Arg278Cys (106)	16	yes, (+) to (−)	*
abbarent peptide (100)	15 – 16	deletion mutant	*
abbarent peptide (100)	15 – 16 premature termination signal	deletion mutant	*

* information is currently not available   (O) = neutral,   (+) = basic,   (−) = acidic

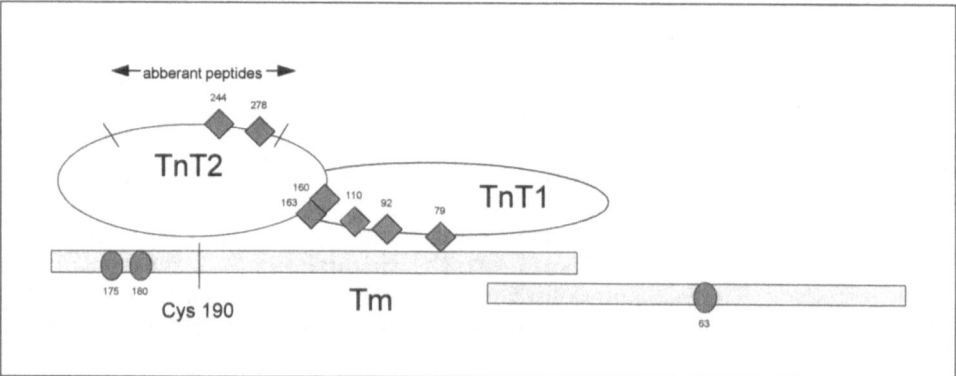

Fig. 3. Schematic representation of TnT-Tm interactions and the mutations in each of these thin filament proteins deemed causal for FHC. Numbers denote amino acid residue. See Tables 2 and 3 for specific information on each mutation. Because FHC is a lethal disease it is important to determine how these point mutations and aberrant peptides (TnT only) contribute to the disruption of myofilament activation and induce the sarcomeric changes characteristic of FHC.

Second, the CB2 region of TnT is undoubtedly involved in the transmission of the Ca^{2+}-induced conformational changes in TnT2 to Tm and/or actin and the N-terminus of the TnT protein. Support for this idea comes from the fact that even though TnT2 and TnT1 fragments do not directly interact (72), TnT2 (in the presence of TnI) strengthens TnT1-Tm interactions (73). This is thought to be the result of conformational changes being transmitted by TnT through action or the Tm coiled-coil.

TnT2

TnT2 (as characterized in fast skeletal muscle), has three functional domains (CB4, 5, and 6) and has been shown to bind, in a Ca^{2+}-dependent manner, to Tm (around cys190) (11, 30, 37), and to actin (29), TnI (10, 34, 76, 77, 96), and TnC (36, 85). It is this region of TnT that is hypothesized to lift off the thin filament upon TnC-Ca^{2+} binding, transmitting the activating signal through TnT1 to Tm-actin (109). Unlike the highly α-helical nature of the CB2 region, circular dichroism studies show very little α-helical or β-sheet structure in the TnT2 domain (78). It was previously thought that the highly basic nature of this domain predisposed this region to interactions with the acidic protein TnC (5). Binding studies confirm that most of the TnT2 region is involved in TnC binding (78). TnT2-TnI interactions have been narrowed to the C-terminal half of CB2 and, more specifically, CB5 (10, 96). The importance of TnT-TnI interactions, with respect to myofilament activation, was recently called into question as Potter et al. (85) proposed a direct regulatory role for TnT by removing 54 amino acids from the N-terminus of skeletal TnI, abolishing TnT-TnI interactions.

As with the N-terminal regions of the TnT protein, there are skeletal TnT isoforms which differ in the carboxy terminal/TnT2 region of the protein. Designated α- and β-, and differing by several amino acids in a 14 amino acid stretch near the C-terminus, these isoforms are expressed in a tissue and developmentally regulated manner (55). Functional characterization of these C-terminal isoforms has been limited to the use of 108 amino acid, genetically expressed fragments, of the C-terminal ends of the protein isoforms (64). Results indicate that the isoforms differ with respect to TnC and Tm binding affinity and, even more interestingly, the α-fragment, in which the C-terminal region is more hydrophobic and less polar, increased TnC-Ca^{2+} affinity three fold over the β-fragment (64). Four mutations in TnT that have been determined as causal for the development of FHC disrupt the C-terminus of TnT. Two of the four C-terminal mutations result in truncated TnT molecules. In one mutant 13 novel nucleotide residues are inserted between the end of exon 15 and the start of exon 16 (100). This encodes a premature termination signal and results in the loss of 14 C-terminal amino acids. The second mutant is one in which seven novel amino acid residues replace the normal 28 amino acids encoded by exons 15 and 16 prior to termination (100). Furthermore, two point mutations, Glu244Asp and Arg278Cys, have been determined to be causal for FHC (106).

While it is likely that the N-terminal mutations, clustered in CB2 domain of TnT, affect myofilament activation by changing how the activating signal is transmitted from one part of the molecule to the other, and subsequently to other thin filament proteins, the C-terminal deletion mutants may disrupt myofilament activation in a number of ways. First, and foremost, transmission of the Ca^{2+} signal by either TnT-TnC or TnT-Tm interactions may change, quite possibly dramatically affecting the level of myofilament activation. In this situation the heart may hypertrophy to compensate for the reduction in the efficacy of Ca^{2+}-induced myofilament activation. Second, these mutations may directly affect TnC-Ca^{2+} affinity as is seen with the C-terminal TnT isoforms. Finally, it is thought that abnormal TnT molecules may act as "poison peptides" destabilizing sarcomeric structure. For example, there is evidence that fruit flies (Drosophila melanogaster) with single point mutations in the TnT proteins of both the flight and jumping muscles cannot fly (25). Interestingly, the point mutations are causal, in this system, for myofibril degeneration (although assembly is not impaired) and a reduction in myofibril lattice diameter. Thus, it appears that TnT mutations may induce sarcomeric disarray and compensatory hypertrophy, the phenotypic hallmark of FHC.

α-Tropomyosin (α-Tm)

α-Tm is one of two Tm isoforms present in striated muscle (40). Tm is approximately 400Å (13) in length and nearly 100 % α-helical (12), except for the extreme N- and C-terminal regions (overlap regions) (81). Amino acid sequence analysis has revealed a series of heptad repeats in which the first and fourth amino acid of a heptad are hydrophobic and from the interface between two α-helices (68, 69). This type of repeating structure allows the two strands to interact in a coiled coil manner (35, 53). Although the coiled-coil motif is very stable, Tm crystals have been found to be flexible and relatively unstable except at the overlap regions (8, 13). Thermal unfolding studies suggest that even at 37 °C the C-terminal half of the molecular is especially unstable (more so than the N-terminal region), with an area around Cys 190 that has been shown to be particularly flexible (83, 86, 104). Furthermore, in both the α- and β-isoforms there is a notch in the α-helical structure near residues 169–172 (81). This is the only area, in both isoforms, where two bulky, hydrophobic residues are sequentially in a row, suggesting that in this region the usual coiled-coil structure is not present. It is well established that TnT binds to this region of Tm in a Ca^{2+} dependent manner (11). Electron density maps and x-ray scattering analysis suggest that in order to accommodate troponin binding and the changes in protein-protein interactions that occur with myofilament activation, the molecule is inherently flexibile (81).

Flexibility is also a necessity with respect to Tm-actin interactions. Phillips et al. (81) suggest that there is one set of seven "α-sites" where weak Tm-actin interactions occur. Therefore, depending on the level of myofilament activation, these sites can be in one of three states. In the off state of the relaxed myofilament the α-sites are not occupied. When Ca^{2+} binds to TnC and the thin filament is switched on, the α-sites become partially occupied and only in the potentiated state, when strong cross-bridges bind, are the α-sites fully saturated.

While the C-terminal regions of Tm are configured to accommodate conformational change, the extreme N- and C-terminal regions involved in end-to-end interactions with other Tm molecules are not. Tm end-to-end interactions were previously thought to be a simple overlap of coiled-coils (54). Yet, electron density mapping has established that the extreme N- and C-terminal regions of Tm interact to form a compact globular structure (81). Additional data suggests that the four strands involved in forming the joint interact in a highly ordered fashion, i.e., as two sets of intertwined N- and C-terminal pairs (81). Truncation of the extreme N- (first nine residues) or C-terminal regions (last 11 residues) which participate in forming the joint have deleterious effects on function. Either type of truncation renders the protein unable to bind to actin, and unable to polymerize (9, 44). Deletion of the Tm overlap regions has also been shown to significantly reduce the Ca^{2+} sensitive, actin-activated myosin ATPase (31) and cooperative actin-S1-ADP binding (66) indicating that disruption of the Tm structure could have a significant effect on myofilament activation.

As illustrated in Table 3, three amino acid substitutions in the Tm protein have been determined to be causal for FHC. Two of the mutations are clustered near Cys 190 and result in the substitution of a neutral amino acid for a positively charged residue (60). Mutations in this already destabilized region of Tm would almost certainly further disrupt the local structure of the protein. This is likely to lead to changes in TnT-Tm interactions that may render the myofilament less sensitive to Ca^{2+}, inducing hypertrophy. On the other hand, local structural disruption may alter the state of Tm-actin interactions in such a way that the myofilament is maintained in an "on" state of activation. This would effectively increase myocardial contractility promoting a state of hyper-contraction and muscle hypertrophy.

Support for these ideas comes from some recent work in transgenic mice which overexpress β-Tm in the heart. In normal mouse cardiac muscle only α-Tm is expressed (59). α- and β-Tm are 88 % homologous at the amino acid level (as determined in rabbit skeletal muscle) (46). In the mouse, isoform switching from α- to β-Tm involves 39 amino acid substitutions (110). Twenty-five of these substitutions occur in the C-terminal half of the molecule. One substitution in β-Tm, conserved across many species, is the presence of a cysteine residue at position 36 (46, 60). Additionally, two distinct amino acid substitutions, Ser229Gln and His276Asn, result in β-Tm having a (-2) charge change relative to α-Tm (110). The substitution at residue 229 could have a significant effect on Tm structure. This replacement occurs in an inner core position of a heptad repeat sequence and would be expected to locally destabilize the coiled-coil structure in the β-isoform. Of major significance, which respect to myofilament activation, is that it has been determined that TnT binds more weakly to β-Tm than to α-Tm (72). While the transgenic animals over expressing β-Tm are phenotypically normal, at the myofilament level they are more sensitive to Ca^{2+}, and to the activating effects of strong cross-bridges (63). Thus, changes at the protein level, even relatively conservative ones, can and do affect myofilament activation.

Although mutations at Tm positions 175 and 180, which occur in regions of flexibility and TnT binding, point clearly to a change in function, effects of mutations at pos-

Table 3. Mutations in the human α-Tm gene causal for famililal hypertrophic cardiomyopathy

Mutation	Exon affected	Charge change	Prognosis
Ala63Val (60)	2	no	*
Asp175Asn (60, 100)	5	yes, ($-$) to (O)	poor prognosis (60)
Glu180Gly (100)	5	yes, ($-$) to (O)	*

* information is currently not available   (O) = neutral,   (+) = basic,   ($-$) = acidic

ition 63 are not clear. The N-terminal region of Tm is structurally more stable than the C-terminal region (71). Furthermore, the sequences around and including residue 63 are completely conserved among different species (60). Substitution of a highly branched valine at this position may significantly disrupt the local structure of this region and could conceivably affect Tm monomer interactions all along the length of the protein. Structural changes resulting from this sort of amino acid substitution could result in any of the previously discussed effects on myofilament activation.

Conclusions

Knowledge that mutations of myofilament proteins are causal in FHC offers new challenges to investigations of structure-function relations of these proteins. One challenge is to understand possible common functional effects of diverse mutations in sarcomeric proteins. Another is to know precisely how any one particular mutation leads to these common functional changes. In the case of myosin mutants it appears that two important functional effects are a slowing of the cross-bridge reaction and a reduced affinity of myosin for actin (16, 93). How a slowing of the cross-bridge reaction might occur with Tm and TnT mutations is uncertain. A possible mechanism might involve changes in the interactions of these proteins with each other and with other thin filament proteins, in a manner similar to that which occurs during isoform switching. Evidence supporting this idea comes from in vitro data obtained in whole-heart preparations from transgenic mice overexpressing β-Tm in the heart (59). Relative to nontransgenic controls, the maximum rate of relaxation and the time to one-half relaxation is increased in hearts containing β-Tm. This is indicative of a slowing of the cross-bridge cycle. Moreover, the differences between the two preparations were increased with low level β-adrenergic stimulation, which has been previously shown to increase the relaxation rate of the heart (112). These changes occur independently of any other changes in thin filament or sarcoplasmic reticulum proteins such as the Ca^{2+}-ATPase or porpholamban (59). Thus, transgenic approaches offer a unique opportunity to probe the constraints on myofilament protein structure necessary for functional viability.

REFERENCES

1. Al-Mahdawi S, Chamberlain S, Cleland J, Nihoyannopoulos P, Gilligan D, French J, Choudhury L, Williamson R, Oakley C (1993) Identification of a mutation in the β-cardiac myosin heavy chain gene in a family with hypertrophic cardiomyopathy. Br Heart J 69: 136–141
2. Anan R, Greve G, Thiefelder L, Watkins H, McKenna WJ, Solomon S, Vecchio C, Shonom H, Nakao S, Tanaka H, Mares A Jr, Towbin JA, Spirito P, Roberts R, Seidman JG, Seidman CE (1994) Prognostic implications of novel β-cardiac myosin heavy chain gene mutations that cause familial hypertrophic cardiomyopathy. J Clin Invest 93: 280–285
3. Breitbart RE, Nadal-Ginard B (1986) Complete nucleotide sequence of the fast skeletal troponin T gene. J Mol Biol 188: 313–324

4. Breitbart RE, Nguyen HT, Medford RM, Destree AT, Mahdavi V, Nadal-Ginard B (1985) Intricate combinatorial patterns of exon splicing generate multiple regulated troponin T isoforms from a single gene. Cell 41: 67–82
5. Brisson JR, Golosinska K, Smillie LB, Sykes BD (1986) Interaction of tropomyosin and troponin T: a proton nuclear magnetic resonance study. Biochemisty 25: 4548–4555
6. Burke AP, Farb A, Virmani R, Goodman J, Smialek JE (1991) Sports-related and non-sports-related sudden cardiac death in young adults. Am Heart J 121: 568–575
7. Carrier L, Hengstenberg C, Beckmann JS, Guicheney P, Dufour C, Bercovici J, Dausse E, Berebbi-Betrand I, Wisnewsky C, Pulvenis D, Fetler L, Vignal A, Weissenbach J, Hillaire D, Feingold J, Bouhour JB, Hagege A, Desnos M, Isnard R, Dubourg O, Komajda M, Schwartz K (1993) Mapping of a novel gene for familial hypertrophic cardiomyopathy to chromosome 11. Nature Genetics 4: 311–313
8. Caspar DLD, Cohen C, Longley W (1969) Tropomyosin: crystal structure, polymorphism and molecular interactions. J Mol Biol 41: 87–107
9. Cho YJ, Liu J, Hitchcock-DeGregori SE (1990) The amino terminus of muscle tropomyosin is a major determinant for function. J Biol Chem 265: 538–545
10. Chong PCS, Hodges RS (1982) Photochemical cross-linking between rabbit skeletal troponin sub-units. J Biol Chem 257: 11667–11672
11. Chong PCS, Hodges RS (1982) Photochemical cross-linking between rabbit skeletal troponin and α-tropomyosin. J Biol Chem 257: 9152–9160
12. Cohen C, Szent-Gyorgyi AG (1957) Optical rotation and helical polypeptide chain configuration in α-proteins. J Amer Chem Soc 79: 248
13. Cohen C, Caspar DLD, Parry DAD, Lucas RM (1971) Tropomyosin crystal dynamics. Cold Spring Harbor Symp Quant Biol 36: 205–216
14. Consevage MW, Salada GC, Baylen BG, Ladda RL, Rogan PK (1994) A new missense mutation, Arg719 Gln, in the β-cardiac heavy chain myosin gene of patients with familial hypertrophic cardio-myopathy. Human Mol Genetics 3: 1025–1026
15. Cotran RS, Kumar V, Robbins SL (eds) (1989) The Heart. In: Pathologic Basis of Disease 4th edition. WB Saunders Company, Philadelphia, pp 642–656
16. Cuda G, Fanananpazir L, Zhu W, Sellers JR, Epstein ND (1993) Skeletal muscle expression and abnormal function of β-myosin in hypertrophic cardiomyopathy. J Clin Invest 91: 2861–2865
17. Durand JB, Anchee AB, Roberts R (1995) Molecular and clinical aspects of inherited cardiomyo-pathies. Annals of Medicine 27: 311–317
18. Epstein ND, Cohn GM, Cyran F, Fananapazir L (1992) Differences in clinical expression of hyper-trophic cardiomyopathy associated with two distinct mutations in the β-myosin heavy chain gene a 908Leu-Val mutation and a 403Arg-Gln mutation. Circulation 86: 345–352
19. Epstein ND, Fananapazir L, Lin HJ, Mulvihill J, White R, Lalouel JM, Lifton RP, Nienhuis AW, Leppert M (1992) Evidence of genetic heterogeneity in five kindreds with familial hypertrophic cardiomyopathy. Circulation 85: 635–647
20. Fananapazir L, Epstein ND (1995) Prevalence of hypertrophic cardiomyopathy and limitations of screening methods. Circulation 92: 700–704
21. Fananapazir L, Dalakas MC, Cyran F, Cohn G, Epstein ND (1993) Missense mutations in the β-myosin heavy-chain gene cause central core disease in hypertrophic cardiomyopathy. Proc Natl Acad Sci USA 90: 3993–3997
22. Fananapazir L, Epstein ND (1994) Genotype-phenotype correlations in hypertrophic cardiomyo-pathy. Circulation 89: 22–32
23. Farah CS, Reinach FC (1995) The troponin complex and regulation of muscle contraction. Faseb J 9: 755–767
24. Flicker PF, Phillips GN JR, Cohen C (1982) Troponin and its interactions with tropomyosin. J Mol Biol 162: 495–501
25. Fryberg E, Fryberg CC, Beall C, Saville DL (1990) Drosophila melanogaster troponin-T mutations engender three distincct syndromes of myofibrillar abnormalities. J Mol Bio 216: 657–675
26. Geisterfer-Lowrance AAT, Kass S, Tanigawa G, Vosberg H, McKenna W, Seidman CE, Seidman JG (1990) A molecular basis for familial hypertrophic cardiomyopathy: a β-myosin heavy chain gene missence mutation. Cell 62: 999–1006
27. Greaves SC, Roche AHG, Meutze JM, Whitlock RML, Veale AMO (1987) Inheritance of hyper-trophic cardiomyopathy: a cross sectional and M mode echocardiographic study of 50 families. Br Heart J 58: 259–66
28. Gusev NB, Barskaya NV, Verin AD, Duzhenkova IV, Khuchua ZA, Zheltova AO (1983) Some properties of cardiac troponin T structure. Biophys J 213: 123–129
29. Heeley DH, Smillie LB (1988) Interaction of rabbit skeletal muscle troponin T and F-actin at physiological ionic strength. Biochemistry 27: 8227–8232

30. Heeley DH, Golosinska K, Smillie LB (1987) The effects of troponin T fragments T1 and T2 on the binding of nonpolymerizable tropomyosin to F-actin in the presence and absence of troponin I and troponin C. J Biol Chem 262: 9971–9978

31. Heeley DH, Smillie LB, Lohmeirer-Vogel EM (1989) Effects of deletion of tropomyosin overlap on regulated actomyosin subfragment 1 ATPase. Biochem J 258: 831–836

32. Hejtmancik JF, Brink PA, Towbin J, Hill R, Brink L, Tapscott T, Trakhtenbroit A, Robert R (1991) Localization of gene for familial hypertrophic cardiomyopathy to chromosome 14q1 in a diverse US population. Circulation 83: 1592–1597

33. Hitchcock SE (1975) Regulation of muscle contraction: binding of troponin and its components to actin and tropomyosin. Eur J Biochem 52: 255–263

34. Hitchcock SE, Zimmerman CJ (1981) Study of the structure of troponin T by measuring the relative reactivities of lysines with acetic anhydride. 147: 125–151

35. Hodges RS, Sodek J, Smillie LB, Jurasek L (1972) Tropomyosin: amino acid sequence and coiled-coil structure. Cold Spring Harbor Symp Quant Biol 37: 299–310

36. Iio T (1985) Conformational changes of troponin T induced by calcium binding to troponin C. J Biochem 98: 261–263

37. Ishii Y, Lehrer SS (1991) Two-site attachment of troponin to pyrene-labelled tropomyosin. J Biol Chem 266: 6894–6903

38. Jarcho JA, McKenna W, Pare P, Solomon SD, Holcombe RF, Dickie S, Levi T, Donis-Keller H, Seidman JG, Seidman CE (1989) Mapping a gene for familial hypertrophic cardiomyopathy to chromosome 14q1. N Engl J Med 321: 1372–1378

39. Jin JP, Lin JJC (1989) Isolation and characterization of cDNA clones encoding embryonic and adult isoforms of rat cardiac troponin T. J Biol Chem 264: 14471–14477

40. Leger J, Bouveret P, Schwartz K, Swynghedauw B (1976) A comparative study of skeletal and cardiac tropomyosins. Pflugers Archiv 362: 271–277

41. Lehman W, Craig R, Vilbert P (1994) Ca^{2+}-induced tropomyosin movement in Limulus thin filaments revealed by three dimensional reconstruction. Nature 368: 65–67

42. Lehrer SS (1994) The regulatory switch of the muscle thin filament: Ca^{2+} or myosin heads? J Muscle Res and Cell Mot 15: 232–236

43. Lowey S, Slayter HS, Weeds AG, Baker H (1969) Substructure of the myosin molecule. J Mol Biol 42: 1–29

44. Mak AS, Smillie LB (1981) Non-polymerizable tropomyosin: preparation, some properties and F-actin binding. 101: 208–214

45. Mak AS, Smillie LB (1981) Structural interpretation of the two site binding of troponin on the muscle thin filament. J Mol Bio 149: 541–550

46. Mak AS, Smillie LB, Stewart GR (1980) A comparison of the amino acid of rabbit skeletal muscle α- and β-tropomyosins. J Biol Chem 255: 3647–3651

47. Marian AJ, Yu QT, Mann DL, Graham FL, Roberts R (1995) Expression of a mutation causing hypertrophic cardiomyopathy disrupts sarcomere assembly in adult feline myocytes. 77: 98–106

48. Marian AJ, Yu QT, Mares A, Hill R, Roberts R, Perryman MB (1992) Detection of a new mutation in the β-myosin heavy chain gene in an individual with hypertrophic cardiomyopathy. J Clin Invest 90: 2156–2165

49. Marion AJ, Robert R (1995) Recent advances in molecular genetics of hypertrophic cardiomyopathy. Circulation 92: 1336–1347

50. Maron BJ, Epstein SE, Roberts WC (1985) Causes of sudden death in competitive athletes. J Am Coll Cardiol 7: 204–214

51. Maron BJ, Nichols PF III, Pickle LW, Wesley YE, Mulvihill JJ (1984) Patterns of inheritance in hypertrophic cardiomyopathy assessment by M mode and two dimensional echocardiography. Am J Cardiol 53: 1087–1094

52. McKenna WJ, Camm AJ (1989) Sudden death in hypertrophic cardiomyopathy. Circulation 80: 1489–1492

53. McLachalan AD, Stewart M, Smillie LB (1975) Sequence repeats in α-tropomyosin. J Mol Biol 98: 281–291

54. McLachalan AD, Stewart M (1975) Tropomyosin coiled-coil interactions: evidence for an unstaggered structure. J Mol Biol 98: 293–304

55. Medford RM, Nguyen HT, Destree AT, Summers E, Nadal-Ginard B (1984) A novel mechanism of alternative RNA splicing for the developmentally regulated generation of troponin T isoforms from a single gene. Cell 38: 409–421

56. Millar NC, Homsher E (1990) The effect of phosphate and calcium on force generation in glycerinated rabbit skeletal muscle fibers. J Biol Chem 265: 20234–20240

57. Morris EP, Lehrer SS (1984) Troponin-tropomyosin interactions. Flourescence studies of the binding of troponin, troponin T, and chymotryptic troponin T fragments to specifically labeled tropomyosin. Biochemistry 23: 2214–2220

58. Moss RL (1992) Ca^{2+} regulation of mechanical properties of striated muscle. Cir Res 70: 865–884

59. Muthuchamy M, Grupp I, Grupp G, O'Toole BA, Kier AB, Boivin GP, Neumann J, Wieczorek DF (1995) Molecular and physiological effects of overexpressing striated muscle β-tropomyosin in the adult murine heart. J Biol Chem: in Press

60. Nakajima-Taniguchi C, Matsue H, Nagata S, Kishmoto T, Yamauchi-Takihara K (1995) Novel missence mutation in α-tropomyosin gene found in japanese patients with hypertrophic cardiomyopathy. J Mol Cell Cardiol 27: 2053–2058

61. Nishi H, Kimura A, Harada H, Toshima H, Sasazuki T (1992) Novel missence mutation in cardiac β-myosin heavy chain gene found in a japanese patient with hypertrophic cardiomyopathy. Biochem Biophys Res Comm 188: 379–387

62. Ohtsuki I (1979) Molecular arrangement of troponin T in the thin filament. J Biochem 86: 491–497

63. Palmiter KA, Kitada Y, Muthuchamy M, Wieczorek DF, Solaro RJ (1996) Exchange of β- for α-tropomyosin in hearts of transgenic mice induces changes in thin filament response to Ca^{2+}, strong cross-bridge binding, and protein phosphorylation. J Biol Chem 271: 11611–11614

64. Pan B, Potter JD (1992) Two genetically expressed troponin T fragments representing α and β isoforms exhibit functional differences. J Biol Chem 267: 23052–23056

65. Pan B, Gordon AM, Potter JD (1991) Deletion of the first 45 NH2-terminal residues of rabbit skeletal troponin T strengthens binding of troponin to immobilized tropomyosin. J Biol Chem 266: 12432–12438

66. Pan BS, Gordon AM, Luo Z (1989) Removal of tropomyosin overlap modifies cooperative binding of myosin S1 to reconstituted thin filaments of rabbit striated muscle. J Biol Chem 264: 8495–8498

67. Parry DAD (1981) Analysis of the amino acid sequence of α-tropomyosin-binding fragment from troponin T. J Mol Biol 146: 259–263

68. Parry DAD (1975) Analysis of the primary sequence of α-tropomyosin from rabbit skeletal muscle. J Mol Biol 98: 519–535

69. Parry DAD (1976) Movement of tropomyosin during regulation of vertebrate skeletal muscle: a simple physical model. Biochem Biophys Res Com 68: 323–328

70. Pato MD, Mak AS, Smillie LB (1981) Fragments of rabbit striated muscle α-tropomyosin. J Biol Chem 256: 602–607

71. Pato MD, Mak AS, Smillie LB (1981) Fragments of rabbit striated muscle α-tropomyosin. J Biol Chem 256: 593–598

72. Pearlstone JR, Smillie LB (1982) Binding of troponin-T fragments to several types of tropomyosin. J Biol Chem 257: 10587–10592

73. Pearlstone JR, Smillie LB (1983) Effects of troponin-I plus -C on the binding of troponin-T and its fragments to α-tropomyosin. J Biol Chem 258: 2534–2542

74. Pearlstone JR, Smillie LB (1981) Identification of a second binding region on rabbit skeletal troponin-T for α-tropomyosin. FEBS Letters 128: 119–122

75. Pearlstone JR, Smillie LB (1977) The binding site of rabbit skeletal α-tropomyosin on troponin T. Can J Biochem 55: 1032–1038

76. Pearlstone JR, Smillie LB (1980) The binding sites of rabbit skeletal troponin-I on troponin-T. Can J Biochem 58: 649–654

77. Pearlstone JR, Smillie LB (1985) The interaction of rabbit skeletal muscle troponin T fragments with troponin I. Can J Biochem Cell Biol 63: 212–218

78. Pearlstone JR, Smillie LB (1978) Troponin T fragments: physical properties and binding to troponin C. Can J Biochem Cell Biol 56: 521–527

79. Pearlstone JR, Carpenter MR, Smillie LB (1977) Primary structure of rabbit skeletal muscle troponin-T. J Biol Chem 252: 971–977

80. Pearlstone JR, Carpenter MR, Johnson P, Smillie LB (1976) Aminoacid sequence of tropomyosin-binding component of rabbit skeletal muscle troponin. Proc Nat Acad Sci USA 73: 1902–1906

81. Phillips GN Jr, Fillers JP, Cohen C (1986) Tropomyosin crystal structure and muscie regulation. J Mol Bio 192: 111–131

82. Phillips GN Jr, Fillers JP, Cohen C (1980) Motions of tropomyosin. Biophys J 32: 485–502

83. Potekhin SA, Privalov PL (1982) Co-operative blocks in tropomyosin. J Mol Biol 159: 519–535

84. Potter JD, Gergely J (1974) Troponin, tropomyosin, and actin interaction in the Ca^{2+} regulation of muscle contraction. Biochemistry 13: 2697–2703

85. Potter JD, Sheng Z, Pan B, Zhao J (1995) A direct regulatory role for troponin T and a dual role for troponin C in the Ca^{2+} regulation of muscle contraction. J Biol Chem 270: 2557–2562

86. Privalov PL (1982) Double-stranded coiled coils: tropomyosin, paramyosin, and the myosin rod. Advan Protein Chem 35: 31–55
87. Rayment I, Holden HM, Whittaker M, Yohn CB, Lorenz M, Holmes KC, Milligan RA (1993) Structure of the actin-myosin complex and its implications for muscle contraction. Science 261: 58–65
88. Risnik VV, Verin AD, Gusev NB (1985) Comparison of the structure of two cardiac troponin T isoforms. Biochem J 225: 549–552
89. Sodek J, Hodges RS, Smillie LB, Jurasek L (1972) Amino-acid sequence of rabbit skeletal tropomyosin and its coiled-coil structure. Proc Nat Sci USA 69: 3800–3804
90. Solaro RJ, VanEyk JI (1996) Altered interactions among thin filament protein modulate cardiac function. J Mol Cell Cardio 28: 217–230
91. Solomon SD, Jarcho JA, McKenna W, Geisterfer-Lowrance A, Germain R, Salerni R, Seidman JG, Seidman CE (1990) Familial hypertrophic cardiomyopathy is a genetically heterogeneous disease. J Clin Invest 86: 993–999
92. Straceski AJ, Geisterfer-Lowrance A, Seidman CE, Seidman JG, Leinwand LA (1994) Functional analysis of myosin missense mutations in familial hypertrophic cardiomyopathy. Proc Nat Acad Sci 91: 589–593
93. Sweeney HL, Straceski AJ, Leinwand LA, Tikunov BA, Faust L (1994) Heterologous expression of a cardiomyopathic myosin that is defective in its actin interaction. J Biol Chem 269: 1603–1605
94. Swynghedauw B (1986) Developmental and functional adaptation of contractile proteins in cardiac and skeletal muscles. Physiol Reviews 66: 710–771
95. Tanigawa G, Jarcho JA, Kass S, Solomon SD, Vosberg H, Seidman JG, Seidman CE (1990) A molecular basis for familial hypertrophic cardiomyopathy: an α/β-cardiac myosin heavy chain hybrid gene. Cell 62: 991–998
96. Tanokura M, Ohtsuki I (1982) Location of troponin I-binding on troponin T sequence. FEBS Letters 145: 147–149
97. Tanokura M, Tawada Y, Onoyama Y, Nakamura S, Ohtsuki I (1981) Primary structure of chymotryptic subfragments from rabbit skeletal troponin T. J Biochem 90: 263–265
98. Tao T, Gong BJ, Leavis PC (1990) Calcium-induced movement of troponin I relative to actin in skeletal muscle thin filaments. Science 2: 1339-1341
99. Theirfelder L, MacRae C, Watkins H, Tomfohrde J, Williams M, McKenna W, Bohm K, Noeske G, Schlepper M, Bowcock A, Vosberg H, Seidman JG, Seidman CE (1993) A familial hypertrophic cardiomyopathy locus maps to chromosome 15q2. Proc Natl Acad Sci 90: 6270–6274
100. Thierfelder L, Watkins H, MacRae C, Lamas R, McKenna W, Vosberg H, Seidman JG, Seidman CE (1994) α-Tropomyosin and cardiac troponin T mutations cause familial hypertrophic cardiomyopathy; a disease of the sarcomere. Cell 77: 701–712
101. Tobacman LS (1988) Structure-function studies of the amino-terminal region of bovine cardiac troponin T. J Biol Chem 263: 2668–2672
102. Tobacman IS, Lee R (1987) Isolation and functional comparison of bovine cardiac troponin T isoforms. J Biol Chem 262: 4059–4064
103. Townsend PJ, Barton PJR, Yacoub MH, Farza H (1995) Molecular cloning of human cardiac troponin T isoforms: expression in developing and failing heart. J Mol Cell Cardiol 27: 2223–2236
104. Ueno H (1984) Local structural changes in tropomyosin detected by a trypsin-probe method. Biochemistry 23: 4791–4798
105. Watkins H, MacRae C, Thierfelder L, Chou YH, Frenneaux M, McKenna W, Seidman JG, Seidman CE (1993) A disease locus for familial hypertrophic cardiomyopathy maps to chromosome 1q3. Nature Genetics 3: 333–337
106. Watkins H, McKenna WJ, Theirfelder L, Suk HJ, Anan R, O'Donoghue A, Spirito P, Matsumori A, Moravec CS, Seidman JG, Seidman CE (1995) Mutations in the genes for cardiac troponin T and α-tropomyosin in hypertrophic cardiomyopathy. N Eng J Med 332: 1058–1064
107. Watkins H, Rosenzweig A, Hwang D, Levi T, McKenna W, Seidman CE, Seidman JG (1992) Characteristics and prognostic implications of myosin missense mutations in familial hypertrophic cardiomyopathy. N Engl J Med 326: 1108–14
108. Watkins H, Theirfelder L, Anan R, Jarcho J, Matsumori A, McKenna W, Seidman JG, Seidman CE (1993) Independent origin of identical β cardiac myosin heavy-chain mutations in hypertrophic cardiomyopathy. Am J Hum Genet 53: 1180–1185
109. White SP, Cohen C, Phillips GN Jr (1987) Structure of co-crystals of tropomyosin and troponin. Nature 325: 826–828
110. Wieczorek DF, Muthuchamy M in production
111. Willadsen KA, Butters CA, Hill LE, Tobacman LS (1992) Effects of the amino-terminal regions of tropomyosin and troponin T on thin filament assembly. J Biol Chem 267: 23746–23752

112. Zhang R, Zhao J, Mandveno A, Potter JD (1995) Cardiac troponin I phosphorylation increases the rate of cardiac muscle relaxation. Cir Res 76: 1028–1035
113. Zot AS, Potter JD (1987) Structural aspects of troponin-tropomyosin regulation of skeletal muscle contraction. Ann Rev Biophys Chem 16: 535–559

Authors' address:
R. John Solaro, PhD
University of Illinois at Chicago
Department of Physiology and Biophysics
901 S. Wolcott (M/C 901)
Chicago, IL 60612, USA

Ca²⁺-dependent and Ca²⁺-independent regulation of contractility in isolated human myocardium

B. Pieske, K. Schlotthauer, J. Schattmann, F. Beyersdorf[1], J. Martin[1], H. Just, G. Hasenfuss

Medizinische Klinik III, Abteilung Kardiologie und Angiologie, Universität Freiburg, Freiburg, Germany
[1] Medizinische Klinik III, Abteilung Herz- und Gefäßchirurgie, Universität Freiburg, Freiburg, Germany

Abstract

Changes in contractile force of the myocardium may depend on changes in the intracellular Ca²⁺ concentration, changes in the responsiveness of the myofibrils for Ca²⁺, or a combination of both. We investigated in isolated muscle strip preparations from human nonfailing and endstage failing hearts the influence of physical (changes in preload, stimulation rate, or rhythm), and pharmacological interventions (α- or β-adrenoceptor-stimulation, endothelin) on developed force of contraction and the corresponding intracellular Ca²⁺ transients.

Methods: Isometric contraction, electrical stimulation, 37 °C. Simultaneous registration of force of contraction and intracellular Ca²⁺ transients (aequorin method).

Results: Increases in preload, α- and endothelin-receptor stimulation resulted in increases in force of contraction without increasing aequorin light emission. Increasing stimulation rate or increasing rest intervals resulted in parallel increases (nonfailing myocardium) or decreases (failing myocardium) of force of contraction and aequorin light emission. β-Adrenoceptor-stimulation exerted inotropic and lusitropic effects in human failing myocardium associated with a large, overproportional increase in aequorin light emission.

Conclusion: The human heart regulates intrinsic contractility via several subcellular mechanisms. Increases in preload (Frank-Starling-mechanism) and α- or endothelin-receptor-stimulation enhance myocardial contractility by increasing the Ca²⁺ responsiveness of the myofilaments; rate- and rhythm-dependent modulation of the contractile state directly depend on changes in the intracellular Ca²⁺-transients; β-adrenoceptor stimulation results in an overproportional large increase in intracellular Ca²⁺ transients, probably due to additional cAMP-dependent Ca²⁺-desensitizing effects on the level of the myofibrils.

Key words Human myocardium – excitation-contraction coupling – Frank-Starling mechanism – endothelin – aequorin

Introduction

Intrinsic myocardial contractility may be regulated via distinct physiological mechanisms: 1) under normal conditions, increases in preload increase intrinsic contractility of the heart (Frank-Starling law of the heart); 2) the sympathetic nervous system with activation of α- and β-adrenoceptors; 3) heart-rate inotropism, i.e., the frequency-dependent increase in intrinsic contractility; 4) circulating or locally generated endogenous peptides such as angiotensin or endothelin. These different mechanisms have been studied in animal models and have been shown to contribute to the regulation of myocardial contractility in humans. However, little is known on the subcellular mode of action of the different interventions in human nonfailing and end-stage failing myocardium.

Contraction and relaxation of the heart depends on cyclic binding and dissociation of Ca^{2+} to troponin C. Inotropic mechanisms may be distinguished by the central role of Ca^{2+} binding to troponin C in excitation-contraction coupling: they are classified as "upstream" if their primary effect is to alter the amplitude of the intracellular Ca^{2+} transient, "central" if they change the affinity of Troponin C for Ca^{2+}, and "downstream" if they change the response of the myofilaments to a given level of Ca^{2+} occupancy at troponin C (3). However, at present, it is difficult to distinguish central from downstream mechanisms, which are therefore often lumped together as "myofibrillar responsiveness to Ca^{2+}" (4).

The goal of the present study was to determine the effects of the different physiological mechanisms for regulation of myocardial contractility on intracellular Ca^{2+} transients. Using the photoprotein aequorin as intracellular Ca^{2+} indicator, we were able to distinguish Ca^{2+}-dependent ("upstream") from Ca^{2+}-independent ("central" and "downstream") modulation of contractile force in isolated human myocardium. The presented work is a synopsis of our recent investigations in human tissue. Part of this work (force-frequency and post-rest behavior) have been published previously, but were included into the paper for comparison and to develop an integrated model of regulation of myocardial contractility in human tissue.

Materials and methods

Experiments were performed in isolated left and right ventricular muscle strip preparations from 12 nonfailing human hearts and 35 end-stage failing human hearts due to either dilated or ischemic cardiomyopathy. Nonfailing donors all had normal left ventricular function prior to explantation; mean ejection fraction in the heart failure group was $22 \pm 2\%$.

Muscle strip preparation

Muscle strips were prepared and attached to an isometric force transducer as described previously (39). Briefly, the explanted hearts were transported to the laboratory in oxygenated modified Tyrode's solution containing 30 mM butanedione-monoxime (BDM) as cardioplegic agent (34). Thin trabeculae (diameter < 0.6 mm^2) were dissected from the ventricular wall with the help of a stereomicroscope and mounted to an isometric force transducer. Muscles were superfused with oxygenated Tyrode's solution (37 °C, pH 7.4) and electrically stimulated (field stimulation, voltage 20 % above threshold, basal pacing frequency 60/min).

Aequorin light emission

After equilibration, muscles were prestretched along their length-tension curve until maximal isometric twitch force was attained. Then, aequorin loading was performed in the nonstimulated muscle using the macroinjection technique (27). After complete stabilization, intracellular Ca^{2+} transients were recorded as aequorin light emission by the help of a photomultiplier tube. Changes in the amplitude of the aequorin light signal (in mV amplifier output) were related to changes in the amplitude in isometric twitch tension (in mN/mm^2 cross-sectional area) of the individual muscle strip preparations as described by Blinks (4).

Interventions

The following interventions were investigated in aequorin-loaded muscle strip preparations:

1) A Ca^{2+} reference concentration-response curve was established for nonfailing and failing myocardium and used for comparison. Ca^{2+} in the superfusing Tyrode's solution was stepwise increased from 1.25 to 5.6 mmol/l and the increases in force and aequorin light were monitored.

2) Frank-Starling mechanism: after aequorin loading, preload was reduced by reducing the stretch of the muscle from its optimal length to 80 % of its optimal length by help of a micromanipulator. Then, the muscle was stretched again to 100 % of its optimal length, and resulting changes in force and aequorin light emission were monitored.

3) Force-frequency-relation: to test for the influence of stimulation rate on force and aequorin light emission, stimulation rate was stepwise increased from 15 to 180 beats/min.

4) Post-Rest-behavior: at a basal stimulation rate of 60/min, the influence of increasing rest intervals (from 2 to 240 s) on isometric force and aequorin light emission of the first beat upon restimulation was tested.

5) α-Adrenoceptor-stimulation: cumulative concentration-response-curves for phenylephrine ($10^{-8} - 10^{-4}$ M) in the presence of the β-adrenoceptor blocker propranolol (10^{-6}).

6) β-Adrenoceptor-stimulation: cumulative concentration-response curves for isoproterenol ($10^{-9} - 10^{-5}$ M).

7) Endothelin-receptor-stimulation: cumulative concentration-response curves for endothelin ($10^{-9} - 3 \times 10^{-7}$).

Results

Ca²⁺ concentration-response curves

Increasing the extracellular Ca^{2+} concentration resulted in a parallel and proportional increase in force of contraction and aequorin light emission in human nonfailing and end-stage failing myocardium. This can be seen from the original tracings of Fig. 1 (left) in a muscle strip from a nonfailing heart. The concentration-dependent proportional increase in force and aequorin light allows to establish a Ca^{2+} reference curve for human nonfailing and end-stage failing myocardium. Fig. 1 (right) depicts the plot of peak twitch tension versus peak aequorin luminescence for increasing extracellular Ca^{2+} from 1.25 mM to 5.6 mM in six muscle strip preparations from six nonfailing hearts. The slope of the regression line is close to unity ($y = -5.3 + 1.09$; $r = 0.99$). Similar results have been obtained for human failing myocardium.

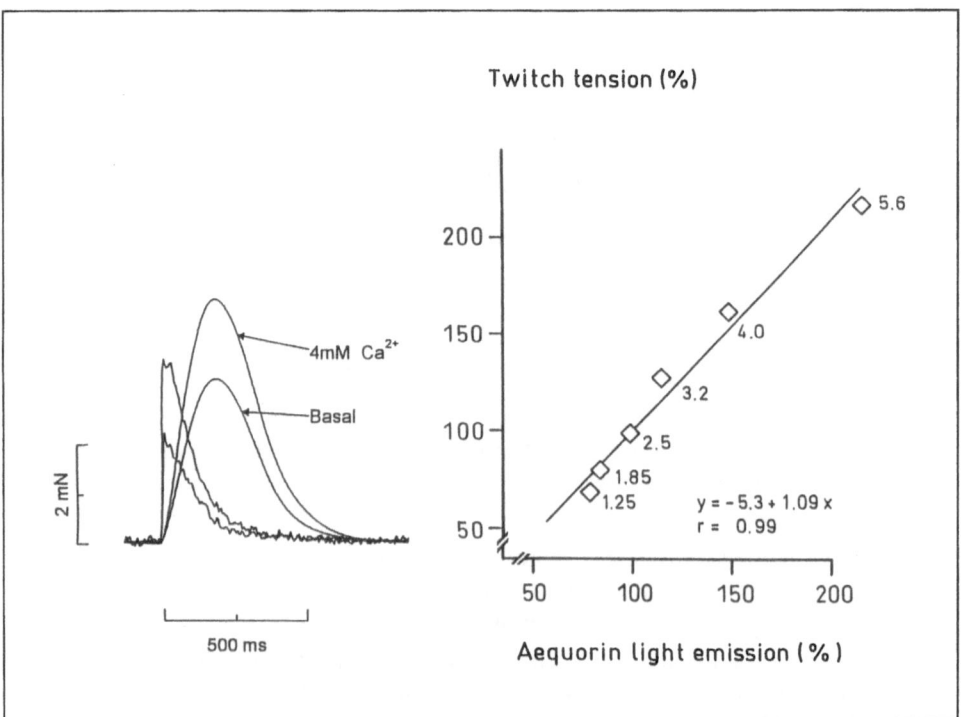

Fig. 1. Left: Original tracing of the effect of a single concentration of $[Ca^{2+}]_o$, 4 mM, on aequorin light transients and the isometric twitch in a muscle strip from a nonfailing heart. Increasing extracellular Ca^{2+} resulted in a similar increase in the amplitude of the aequorin transient and the isometric twitch.
Right: Plot of average increase in isometric twitch tension (ordinate) versus average increase in aequorin light emission (abscissa). Average values from six concentration-response curves from six nonfailing hearts. The slope of the regression line is close to unity (modified from reference (40), with permission).

Frank-Starling-Mechanism

To investigate the intracellular mechanism of action underlying the preload-dependent increase in myocardial contractility, aequorin-loaded muscle strip preparations from human end-stage failing hearts were stretched from 80 % of their optimal length to 100 % of their optimal length (l_{max}). Fig. 2 (left) shows the original registration from a typical experiment. Stretching the muscle strip preparation from a heart with dilated cardiomyopathy resulted in a remarkable increase in isometric twitch tension and a prolongation of total twitch time, mainly due to delayed relaxation. However, aequorin light transients did not change upon stretch (upper part of the figure). Fig. 2 (right) shows the average results from seven muscle strip preparations from failing hearts with dilated cardiomyopathy. It can be seen that isometric force of contraction increased significantly upon stretch with no significant change in aequorin light emission.

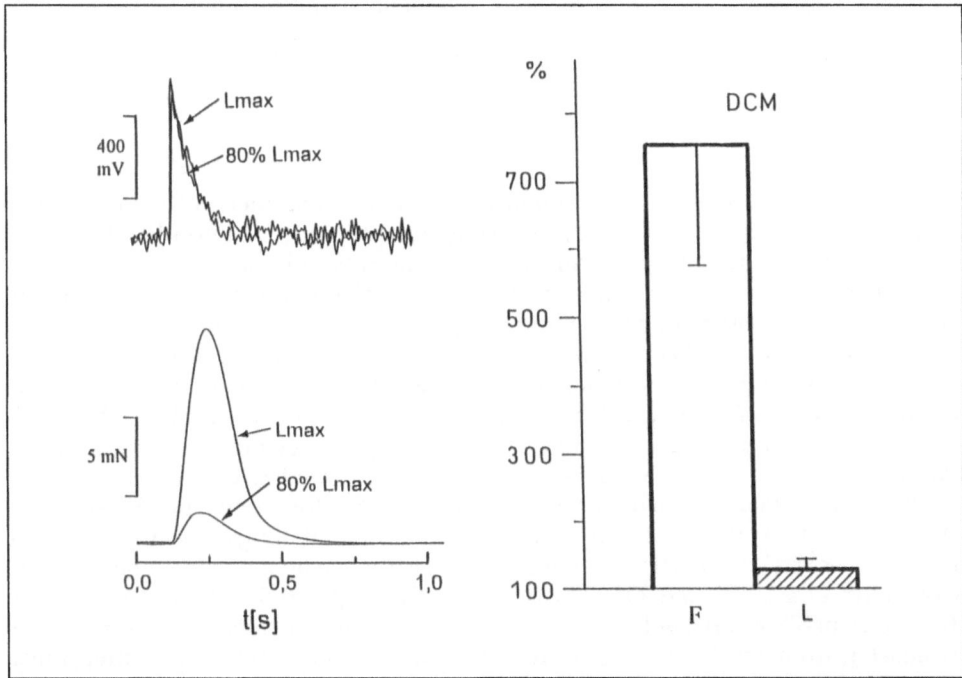

Fig. 2. Left: Original tracing of the influence of stretching a muscle strip from a failing heart from 80 % of its optimal length (80 % Lmax) to its optimal length (Lmax) on isometric twitch and aequorin light transient (noisy lines). The substantial increase in force and the delayed relaxation was associated with no changes in aequorin light emission.
Right: Average values from eight muscles from failing hearts due to ischemic cardiomyopathy. Muscles length was increased from 80 % Lmax to 100 % Lmax. Changes in force (open bar) and aequorin light emission (dashed bar) in % of their value at 80 % Lmax are indicated. F, Force. L, Light.

Force-Frequency-Relationship

Fig. 3 (left) shows original tracings of the typical effect of an increase in stimulation rate from 30 to 120 beats/min on the isometric twitch and the aequorin light transient in a muscle strip from a nonfailing and an end-stage failing human heart. In the non-failing myocardium, isometric force and aequorin light emission increased with higher stimulation rates (2.0 Hz), while both parameters declined in the failing myocardium. The frequency-dependency of isometric force of contraction and aequorin light emission over the whole physiological frequency range is shown in Fig. 3 (right). In seven muscle strip preparations from five nonfailing hearts, isometric force and aequorin light emission continuously increased with increasing pacing rates (positive force-frequency relationship). Isometric force was maximum at a stimulation rate of 150 beats/min (increase to 212 ± 34 % of the basal value at 15/min; $p < 0.05$). Aequorin light emission rose in parallel and was maximum at a stimulation rate of 180/min (increase to 218 ± 39 % of the basal value at 15/min; $p < 0.05$). However, in end-stage failing myocardium, force of contraction and aequorin light emission declined with higher stimulation rates (negative force-frequency relationship): in 12 muscle strip preparations from nine failing hearts due to dilated cardiomyopathy, isometric twitch tension declined to 62 ± 9 % of the basal value at 180/min ($p < 0.05$). Aequorin light emission declined in parallel to 71 ± 7 % at 180/min ($p < 0.05$). For both types of myocardium there was a close relationship between the stimulation rate at which maximum isometric force and maximum aequorin light emission were reached.

Post-Rest-Behavior

Post-rest potentiation or decay of isometric force of contraction is believed to reflect intracellular Ca^{2+} uptake and release from the sarcoplasmic reticulum (40). The influence of a rest period of 120 s on aequorin light transients and isometric twitch tension of the first beat upon restimulation is depicted in original tracings in Fig. 4 (upper panel). In a muscle strip from a nonfailing heart, aequorin light emission and force of contraction of the first beat upon restimulation was potentiated after a 120 s rest period as compared to pre-rest steady state level, showing the Ca^{2+}-dependency of rest potentiation of isometric force in human nonfailing myocardium. However, force of contraction and aequorin light emission slightly declined (rest decay) after 120 s rest in a muscle strip from a failing heart due to dilated cardiomyopathy. These parallel changes in aequorin light emission and isometric force could be seen over the whole range of rest intervals (Fig. 4, lower panel). In nonfailing myocardium (n = 3 from three hearts), isometric twitch tension and aequorin light emission increased to maximally 217 ± 23 % and 207 ± 57 %, respectively ($p < 0.05$) at a rest interval of 60 s and remained stable at longer rest intervals. In failing myocardium (n = 6 from six hearts), isometric twitch tension increased to maximally 166 ± 8 % after a rest interval of 20 s ($p < 0.05$) and aequorin light emission rose in parallel to 145 ± 11 % after a rest interval of 15 s ($p < 0.05$). However, both parameters significantly declined at longer rest intervals (to 55 ± 14 % and 64 ± 10 %, respectively, after a rest interval of 240 s ($p < 0.05$ vs. pre-rest levels; rest decay).

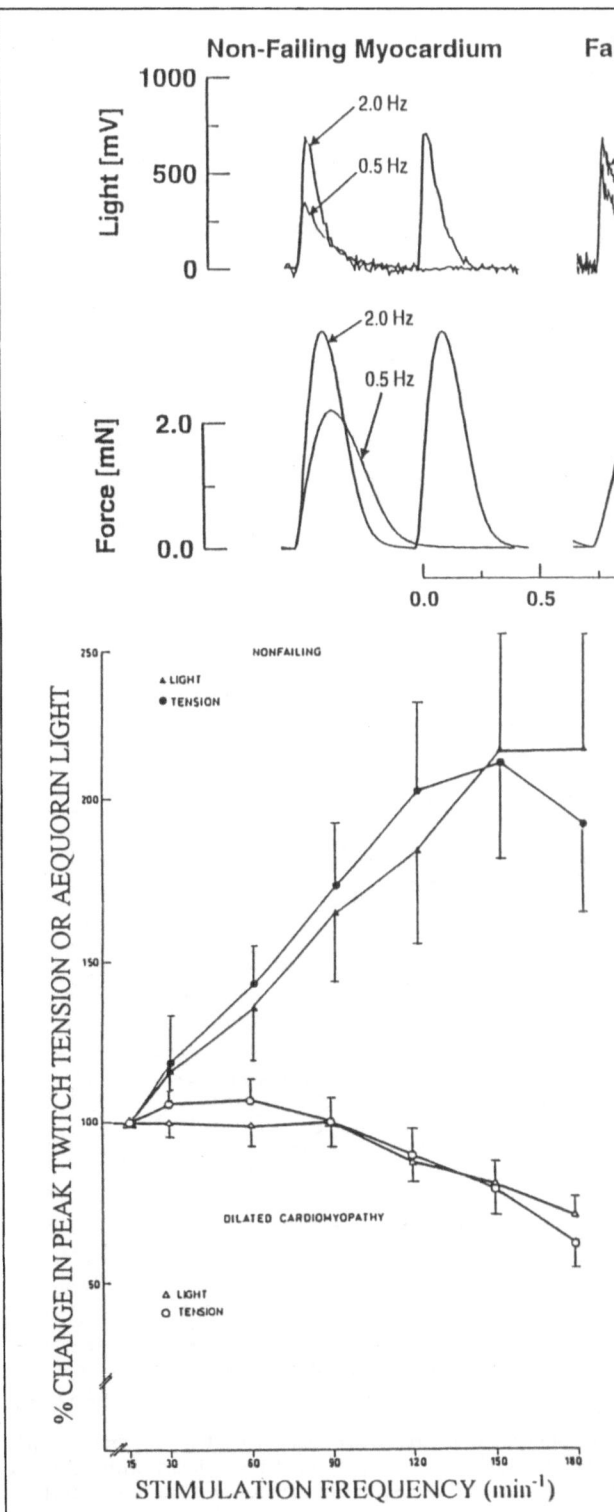

Fig. 3. Left: Influence of an increase in stimulation rate from 30 to 120 beats/min [0.5 – 2.0 Hz] on isometric force (mN) and aequorin light emission (in mV amplifier output) in a muscle strip from a nonfailing and an end-stage failing heart. Increasing stimulation rate resulted in a similar increase of force and aequorin light in nonfailing, but similar decrease in failing tissue.

Right: Average change in force and aequorin light emission (in % of the basal value at 15 beats/min; ordinate) in seven muscle strips from five nonfailing hearts and in 12 muscle strips from nine end-stage failing hearts upon stepwise increasing stimulation frequency from 15 to 180 beats/min (Abscissa). Force and aequorin light increased in parallel in nonfailing, and decreased in parallel in failing tissue (modified from reference (39), with permission).

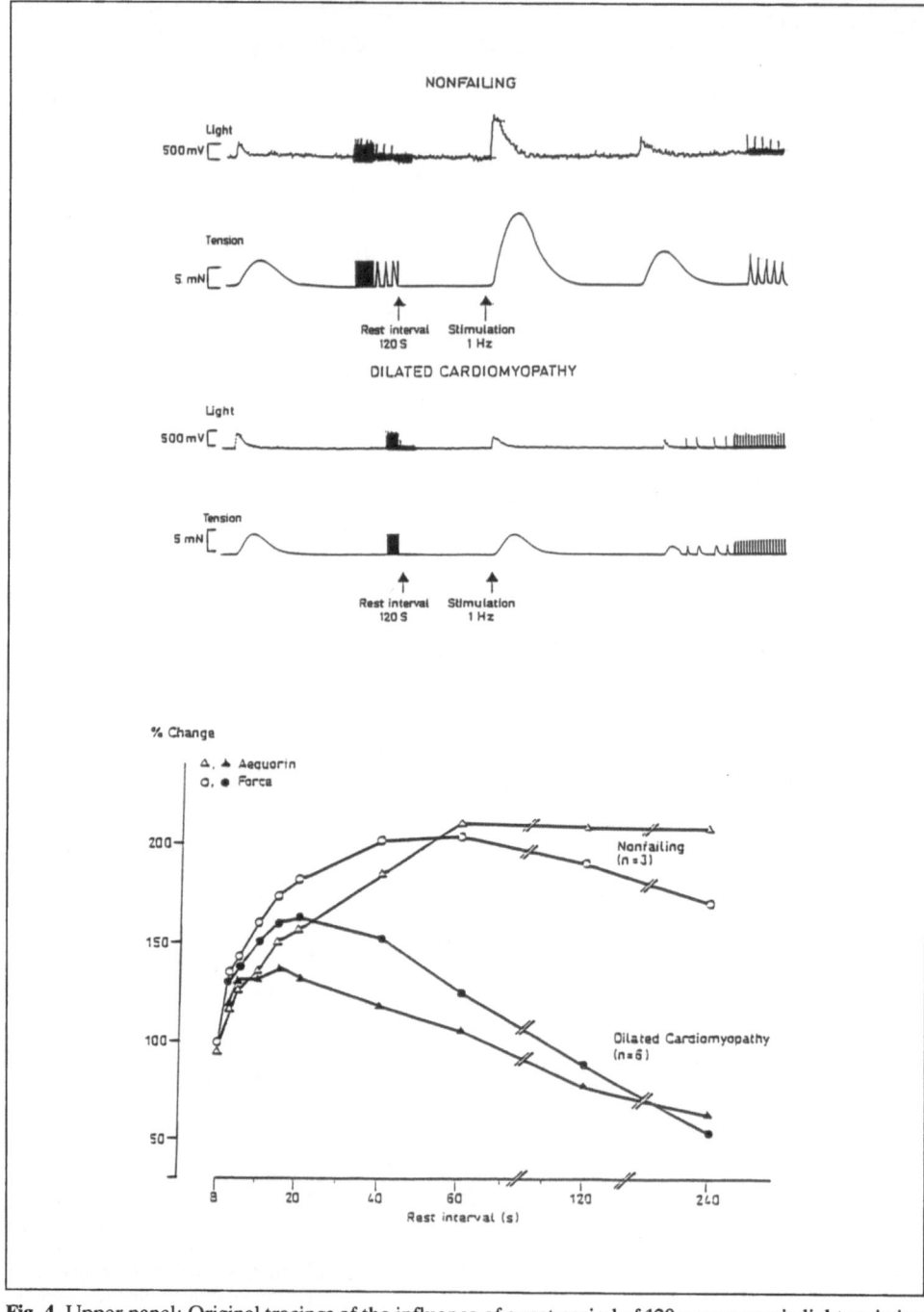

Fig. 4. Upper panel: Original tracings of the influence of a rest period of 120 s on aequorin light emission and isometric force of the first beat upon restimulation in a muscle strip from a nonfailing and a failing heart. Basal stimulation frequency, 1 Hz.
Lower panel: Change in aequorin light emission and isometric force of the first beat upon restimulation in three muscle strips from three nonfailing hearts and six muscle strips from six failing hearts with increasing rest intervals. Values are given in % of the steady-state value prior to the individual rest interval (from reference (40), with permission).

α-Adrenoceptor stimulation, endothelin receptor stimulation and β-adrenoceptor stimulation

Figure 5 shows typical tracings of the effects of β-adrenoceptor stimulation (left; iso-proterenol 10^{-6} M), α-adrenoceptor stimulation (middle; phenylephrine 10^{-4} M in the presence of propranolol 10^{-6} M) and endothelin-receptor stimulation (right; endothelin-1, 10^{-7} M) in aequorin-loaded muscle strips from three end-stage failing hearts. It becomes evident that phenylephrine and endothelin exert positive inotropic and negative lusitropic effects without changing the amplitude of the aequorin light transients; after isoproterenol, however, a marked positive inotropic and positive lusi-tropic effect and a large, overproportional increase in aequorin light emission can be seen.

Figure 6 shows the corresponding cumulative concentration-response curves in human end-stage failing myocardium. The positive inotropic effect of phenylephrine in the presence of propranolol (middle) starts at a concentration of 10^{-7} M and is maximum at a concentration of 10^{-5} M. However, aequorin light emission does not increase. ET-1 concentration-dependently increases force of contraction with even slight decreases in aequorin light emission in the lower concentration range (right). The maximal positive inotropic effect of ET-1 is similar to the maximal inotropic effect of phenylephrine. These data suggest that α-adrenoceptor stimulation with phenylephrine and endothelin-receptor stimulation exert positive inotropic effects inhuman myocardium without increasing intracellular Ca^{2+} transients. In contrast, the pronounced and overproportional increase of aequorin light emission as compared to force development after β-adrenoceptor stimulation can be seen over the

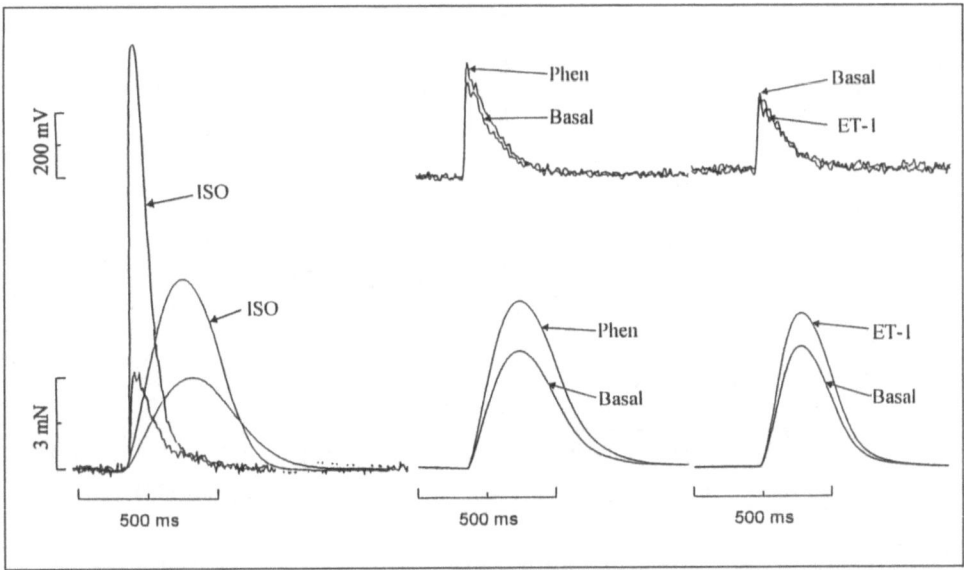

Fig. 5. Original tracings of the typical effects of isoproterenol (10^{-6} M; left), phenylephrine (10^{-4} M, in the presence of propranolol 10^{-6} M; middle), and endothelin-1 (10^{-7} M; right) on aequorin light emission and isometric force. Muscle strip preparations from three end-stage failing hearts.

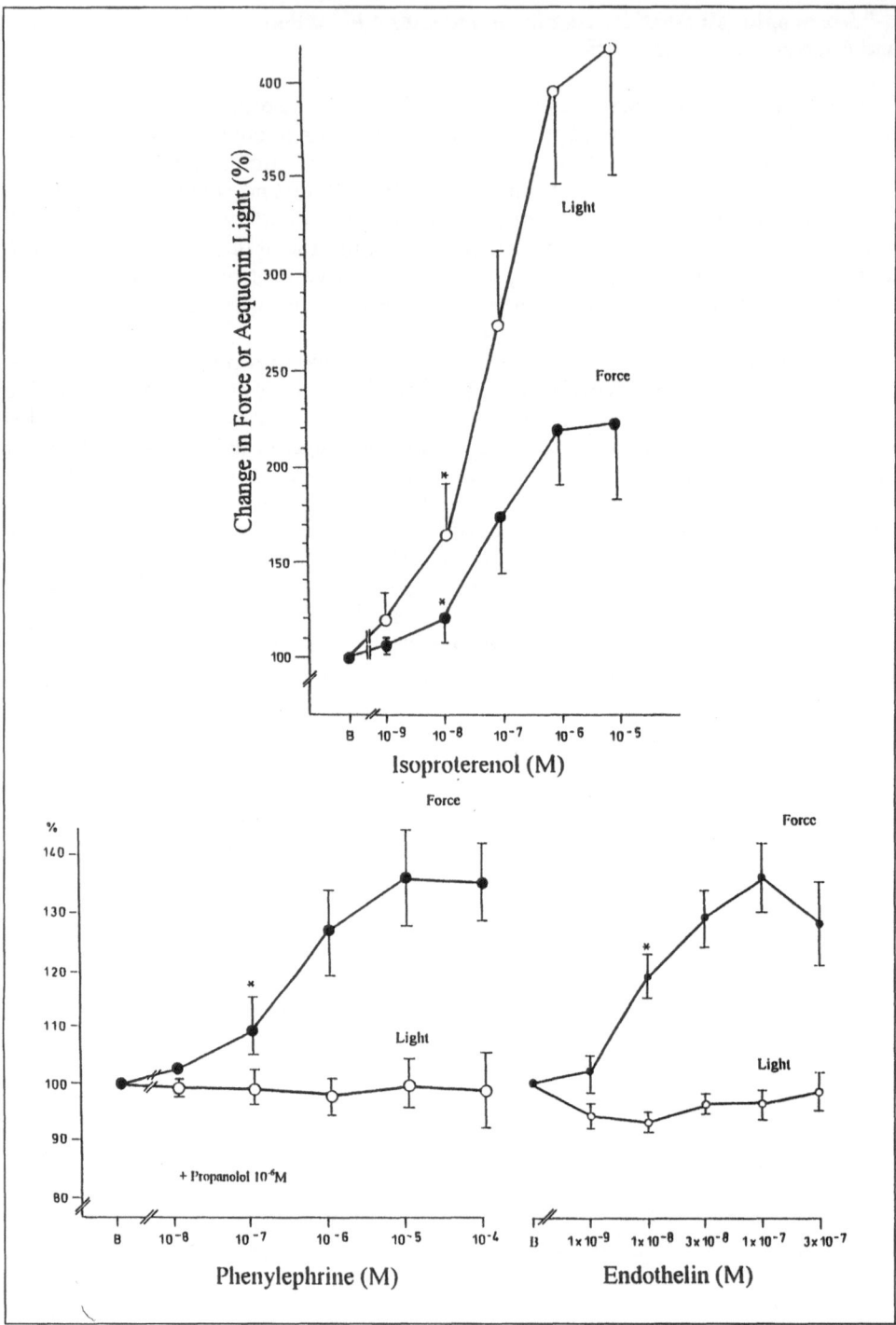

Fig. 6. Cumulative concentration-response curves for isoproterenol (10^{-9} – 10^{-5} M; left), phenylephrine (10^{-8} – 10^{-4} M in the presence of propranolol; middle), and endothelin-1 (10^{-9} – 3×10^{-7} M; right) in aequorin loaded muscle strips from failing human hearts. Change in force of contraction and aequorin light emission are given in % of the basal value before the intervention (ordinate).

whole concentration range of isoproterenol (10^{-9} – 10^{-5} M) in human failing myocardium (Fig. 6, left). Of note, even in failing myocardium, the inotropic effect of isoproterenol is significantly larger than the inotropic effect of α- or endothelin receptor stimulation.

Comparison of the different regulatory mechanisms of myocardial contractility with respect to their influence on intracellular Ca^{2+} transients

To test for influences of inotropic mechanisms on the responsiveness of the myofilaments for Ca^{2+}, a plot of the relative increase in isometric force versus the relative increase in aequorin light emission has been established for each intervention according to Blinks (4). The results are shown in Fig. 7. The slope of the regression line of the Ca^{2+} concentration response curve from Fig. 1 has been taken for comparison. This allows to characterize the different inotropic interventions with respect to their

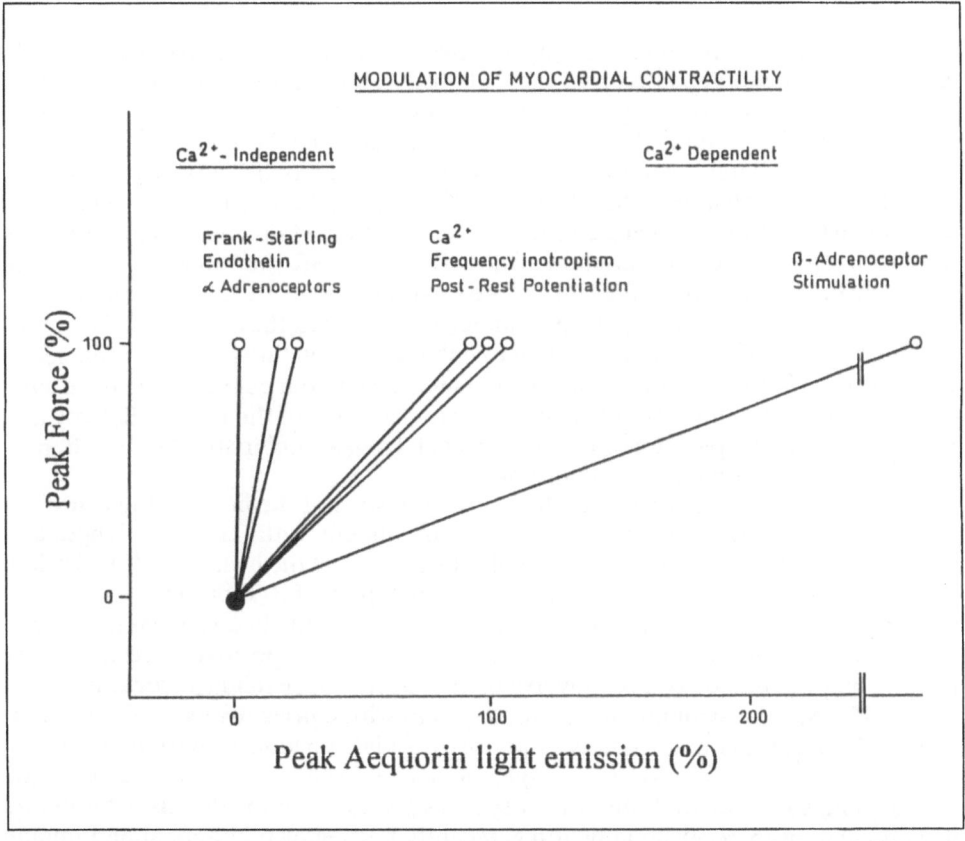

Fig. 7. Plot of the relative change in peak isometric force (in %; ordinate) versus peak aequorin light emission (in %; abscissa) for all interventions tested. Data from the Ca^{2+} reference curve from Fig. 1 have been taken for comparison.

intracellular mechanism of action. Inotropic interventions may be divided into Ca^{2+}-independent (left of the Ca^{2+} reference curve) or Ca^{2+} dependent (close to or right of the Ca^{2+} reference curve). It becomes evident that prestretch, α-adrenoceptor stimulation and endothelin receptor stimulation act mainly Ca^{2+}-independently, whereas the positive inotropic effect of β-adrenoceptor stimulation depends on an over-proportional increase in intracellular Ca^{2+} transients. Frequency-modulation and post-rest modulation of myocardial contractility directly depend on proportional changes in the intracellular Ca^{2+} transients.

Discussion

The major results of the present study were that 1) the Frank-Starling-mechanism and α- and endothelin receptor stimulation increase contractility without increasing intracellular Ca^{2+} transients, 2) force-frequency and post-rest modulation of myocardial contractility depend on parallel and proportional changes in intracellular Ca^{2+} transients, and 3) β-adrenoceptor stimulation results in an overproportional increase in intracellular Ca^{2+}.

Since the crucial experiment of Ringer in 1883 (43), it is well known that contractile function of the heart depends on extracellular Ca^{2+}. It has since been established that Ca^{2+} enters the cell during depolarization through voltage dependent Ca^{2+} channels. For the human heart, it is believed that the transsarcolemmal Ca^{2+} influx induces the release of a much larger amount of Ca^{2+} ions from the sarcoplasmic reticulum via the ryanodine release channels ("Ca^{2+}-induced Ca^{2+} release", Ref. 16). Ca^{2+} then binds to troponin C, thereby inducing contraction. Relaxation is initiated by dissociation of Ca^{2+} from Troponin C and reuptake to the SR via the SR Ca^{2+} pumps. Part of the Ca^{2+} may be extruded from the cell via the sarcolemmal Na^+/Ca^{2+} exchanger.

Myocardial contractility may be modulated by increasing the amount of Ca^{2+} available for binding to Troponin C, leading to enhanced activation of the myofilaments. Alternatively, force of contraction can be increased without changing the intracellular Ca^{2+} concentrations by enhancing the responsiveness of the myofibrils for Ca^{2+}. Some positive inotropic interventions may result from a combination of Ca^{2+}-dependent and Ca^{2+}-independent mechanisms (3).

Four basic mechanisms regulate the contractile state of the heart in the acute setting. First, muscle force and stroke volume vary directly with sarcomere length and preload, respectively, referred to as Frank-Starling law of the heart (19, 46). Furthermore, heart rate inotropism has been shown to be a powerful determinant of the contractile state of the heart (18, 21). However, it has recently been shown in isolated human myocardium and patients with heart failure, that the positive force-frequency relation may be blunted or even inverse in human end-stage failing myocardium (17, 18, 21, 35, 38). The sympathetic nervous system with consecutive stimulation of α- and β-adrenoceptors may acutely adapt myocardial function to peripheral needs; however, the sympathetic system is highly activated in chronic congestive heart failure, leading to substantial alterations such as β-adrenoceptor desensitization and downregulation (5, 7–9). Finally, it has recently been shown in animal and human tissue that circulating or locally generated endogenous peptides may enhance myocardial contractility (41, 51).

However, the intracellular mechanism of action of these basic determinants of myocardial contractility in the human myocardium is not fully evaluated. Since regulation of the intracellular Ca^{2+} transients has major impact on cardiac contractility, intracellular Ca^{2+} transients and contractility were simultaneously assessed in human isolated tissue.

Frank-Starling mechanism

The relative importance of the Frank-Starling mechanism for regulation of cardiac output increases in the elderly due to a reduced effectiveness of catecholamines and heart rate inotropism (30). This might also be the case in patients with congestive heart failure, where catecholamine response (7, 9) and heart rate inotropism (17, 21) is blunted. However, recent studies have suggested that the Frank-Starling mechanism is absent in conscious dogs with heart failure (29) and in isolated human myocardium from patients with end-stage heart failure (45). In contrast, using skinned fiber preparations under sarcomere-length control, isolated muscle strip preparations, and human whole heart preparations, Holubarsch et al. (25) described a preserved stretch- and preload-dependent increase in contractility in the failing human heart. Accordingly, in the present study, muscle strips from end-stage failing human hearts showed a substantial length-dependent increase in isometric twitch tension.

Length-dependent activation of contractile force may result from changes in the responsiveness of the myofilaments for Ca^{2+}, or by changes in the intracellular Ca^{2+} concentrations. Allen and Kurihara (1) reported from aequorin-loaded cat papillary muscle experiments that the length-dependent increase in force of contraction has a Ca^{2+}-independent and a Ca^{2+} dependent component. The reported increase in the amplitude of the Ca^{2+} transients might result from the effect of stretch on the physical properties of the membraneous structure of the sarcolemma (32), increased inward currents from stretch-activated receptors (10, 28), or increased release of Ca^{2+} from the SR (15). However, using skinned fiber preparations from several animal species, a stretch-induced increase in the Ca^{2+} sensitivity of the myofilaments has been reported (26). Accordingly, Hoffmann und Fuchs (24) could directly demonstrate stretch-induced increased binding of Ca^{2+} to troponin C. Therefore, length-dependence of contractile force in isolated muscle strip preparations has been partially attributed to length-dependence of Ca^{2+} sensitivity of the myofilaments (2, 20). Holubarsch et al. (25) demonstrated in human myocardium a significant leftward shift of the pCa-force relationship in skinned fiber preparations with increasing sarcomere lengths compatible with the concept of a sarcomere length-dependent change in Ca^{2+} sensitivity of the myofilaments. However, the intracellular mechanism underlying the observed length-dependent increase in contractility in the human heart has not been investigated in intact human tissue. Therefore, we assessed the effects of muscle length on the transient change of the myoplasmic Ca^{2+} transient, represented by the amplitude of the aequorin light signal. We could demonstrate a significant length-dependent increase in isometric twitch tension with only minor increases in aequorin light emission. Furthermore, stretching the muscle strips resulted in a remarkable slowing of relaxation. Both findings are compatible with the conclusion that length-dependent activation of contractile force in isolated human myocardium predominantly results from increased Ca^{2+} responsiveness of the myofilaments.

However, using the fluorescent indicator Indo-1, Le Guennec et al. (31) described a length-dependent increase in diastolic Ca^{2+} levels in isolated guinea-pig myocytes. It has to be kept in mind that due to its Ca^{2+} binding kinetics, aequorin is a rather insensitive indicator for low diastolic Ca^{2+} concentrations. Therefore, small diastolic changes in intracellular Ca^{2+} upon stretch might have gone unrecognized in this study. Furthermore, it cannot be excluded that in addition to the increased affinity of Ca^{2+} for troponin C, some increase in intracellular Ca^{2+} transients had occurred in human tissue upon stretch without an increase in aequorin luminescence due to enhanced binding of Ca^{2+} to troponin C.

The use of the Frank-Starling mechanism with increased responsiveness of the myofilaments for Ca^{2+} may be important for the failing heart for several reasons: a) increased Ca^{2+} results in increased energy and oxygen expenditure; b), Ca^{2+} overload may impair diastolic function and trigger arrhythmias. Therefore, optimizing preload in patients with heart failure may be a favorable way to improve myocardial contractility without increased risk of deficient oxygen or energy supply or increased risk of ventricular arrhythmias.

alpha- and endothelin-receptor stimulation

Similar to length-dependent activation, α-adrenoceptor and endothelin-receptor stimulation resulted in a positive inotropic and negative lusitropic effect without increasing intracellular Ca^{2+} transients. Interestingly, both receptors share the same postreceptor signaling cascade, i.e., phospholipid breakdown with subsequent inositoltriphosphate and diacylglycerol formation (14). Diacylglycerol has been shown to activate protein kinase C, ultimately leading to intracellular alkalinization due to enhanced activity of the Na^+/H exchanger. It has been shown in animal experiments that reduced intracellular H^+ concentrations increase the responsiveness of the myofilaments for Ca^{2+}, possibly due to reduced competition of H^+ for binding sites on troponin C (13). Using the Ca^{2+} indicator aequorin, Wang et al. (51) described an endothelin-induced increased Ca^{2+}-responsiveness of the myofilaments in aequorin-loaded ferret papillary muscles. Similarly, Endoh and Blinks (12) described a Ca^{2+}-independent inotropic effect of phenylephrine in isolated rabbit papillary muscle; similar to the results obtained in this study, the authors opposed the Ca^{2+}-sensitizing effect of α-adrenoceptor stimulation to the overproportional increase in intracellular Ca^{2+} transients after β-adrenoceptor stimulation. However, the functional relevance of α- or endothelin receptor stimulation in human congestive heart failure has not yet been demonstrated. In the present *in vitro* investigation, the positive inotropic effect of β-adrenoceptor stimulation or length dependent activation was more pronounced than α- or ET-receptor stimulation in failing human myocardium despite reduced β-adrenoceptor densities. In contrast, α- and ET receptors seem to be unchanged or even upregulated in the failing human heart (6, 41, 50) despite increased norepinephrine and endothelin (52) plasma levels. Furthermore, Sakai et al. (44) recently reported the functional relevance of an activated ET system in a rat model of ischemic heart failure. Taken together, both alpha- and ET receptor stimulation results in a small to intermediate positive inotropic effect in failing human myocardium due to increased responsiveness of the myofilaments for Ca^{2+}. This might be of potential energetical benefit in heart failure patients. However, the functional relevance of this direct inotropic effect in patients with heart failure remains to be elucidated.

Changes in stimulation rate and rest intervals

In contrast to the increase in force without changes in the amplitude of the intracellular Ca^{2+} transients, heart rate inotropism directly results from parallel changes in the intracellular Ca^{2+} transients (39). We have shown that the positive force-frequency relation in isolated human myocardium is associated with a parallel frequency-dependent increase in intracellular Ca^{2+} transients. This has been attributed to a frequency-dependent increase in transsarcolemmal Ca^{2+} influx per unit of time with subsequent increased loading, and hence release, of Ca^{2+} from the SR for activation of the myofilaments. In contrast, in failing human myocardium, the force-frequency relation is blunted or even inverse (35, 38). Again, frequency-dependent changes in force were paralleled by frequency-dependent changes in intracellular Ca^{2+} transients (this study; ref. 39). This may be due to a reduced frequency-enhancement of transsarcolemmal Ca^{2+} influx (42) in association with a reduced SR Ca^{2+} ATPase uptake capacity (22, 33, 39) and an enhanced expression and activity of the sarcolemmal Na^{+}/Ca^{2+} exchanger (47). At higher stimulation rates, diastole, i.e., time for SR Ca^{2+} uptake, shortens, and less Ca^{2+} may be stored within the SR for subsequent release. Similarily, post-rest potentiation of intracellular Ca^{2+} transients and force of contraction in human nonfailing myocardium is converted to post-rest decay in failing myocardium (this study; ref. 40). Again, this may be attributed to a reduced SR Ca^{2+} pump capacity and enhanced activity of the Na^{+}/Ca^{2+} exchanger. Ca^{2+} which continuously leaks from the SR during the rest interval may not be taken up back to the SR, but eliminated from the cytosol by the Na^{+}/Ca^{2+} exchanger (48). In conclusion, changes in contractile stength due to changes in rate and rhythm directly depend on parallel changes in the amplitude of the intracellular Ca^{2+} transients. In the failing human myocardium, significant alterations occur with respect to intracellular Ca^{2+} handling leading to profound alterations of cardiac contractile performance.

β-Adrenoceptor stimulation

As opposed to the Ca^{2+}-independent pathways and the rate-dependent parallel changes in force and Ca^{2+} transients, the positive inotropic effect of β-adrenoceptor stimulation is associated with a large, overproportional increase in intracellular Ca^{2+} transients. Similar results have been obtained in aequorin-loaded rabbit (12) and ferret (36) papillary muscle. A large increase in Ca^{2+} cycling after isoproterenol stimulation has also been observed by Hasenfuss et al. (23) in isolated human myocardium using a myothermal method. The pronounced increase in intracellular Ca^{2+} cycling after isoproterenol may be attributed to the cAMP-dependent phosphorylation of sarcolemmal Ca^{2+} channels and phospholamban, leading to enhanced Ca^{2+} influx and increased SR Ca^{2+} pump activity. In addition to enhanced Ca^{2+} reuptake to the SR, the positive lusitropic effect of isoproterenol observed in this study has been attributed to an cAMP-dependent decrease in the affinity of troponin C for Ca^{2+}. The overproportional increase in intracellular Ca^{2+} after β-adrenoceptor stimulation and subsequent cAMP formation may explain the disappointing results from clinical trials investigating the effects of catecholamines and phosphodiesterase inhibitors in patients with chronic congestive heart failure (11, 37, 49). These trials showed increased mortality of patients due to increased incidence of ventricular arrhythmias and enhanced progression of cardiac disease. These findings may be explained by the overproportional increase in intracellular Ca^{2+}, possibly resulting in increased energy expenditure, oxygen demand, and enhanced susceptibility to ventricular arrhythmias.

In conclusion, physiologic modulation of intrinsic myocardial contractility may be mediated via Ca^{2+}-dependent and Ca^{2+}-independent pathways. Due to well described alterations in Ca^{2+} handling in human heart failure, Ca^{2+} independent mechanisms for maintaining myocardial contractility may become more effective. Further benefit for activating Ca^{2+}-independent mechanisms might result from decreased oxygen and energy demands and reduced incidence of malignant arrhythmias. However, the functional role of some of these mechanisms in heart failure and their possibly detrimental effects on diastolic function due to delayed relaxation remain to be elucidated.

Acknowledgements   This grant was supported by DFG grant HA 1233/3-2. The excellent technical assistance of Thomas Weber is appreciated.

REFERENCES

1. Allen DG, Kurihara S (1982) The effects of muscle length on intracellular calcium transients in mammalian cardiac muscle. J Physiol 327: 79–94
2. Allen DG, Kentish JC (1988) Calcium concentration in the myoplasm of skinned ferret ventricular muscle following changes in muscle length. J Physiol 407: 489–503
3. Blinks JR, Endoh M (1986) Modification of myofibrillar responsiveness to Ca^{2+} as an inotropic mechanism. Circulation 73 (Suppl III): 85–98
4. Blinks JR (1993) Analysis of the effects of drugs on myofibrillar Ca^{2+} sensitivity in intact cardiac muscle. In: Modulation of Cardiac Ca^{2+} Sensitivity. Lee JA and Allen DG, editors. Oxford University Press, Oxford, UK: 242–282
5. Böhm M, Gierschik P, Jakobs K, Pieske B, Schnabel P, Ungerer M, Erdmann E (1990) Increase of $G_{i\alpha}$ in human hearts with dilated but not ischemic cardiomyopathy. Circulation 82: 1249–1265
6. Böhm M, Diet F, Feiler G, Kemkes B, Erdmann E (1988) α-Adrenoceptors and α-adrenoceptor-mediated positive inotropic effects in failing human myocardium. J Cardiovasc Pharm 12: 357–364
7. Bristow MR, Ginsberg K, Minobe WA, Cubicciotti RS, Sageman WS, Lurie K, Billingham MR, Harrison DL, Stinson EB (1982) Decreased catecholamine sensitivity and β-adrenergic density in failing human hearts. N Engl J Med 307: 205–211
8. Bristow MR, Hershberg RE, Port JD, Minobe WA, Rasmussen R (1988) β_1- and β_2-Adrenergic receptor-mediated adenylate cyclase stimulation in non-failing and failing ventricular myocardium. Mol Pharmacol 35: 295–303

9. Brodde OE (1994) Beta-adrenoceptors in cardiac disease. Pharmacol Ther 60: 405–430
10. Craelius W, Chen V, El-Sherif N (1988) Stretch-activated ion channels in ventricular myocytes. Biosci Rep 8: 407–414
11. Dies F, Krell MJ, Whitlow P et al. (1986) Intermittent dobutamine in ambulatory outpatients with chronic cardiac failure. Circulation 80: 74–83
12. Endoh M, Blinks JR (1988) Actions of sympathomimetic amines on the Ca^{2+} transients and contractions of rabbit myocardium: reciprocal changes in myofibrillar responsiveness to Ca^{2+} mediated through alpha- and β-adrenoceptors. Circ Res 62: 247–265
13. Endoh M (1991) Signal transduction of myocardial alpha$_1$-adrenoceptors: regulation of ion channels, intracellular calcium, and force of contraction – a review. J Appl Cardiol 6: 379–399
14. Endoh M, Morita H, Kimura J (1996) The role of phosphoinositide hydrolysis in the regulation of cardiac function via alpha-adrenergic, endothelin, and angiotensin receptors. In: Molecular and Cellular Mechanisms of Cardiovascular Regulation, Eds: Endoh M, Morad M, Scholz H, Ijima T. Springer Verlag Tokyo, Berlin, Heidelberg, New York: 327–351
15. Fabiato A, Fabiato F (1975) Dependence of the contractile activation of skinned cardiac cells on the sarcomere length. Nature 256: 54–56
16. Fabiato A (1985) Simulated calcium current can both cause calcium loading and trigger calcium release from the sarcoplasmic reticulum of a skinned cardiac Purkinje fiber. J Gen Physiol 85: 291–320
17. Feldman MD, Gwathmey JK, Phillips P, Schoen F, Morgan JP (1988) Reversal of the force-frequency relationship in working myocardium from patients with end-stage heart failure. J Appl Cardiol 3: 273–283
18. Feldman MD, Alderman JR, Aroesty JM, Royal HD, Ferguson JJ, Owen RM, Grossman W, McKay RG (1988) Depression of systolic and diastolic myocardial reserve during atrial pacing tachycardia in patients with dilated cardiomyopathy. J Clin Invest 82: 1661–1669
19. Frank O (1895) Zur Dynamik des Herzmuskels. J Biol 32: 370–447. Translation from German: Chapman CP, Wasserman EB (1959) On the dynamics of cardiac muscle. Am Heart J 58: 282–317
20. Gulati J (1992) Length-sensing function of troponin C and Starling's law. Circulation 85: 1954–1955
21. Hasenfuss G, Holubarsch C, Hermann HP, Astheimer K, Pieske B, Just H (1994) Influence of the force-frequency relation on hemodynamics and left ventricular function in patients with nonfailing hearts and in patients with dilated cardiomyopathy. Eur Heart J 15: 164–170
22. Hasenfuss G, Reinecke R, Studer H, Meyer M, Pieske B, Holtz J, Holubarsch C, Posival H, Just H, Drexler H (1994) Relation between myocardial function and expression of sarcoplasmic reticulum Ca^{2+}-ATPase in failing and nonfailing human myocardium. Circ Res 75: 434–442
23. Hasenfuss G, Mulieri LA, Leavitt BJ, Alpert NR (1994) Influence of isoproterenol on contractile function, excitation-contraction coupling, and energy turnover of isolated nonfailing human myocardium. J Mol Cell Cardiol 26: 1461–1469
24. Hofmann PA, Fuchs F (1988) Bound calcium and force development in skinned cardiac muscle bundles: Effect of sarcomere length. J Mol Cell Cardiol 20: 667–677
25. Holubarsch C, Ruf T, Goldstein D, Ashton RC, Nickl W, Pieske B, Pioch K, Lüdemann J, Wiesner S, Hasenfuss G, Posival H, Just H, Burkhoff D (1996) Existence of the Frank-Starling mechanism in the failing human heart. Investigations on the organ, tissue, and sarcomere level. Circulation 94: 683–689
26. Kentish JC, ter Keurs H, Ricciardi L, Bucx J, Noble MIM (1986) Comparison between the sarcomere length-force relations of intact and skinned trabeculae from rat right ventricle. Circ Res 58: 755–768
27. Kihara Y, Morgan JP (1989) A comparative study of three methods for intracellular loading of the calcium indicator aequorin in ferret papillary muscles. Biochem Biophys Res Commun 162: 402–407
28. Kirber MT, Walsh JV, Singer JJ (1988) Stretch-activated ion channels in smooth muscle: A mechanism for the initiation of stretch-induced contraction. Pflugers Arch 412: 339–345
29. Komamura K, Shannon RP, Ihara T, Shen YT, Mirsky I, Bishop SP, Vatner SF (1993) Exhaustion of the Frank-Starling mechanism in conscious dogs with heart failure. Am J Physiol 265: H1119–H1131
30. Lakatta EG (1983) Determinants of cardiovascular performance: Modifications due to aging. J Chronic Dis 36: 15–30
31. Le Guennec JY, White E, Gannier F, Argibay JA, Garnier D (1991) Stretch-induced increase of intracellular calcium concentration in single guinea-pig ventricular myocytes. Exp Physiol 76: 975–978
32. Levin KR, Page E (1980) Quantitative studies on plasmalemmal folds and caveolae of rabbit ventricular myocardial cells. Circ Res 46: 244–255
33. Meyer M, Schillinger W, Pieske B, Holubarsch C, Heilmann C, Posival H, Kuwajima G, Mikoshiba K, Just H, Hasenfuss G (1995) Alterations of sarcoplasmic reticulum proteins in failing human dilated cardiomyopathy. Circulation 92: 778–784
34. Mulieri LA, Leavitt BJ, Hasenfuss G, Allen PD, Alpert NR (1989) Protection of human left ventricular myocardium from cutting injury with 2,3 butanedione monoxime. Circ Res 65: 1441–1444
35. Mulieri LA, Hasenfuss G, Ittleman F, Leavitt B, Allen PD, Blanchard EM, Alpert NR (1992) Altered myocardial force-frequency relation in human heart failure. Circulation 85: 1743–1750

36. Okazaki O, Suda N, Hongo K, Konishi M, Kurihara S (1990) Modulation of Ca^{2+} transients and contractile properties by β-adrenoceptor stimulation in ferret ventricular muscles. J Physiol (Lond) 423: 221–240
37. Packer M (1991) The PROMISE Study Research Group. Effects of oral milrinone on mortality in severe chronic heart failure. N Engl J Med 325: 1468–1475
38. Pieske B, Hasenfuss G, Holubarsch C, Schwinger R, Böhm M, Just H (1992) Alteration of the force-frequency relationship in the failing human heart depends on underlying cardiac disease. Basic Res Cardiol 87 (I): 213–221
39. Pieske B, Kretschmann B, Meyer M, Holubarsch C, Weirich J, Posival H, Minami K, Just H, Hasenfuss G (1995) Alterations in intracellular calcium handling associated with the inverse force-frequency relation in human dilated cardiomyopathy. Circulation 92: 1169–1178
40. Pieske B, Sütterlin M, Schmidt-Schweda S, Minami K, Meyer M, Olschewski M, Holubarsch C, Just H, Hasenfuss G (1996) Diminished post-rest potentiation of contractile force in human dilated cardiomyopathy: functional evidence for alterations in intracellular Ca^{2+} handling. J Clin Invest 98: 764–776
41. Pieske B, Beyermann B, Duis J, Clozel M, Breu V (1996) Endothelin-1 increases contractility in human dilated cardiomyopathy via an upregulated ET_A receptor subtype. Circulation 94 (Suppl): I-406
42. Piot C, Lemaire S, Albat B, Seguin J, Nargeot J, Richard S (1996) High frequency-induced upregulation of human cardiac calcium currents. Circulation 93: 120–128
43. Ringer S (1883) A further contribution regarding the influence of the different constituents of the blood on the contractions of the heart. J Physiol 4: 29–42
44. Sakai S, Miyauchi T, Sakurai T, Kasuya Y, Ihara M, Yamaguchi I, Goto K, Sigisthita Y (1996) Endogenous Endothelin-1 participates in the maintenance of cardiac function in rats with congestive heart failure. Marked increase in Endothelin-1 production in the failing heart. Circulation 93: 1214–1222
45. Schwinger RHG, Böhm M, Koch A, Schmidt U, Morano I, Eissner HJ, Überfuhr R, Reichart B, Erdmann E (1994) The failing human heart is unable to use the Frank-Starling mechanism. Circ Res 74: 959–969
46. Starling EH (1918) Linacre lecture on the law of the heart. London, England: Longmanns
47. Studer R, Reinecke H, Bilger J, Eschenhagen T, Böhm M, Hasenfuss G, Just H, Holtz J, Drexler H (1994) Gene expression of the Na^+/Ca^{2+} exchanger in end-stage human heart failure. Circ Res 75: 443–453
48. Sutko JL, Bers DM, Reeves JP (1986) Postrest inotropy in rabbit ventricle: Na^+/Ca^{2+} exchange determines sarcoplasmic reticulum Ca^{2+} content. Am J Physiol 250: H654–H661
49. Uretsky BF (1990) The ENOXIMONE Multicenter Trial Group. Multicenter trial of oral enoximone in patients with moderate to moderately severe congestive heart failure. Lack of benefit compared to placebo. Circulation 82: 774–780
50. Vago T, Bevilacqua M, Norbiato G, Baldi G, Chebat E, Bertora P, Baroldi G, Accinni R (1989) Identification of $\alpha 1$-adrenergic receptors on sarcolemma from normal subjects and patients with idiopathic dilated cardiomyopathy: Characteristics and linkage to GTP-binding proteins. Circ Res 64: 474–481
51. Wang J, Paik G, Morgan JP (1991) Endothelin-1 enhances myofilament Ca^{2+} responsiveness in aequorin-loaded ferret myocardium. Circ Res 69: 582–589
52. Wei C, Lerman A, Rodeheffer RJ, McGregor CGA, Brandt RR, Wright S, Heublein DM, Kao PC, Edwards WD, Burnett JC (1994) Endothelin in human congestive heart failure. Circulation 89: 1580–1586

Authors' address:
Dr. med. Burkert Pieske
Medizinische Klinik III
Abteilung Kardiologie und Angiologie
Universität Freiburg
Hugstetter Str. 55
79106 Freiburg, Germany

Calcium handling proteins in the failing human heart

G. Hasenfuss, M. Meyer, W. Schillinger, M. Preuss, B. Pieske, H. Just

Medizinische Klinik III, Universität Freiburg, Freiburg, Germany

Abstract

There is accumulating evidence that disturbed calcium homeostasis may play a key role in the pathophysiology of human heart failure. Because disturbed calcium handling could result from altered protein expression, levels of calcium handling proteins were quantitated by Western Blot analysis in failing and nonfailing human myocardium from hearts with endstage failing dilated or ischemic cardiomyopathy. Protein levels of the sarcoplasmic reticulum calcium release channel (ryanodine receptor) and of calcium storage proteins (calsequestrin and calreticulin) were similar in failing and nonfailing human myocardium. However, proteins involved in calcium removal from the cytosol were significantly altered in the failing human heart: 1) SR-Ca^{2+}-ATPase, relevant for removal of calcium from the cytosol into the lumen of the sarcoplasmic reticulum, was decreased; 2) phospholamban, which inhibits the SR-Ca^{2+}-ATPase in the basal unphosphorylated state, was slightly decreased; 3) the ratio of SR-Ca^{2+}-ATPase to phospholamban was decreased; 4) the sarcolemmal Na^+-Ca^{2+}-exchanger, relevant for transsarcolemmal calcium extrusion was increased in the failing hearts. In summary, altered levels of proteins involved in calcium removal from the cytosol suggest an increase in transsarcolemmal calcium elimination relative to sarcoplasmic reticulum calcium removal. These findings support the concept that reduced function of the sarcoplasmic reticulum to accumulate calcium may reflect a major defect in excitation-contraction coupling in human heart failure.

Key words Calcium – heart failure – sarcoplasmic reticulum – gene expression – human myocardium

Introduction

Previous studies have shown that myocardial hypertrophy and failure are associated with altered gene expression including isoform shifts and quantitative changes of transcription (for review see (2, 48)). Altered gene expression of calcium handling proteins may underlie disturbed excitation-contraction coupling which is considered to be of major pathophysiological relevance in human heart failure. Disturbed excitation-contraction coupling is suggested from the following findings: 1) Myothermal studies indicated that the total amount of calcium cycling and the rate of calcium removal are reduced in the failing human myocardium (20). 2) Systolic free calcium concentration was reduced and diastolic calcium levels were elevated when fura-2 was used to measure free intracellular calcium concentrations in isolated myocytes from failing human hearts (7). 3) Prolongation of calcium transients has been observed in isolated myocytes using fura-2 (7) and in ventricular muscle strip preparations using the calcium indicator aequorin (18). 4) The frequency-dependent rise of the calcium transients was found to be blunted and an inversion of the calcium-frequency relation (aequorin light emission) was observed in isolated ventricular muscle strip preparations from end-stage failing human hearts (41). 5) Post-rest potentiation of calcium transients was diminished, as indicated from aequorin light measurements in isolated muscle strip preparations (42). 6) Frequency-dependent upregulation of L-type calcium currents was shown to be blunted or absent in ventricular myocytes from failing compared to nonfailing human hearts (43).

In the present paper, we review our own findings and data from the literature available on expression of myocardial proteins relevant for calcium handling in the failing and nonfailing human heart. The data indicate that in the failing heart decreased SR-Ca^{2+}-uptake due to decreased expression and activity of the calcium pump results in decreased systolic calcium availability to contractile proteins. Increased expression of the sarcolemmal Na^+-Ca^{2+}-exchanger may compensate for diastolic calcium removal to preserve diastolic function but may further decrease intracellular systolic calcium availability and thus systolic performance.

Sarcolemmal L-type calcium channel

Calcium entry through voltage-gated L-type calcium channels is the key event causing the transition from the resting state of the myocardium to contraction (12). This calcium channel is a multimeric protein complex. The α_1-subunit contains the calcium conducting pore and the binding sites for calcium channel blockers (24). Three genes code for the dihydropyridine-sensitive α_1-subunits in skeletal, neuronal and cardiac/smooth muscle tissue. The cardiac and smooth muscle L-type calcium channel α_1-subunits are splice variants of the same gene (24). Abundance of the L-type calcium channel α_1-subunit in failing and nonfailing human myocardium has been studied by Northern blot analysis and by dihydropyridine binding. Takahashi et al. reported a significant decrease in mRNA levels encoding the dihydropyridine receptor as well as a decrease in dihydropyridine binding sites in failing human hearts with dilated and ischemic cardiomyopathy (49). This is in contrast to findings by Rasmussen et al. which indicate that dihydropyridine binding sites are not significantly altered in the human ventricular tissue from hearts with end-stage dilated cardiomyopathy (44).

Unaltered levels of the α_1-subunit of L-type calcium channels would be consistent with functional measurements by Beuckelmann et al. They showed that calcium current densities, measured during basal conditions, are similar in isolated myocytes from failing hearts with dilated cardiomyopathy and from nonfailing hearts (8). However, more recent measurements by Piot et al. suggest that function of L-type calcium channels may be altered in human heart failure (43). They observed that increasing frequencies augment calcium currents in myocytes from nonfailing hearts whereas high frequency upregulation of calcium currents was lost or attenuated in myocytes from hearts with reduced left ventricular function. This finding may indicate that quantitative or qualitative changes of other subunits of the multimeric L-type calcium channel occur in the failing human heart.

Sarcoplasmic reticulum calcium release channel

The calcium sensitive SR calcium release channel (ryanodine receptor) is regulated by calcium which enters the cell through voltage gated calcium channels in the sarcolemma. Once activated by calcium influx, the channel opens and releases calcium for activation of contractile proteins (4, 11, 50). This process is termed calcium-induced calcium release (12). The ryanodine receptor forms a tetrameric structure comprised of four monomers (50). Molecular cloning analysis has revealed that two distinct genes encode the cardiac and skeletal muscle specific receptors (31, 39).

Several groups have studied mRNA expression of the ryanodine receptor in human heart failure and results have not been consistent (Table 1). Using a radioligand binding assay, Go et al. in a small number of samples found that high affinity binding sites for [^{3}H]ryanodine were decreased by about 30 % in left ventricular myocardium from failing human hearts (17). When we studied protein levels of the ryanodine receptor in failing and nonfailing human hearts from patients with dilated or ischemic cardiomyopathy, there was no significant difference between nonfailing and failing myocardium (Fig. 1, Table 1) (33, 45). Of course, unaltered protein

Table 1. Quantification of SR-Ca^{2+}-release channel (RYR) in human heart failure

Quantity	Disease	Method	Reference
28 % ↓	ICM	Northern Blot	Brillantes et al. Circ Res 71; 1992 (9)
n.s.	DCM	Northern Blot	idem
31 % ↓	DCM, ICM	Northern Blot	Go et al. J Clin Invest 95; 1995 (17)
Inverse Relation with ANF	DCM	Northern Blot	Arai et al. Circ Res 72; 1993 (3)
n.s.	DCM	Western Blot	Meyer et al. Circulation 92; 1995 (33)
n.s.	ICM	Western Blot	Schillinger et al. Moll Cell Biochem 160/161; 1996 (45)

ANF = atrial natriuretic factor; DCM = dilated cardiomyopathy; ICM = ischemic cardiomyopathy; RYR = ryanodine receptor; n.s. = no significant change versus nonfailing human myocardium levels of the ryanodine receptor do not exclude that altered function of the normally expressed ryanodine receptor may be involved in disturbed excitation-contraction coupling in the failing human heart. D'Agnolo et al. recently found that caffeine threshold of the ryanodine receptor was increased, suggesting impaired gating mechanism of the calcium release channel in dilated cardiomyopathy (10). Nimer et al. reported differences in response to ryanodine between failing and nonfailing myocardium which may also reflect altered function of the ryanodine receptor (38). In contrast, Holmberg and Williams reported normal basal properties of the ryanodine receptor from failing human hearts in single-channel recordings under voltage-clamp conditions (23).

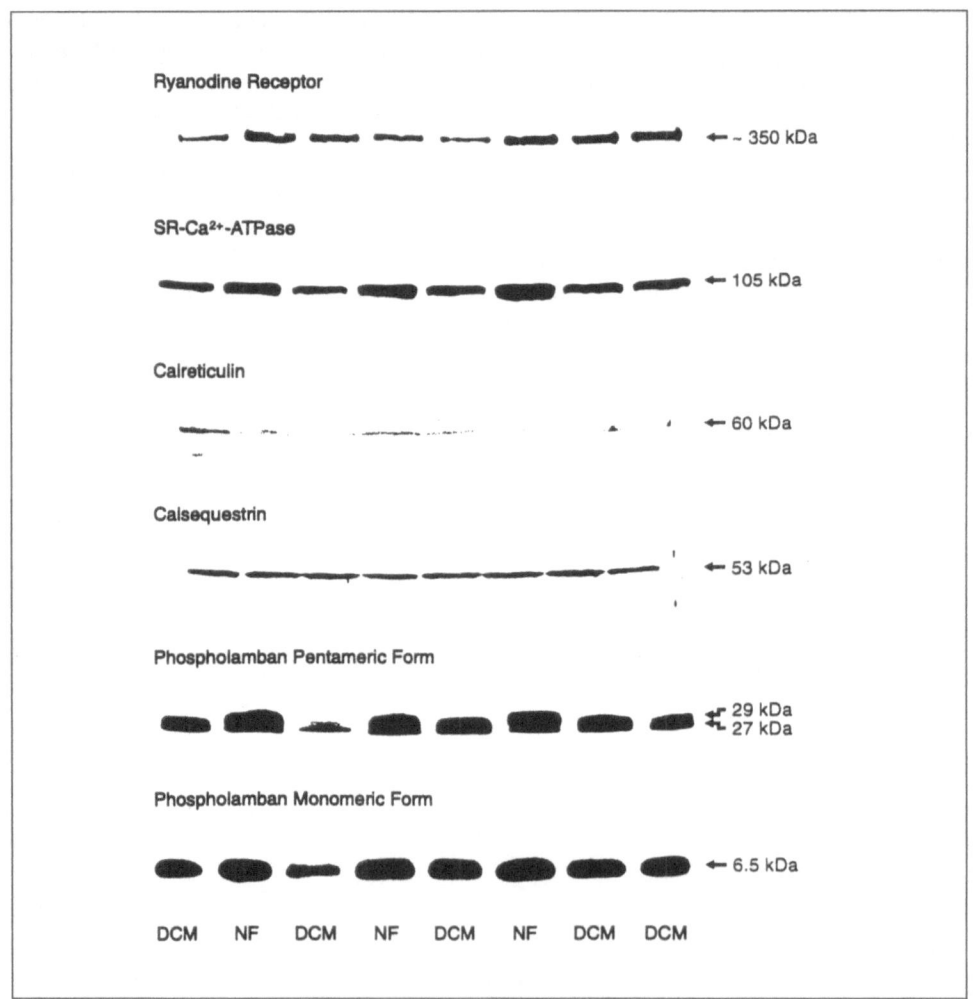

Fig. 1. Western Blot analysis of sarcoplasmic reticulum (SR) proteins in myocardium from nonfailing human hearts (NF) and from hearts with end-stage failing dilated cardiomyopathy (DCM). With permission from reference (33).

Sarcoplasmic reticulum calcium storage proteins

Calsequestrin and calreticulin are located within the lumen of the SR (29, 30, 34). Calsequestrin, a high-capacity moderate affinity calcium-binding protein is primarily responsible for the calcium storage capacity of the SR in cardiac muscle (29). Two distinct isoforms of calsequestrin have been identified. The skeletal muscle isoform expressed in both fast- and slow-twitch skeletal muscle, and the cardiac isoform, expressed predominantly in the heart (1, 15). Our finding (33) of unchanged calsequestrin protein levels in dilated cardiomyopathy (Fig. 1) is consistent with recent mRNA as well as protein measurements (3, 35, 49). Furthermore, several studies performed in animal models of myocardial hypertrophy and failure indicate that calsequestrin levels remain unchanged (2, 36). Calreticulin is a major calcium binding protein of non-muscle endoplasmic reticulum membranes (29, 34). In addition to its apparent calcium storage role, evidence is accumulating which suggests that calreticulin has other regulatory functions within the cell. It may be involved in regulation of DNA-synthesis and protein-synthesis (34). Western blot analysis shows that calreticulin is present in nonfailing and failing human hearts, and that levels of this protein are similar in both types of human myocardium (Fig. 1) (33).

Sarcoplasmic reticulum calcium pump and phospholamban

Calcium transport into the SR occurs by SR-Ca^{2+}-ATPase, which transports two calcium ions per molecule of high-energy phosphate hydrolyzed against a high ion gradient (29). This pump, together with the Na^+-Ca^{2+}-exchanger and the sarcolemmal calcium-ATPase, eliminates calcium from the cytosol in order to facilitate relaxation of the myocardium (4). Moreover, SR-Ca^{2+}-ATPase is crucial for calcium accumulation within the SR and thus, for the availability of calcium for systolic release through the ryanodine receptor (4). Sarco-endoplasmic reticulum Ca^{2+}-ATPases are encoded by three genes and five different isoforms are expressed: the adult fast-twitch skeletal muscle isoform (SERCA1a), its alternatively spliced neonatal isoform (SERCA1b), the cardiac/slow-twitch skeletal muscle isoform (SERCA2a), its alternatively spliced smooth muscle/nonmuscle isoform (SERCA-2b), and an isoform expressed in a broad variety of muscle and nonmuscle tissues (SERCA3) (for review see (2)). No isoform shift has been detected in the failing human heart (2). Abundance of SR-Ca^{2+}-ATPase at the level of the mRNA, has been consistently shown to be reduced in the failing human compared to the nonfailing heart (Table 2).

At the level of the protein, findings have been controversial (Table 2). Studies performed by our own group showed a decrease in SR-Ca^{2+}-ATPase protein levels in failing human myocardium from hearts with end-stage dilated or ischemic cardiomyopathy by about 40 % (Fig. 2) (21, 33, 45, 47).

The SR-Ca^{2+}-ATPase is regulated by phospholamban (26, 27, 29). Dephosphorylated phospholamban is an inhibitor of the SR-Ca^{2+}-ATPase activity and phosphorylation relieves this inhibition. The inhibition has been suggested to involve direct protein-protein interaction followed by conformational changes in the SR-Ca^{2+}-ATPase resulting in a decrease in the affinity of the calcium pump for calcium (25, 27). There are no isoforms of phospholamban, and the same proteins are expressed in cardiac and slow twitch skeletal muscle (16). Previous reports on mRNA and protein levels in failing versus nonfailing human hearts are not consistent (Table 3). Using quantitative Western blot analysis, our group showed that phospholamban protein levels are significantly decreased relative to total protein in failing dilated cardiomyopathy. When phospholamban was normalized to calsequestrin, however, there was no significant difference between failing and nonfailing myocardium (33).

Interestingly, SR-Ca^{2+}-ATPase protein levels were decreased to a greater proportion than protein levels of phospholamban in the failing myocardium (Fig. 2). If we assume that the stoichiometry of phospholamban to SR-Ca^{2+}-ATPase determines the level of SR-Ca^{2+}-ATPase inhibition, this finding may indicate that in the basal low phosphorylated state depression of SR calcium uptake is even more pronounced than would be expected from the decrease of SR-Ca^{2+}-ATPase protein levels in the failing myocardium.

Decreased protein levels of SR-Ca^{2+}-ATPase could result from a decreased content of SR within the myocytes from failing hearts or from a reduced density of the

Table 2. Quantification of SR-Ca^{2+}-ATPase in human heart failure

Quantity	Disease	Method	Reference
48 % ↓	DCM, ICM	Northern Blot	Mercadier et al. J Clin Invest 85; 1990 (32)
50 % ↓	DCM, ICM	Northern Blot	Takahashi et al. Circ Res 71; 1992 (49)
Inverse Relation with ANF	DCM	Northern Blot	Arai et al. Circ Res 72; 1993 (3)
50 % ↓	DCM, ICM	Northern Blot	Studer et al. Circ Res 75; 1994 (47)
50–60 % ↓	DCM, ICM	Northern Blot	Linck et al. Cardiovasc Res 31; 1996 (28)
54 % ↓	DCM	Northern Blot	Schwinger et al. Circulation 92; 1995 (46)
40 % ↓	DCM, ICM	Western Blot	Studer et al. Circ Res 75; 1994 (47)
36 % ↓	DCM, ICM	Western Blot	Hasenfuss et al. Circ Res 75; 1994 (21)
33 % ↓	DCM	Western Blot	Meyer et al. Circulation 92; 1995 (33)
n.s.	DCM	Western Blot	Movsesian et al. Circulation 90; 1994 (35)
n.s.	DCM	Western Blot	Schwinger et al. Circulation 92; 1995 (46)
n.s.	DCM, ICM	Western Blot	Linck et al. Cardiovasc Res 31; 1996 (28)

ANF = atrial natriuretic factor; DCM = dilated cardiomyopathy; ICM = ischemic cardiomyopathy; n.s. = no significant change versus nonfailing human myocardium

Table 3. Quantification of phospholamban in human heart failure

Quantity	Disease	Method	Reference
↓	DCM	PCR	Feldman et al. Circulation 83; 1991 (13)
27–35 % ↓	DCM, ICM	Northern Blot	Linck et al. Cardiovasc Res 31; 1996 (28)
Inverse Relation with ANF	DCM, ICM	Northern Blot	Arai et al. Circ Res 72; 1993 (3)
40 % ↓	DCM	Northern Blot	Schwinger et al. Circulation 92; 1995 (46)
n.s.	DCM	Western Blot	Movsesian et al. Circulation 90; 1994 (35)
18 % ↓	DCM	Western Blot	Meyer et al. Circulation 92; 1995 (33)
n.s.	DCM, ICM	Western Blot	Linck et al. Cardiovasc Res 31; 1996 (28)
n.s.	DCM	Western Blot	Schwinger et al. Circulation (46) 92; 1995

ANF = atrial natriuretic factor; DCM = dilated cardiomyopathy; ICM = ischemic cardiomyopathy; n.s. = no significant change versus nonfailing human myocardium; PCR = polymerase chain reaction

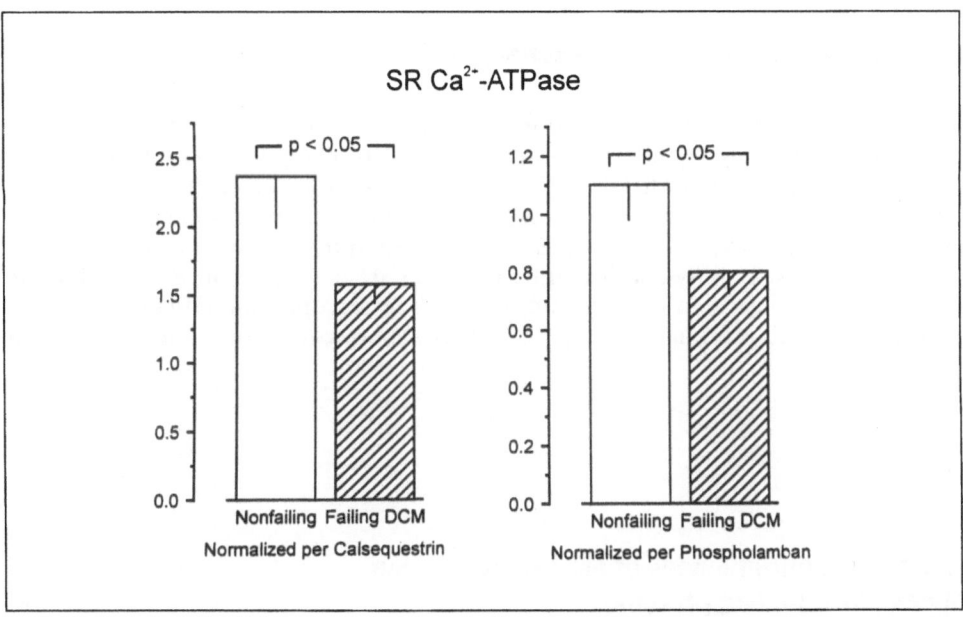

Fig. 2. Bar graph showing protein levels of sarcoplasmic reticulum (SR) Ca^{2+}-ATPase in nonfailing myocardium (NF) and in end-stage failing myocardium from hearts with dilated cardiomyopathy. Left, normalization was performed per protein levels of calsequestrin. Right, normalization was performed per protein levels of phospholamban. Decreased SR-Ca^{2+}-ATPase to phospholamban ratio may indicate decreased pump activity, because phospholamban inhibits the pump.

calcium pump within the SR membrane. The findings of unchanged protein levels of ryanodine receptor, calsequestrin, and calreticulin and decreased SR-Ca^{2+}-ATPase protein levels relative to calsequestrin, ryanodine receptor and phospholamban support the latter possibility. The present data do not allow to decide whether decreased levels of SR-Ca^{2+}-ATPase result from a selective down-regulation of the expression of this protein or from a lack of upregulation in the presence of a hypertrophy-associated increased expression of other myocyte and nonmyocyte proteins in the failing myocardium.

Sarcolemmal calcium pump

The sarcolemmal calcium pump is not homologous with the SR-Ca^{2+}-ATPase and has a different ATP to calcium stoichiometry (19, 37). Rate of calcium transport by this pump seems to be small compared to that of SR-Ca^{2+}-ATPase, and therefore, this pump is not considered to quantitatively contribute to beat to beat calcium elimination and myocardial relaxation (6). Data on expression or function of the sarcolemmal calcium pump in human myocardium are not available.

Sarcolemmal sodium-calcium exchanger

The Na^+-Ca^{2+}-exchanger is the dominant myocardial calcium efflux mechanism which may contribute significantly to relaxation. However, it can also promote calcium influx into the cytosol. The Na^+-Ca^{2+}-exchanger transports three sodium ions for one calcium ion resulting in a net inward current. It has been shown that mRNA as well as protein levels are significantly increased in the failing human heart (47). This finding was recently confirmed by Flesch et al. (14). It is conceivable that the Na^+-Ca^{2+}-exchanger can compensate for reduced sarcoplasmic reticulum calcium removal since this protein has been shown to be a powerful extrusion mechanism for calcium (5, 40).

Functional consequences of altered expression of calcium handling proteins

There is considerable evidence that altered levels and function of proteins relevant for calcium elimination from the cytosol are of pathophysiological relevance in human heart failure. It was shown recently that decreased SR-Ca^{2+}-ATPase protein levels are closely related to altered force-frequency relation and altered post-rest potentiation of the failing human heart (21, 41, 42). This relation between protein levels and myocardial function may be explained by the following mechanisms: In myocardium with a high expression of the SR-Ca^{2+}-ATPase the increase in contractile force at higher stimulation rates may result from an increased amount of calcium released from the sarcoplasmic reticulum. This may be the consequence of a larger amount of calcium entering the cell at higher heart rates and of an increased loading of the SR in the presence of a high capacity for SR calcium accumulation. This may also be associated with post-rest potentiation (42). In myocardium with a low expression of the SR-Ca^{2+}-ATPase, the decrease in twitch tension at higher rates of stimulation may result from a decreased amount of calcium released from the SR. The decreased calcium release may occur because the higher stimulation frequency reduces the time available for calcium transport, which in presence of a reduced calcium transport capacity may cause SR calcium depletion. Likewise, decreased calcium accumulation during rest may explain blunted post-rest potentiation of the failing human heart (42). In addition to decreased SR-Ca^{2+}-ATPase protein levels, altered function of the pump or of other calcium handling proteins may be involved in altered force-frequency relation, altered post-rest potentiation, and reduced myocardial function in failing human myocardium.

In the failing heart with increased expression of the sarcolemmal Na^+-Ca^{2+}-exchanger, transsarcolemmal calcium elimination may compete with SR calcium removal. Calcium elimination by the Na^+-Ca^{2+}-exchanger may preserve low diastolic calcium levels and prevent the rise of diastolic force. Accordingly, it was shown recently that diastolic function in myocardium from end-stage failing human hearts is closely related to protein levels of Na^+-Ca^{2+}-exchanger; in failing hearts with high Na^+-Ca^{2+}-exchanger protein levels diastolic function was normal (22). Of course, calcium extruded by Na^+-Ca^{2+}-exchanger is no longer available for activation of contractile proteins during systole. Further studies are warranted to evaluate the regulatory mechanisms which decrease SR-Ca^{2+}-ATPase and increase Na^+-Ca^{2+}-exchanger protein levels in the failing heart.

Acknowledgements This study was supported by DFG grant HA 1233/3-2. G. Hasenfuss is an Established Investigator of the German Research Foundation (DFG, Heisenberg-Stipendium HA 1233/4-1).

REFERENCES

1. Arai M, Alpert NR, Periasamy M (1991) Cloning and characterization of the gene encoding rabbit cardiac calsequestrin. Gene 109: 275–279
2. Arai M, Hirosuke M, Periasamy M (1994) Sarcoplasmic reticulum gene expression in cardiac hypertrophy and heart failure. Circ Res 74: 555–564
3. Arai M, Alpert NR, MacLennan DH, Barton P, Periasamy M (1993) Alterations in sarcoplasmic reticulum gene expression in human heart failure: a possible mechanism for alterations in systolic and diastolic properties of the failing myocardium. Circ Res 72: 463–469
4. Barry WH, Bridge JHB (1993) Intracellular calcium homeostasis in cardiac myocytes. Circulation 87: 1806–1815
5. Bers DM, Christensen DM, Nguyen TX (1988) Can Ca^{2+} entry via Na^+-Ca^{2+}-exchange directly activate cardiac muscle contraction? J Mol Cell Cardiol 20: 405–414

6. Bers DM (1993) Na^+/Ca^{2+} exchange and the sarcolemmal calcium pump. In: Bers DM, ed. Excitation-Contraction Coupling and Cardiac Contractile Force. Dordrecht: Kluwer Academic Publishers: 71–92

7. Beuckelmann DJ, Näbauer M, Erdmann E (1992) Intracellular calcium handling in isolated ventricular myocytes from patients with terminal heart failure. Circulation 85: 1046–1055

8. Beuckelmann DH, Erdmann E (1992) Ca^{2+}-currents and intracellular $(Ca^{2+})_i$-transients in single ventricular myocytes isolated from terminally failing human myocardium. Bas Res Cardiol (Suppl) 87: 235–243

9. Brillantes AM, Allen P, Takahashi T, Izumo S, Marks AR (1992) Differences in cardiac calcium release channel (ryanodine receptor) expression in myocardium from patients with end-stage heart failure caused by ischemic versus dilated cardiomyopathy. Circ Res 71: 18–26

10. D'Agnolo A, Luciani GB, Mazzucco A, Gallucci V, Salviati G (1992) Contractile properties and Ca^{2+} release activity of the sarcoplasmic reticulum in dilated cardiomyopathy. Circulation 85: 518–525

11. Endo M (1977) Calcium release from the sarcoplasmic reticulum. Physiol Rev 57: 71–108

12. Fabiato A (1983) Calcium-induced release of calcium from the cardiac sarcoplasmic reticulum. Am J Physiol 245: C1–C14

13. Feldman AM, Ray PE, Silan CM, Mercer JA, Minobe W, Bristow MR (1991) Selective gene expression in failing human heart. Circulation 83: 1866–1872

14. Flesch M, Schwinger RHG, Schiffer F, Frank K, Süßkamp M, Kuhn-Regnier F, Arnold G, Böhm M (1996) Evidence for functional relevance of an enhanced expression of the Na^+-Ca^{2+}-exchanger in failing human myocardium. Circulation 94: 992–1002

15. Fliegel L, Ohnishi M, Carpenter MR, Khanna VK, Reithmeir RAF, MacLennan DH (1987) Amino acid sequence of fast-twitch skeletal muscle calsequestrin deduced from cDNA and peptide sequencing. Proc Natl Acad Sci USA 84: 1167–1171

16. Fujii J, Lytton J, Tada M, MacLennan DH (1987) Rabbit cardiac and slow-twitch muscle express the same phospholamban gene. FEBS Lett 227: 51–55

17. Go LO, Moschella MC, Watras J, Handa KK, Fyfe BS, Marks AR (1995) Differential regulation of two types of intracellular calcium release channels during end-stage heart failure. J Clin Invest 95: 888–894

18. Gwathmey JK, Copelas L, MacKinnon R, Schoen FJ, Feldman MD, Grossman W, Morgan JP (1987) Abnormal intracellular calcium handling in myocardium from patients with end-stage heart failure. Circ Res 61: 70–76

19. Hasenfuss G, Mulieri LA, Holubarsch C, Pieske B, Just H, Alpert NR (1992) Energetics of calcium cycling in nonfailing and failing human myocardium. In: Holtz J, Drexler H, Just H, eds. Cardiac Adaption in Heart Failure. Darmstadt: Steinkopff Verlag: 81–92

20. Hasenfuss G, Mulieri LA, Leavitt JB, Allen PD, Haeberle JR, Alpert NR (1992) Alteration of contractile function and excitation-contraction coupling in dilated cardiomyopathy. Circ Res 70: 1225–1232

21. Hasenfuss G, Reinecke H, Studer R, Meyer M, Pieske B, Holtz J, Holubarsch C, Posival H, Just H, Drexler H (1994) Relation between myocardial function and expression of sarcoplasmic reticulum Ca^{2+}-ATPase in failing and nonfailing human myocardium. Circ Res 75: 434–442

22. Hasenfuss G, Preuss M, Lehnart S, Prestle J, Meyer M, Just H (1996) Relationship between diastolic function and protein levels of sodium-calcium-exchanger in end-stage failing human hearts. Circulation (Suppl 8) 94: I-433

23. Holmberg SRM, Williams AJ (1989) Single channel recordings from human cardiac sarcoplasmic reticulum. Circ Res 65: 1445–1449

24. Hullin R, Biel M, Flockerzi V, Hofmann F (1993) Tissue-specific expression of calcium channels. Trends Cardiovasc Med 3: 48–53

25. James P, Inui M, Tada M, Chiesi M, Carofoli E (1989) Nature and site of phospholamban regulation of the Ca^{2+} pump of sarcoplasmic reticulum. Nature 342: 90–92

26. Kranias EG, Garvey JL, Srivastava RD, Solaro RJ (1985) Phosphorylation and functional modifications of sarcoplasmic reticulum and myofibrils in isolated rabbit hearts stimulated with isoprenaline. Biochem J 226: 113–121

27. Kim HW, Steenaart NAE, Ferguson DG, Kranias EG (1990) Functional reconstitution of the cardiac sarcoplasmic reticulum Ca^{2+}-ATPase with phospholamban in phospholipid vesicles. J Biol Chem 265: 1702–1709

28. Linck B, Boknik P, Eschenhagen T, Müller FU, Neumann J, Nose M, Jones LR, Schmitz W, Scholz H (1996) Messenger RNA expression and immunological quantification of phospholamban and SR-Ca^{2+}-ATPase in failing and nonfailing human hearts. Cardiovasc Res 31: 625–632

29. Lytton J, MacLennan DH (1991) Sarcoplasmic reticulum. In: Fozzard HA, Hennings RB, Haber E, Katz AM (eds) The Heart and Cardiovascular System. New York, NY: Raven Press Inc; 1203–1222

30. MacLennan DH, Wong PTS (1971) Isolation of a calcium sequestering protein from sarcoplasmic reticulum. Proc Natl Acad Sci USA 68: 1231–1235
31. Marks AR, Tempst P, Hwang KS, Taubman MB, Inui M, Chadwick C, Fleischer S, Nadal-Ginard B (1989) Molecular cloning and characterization of the ryanodine receptor/junctional channel complex cDNA from skeletal muscle sarcoplasmic reticulum. Proc Natl Acad Sci USA 86: 8683–8687
32. Mercadier JJ, Lompre AM, Duc P, Boheler KR, Fraysse JB, Wisnewsky C, Allen PD, Komajda M, Schwartz K (1990) Altered sarcoplasmic reticulum Ca^{2+}-ATPase gene expression in the human ventricle during end-stage heart failure. J Clin Invest 85: 305–309
33. Meyer M, Schillinger W, Pieske B, Holubarsch C, Heilmann C, Posival H, Kuwajima G, Mikoshiba K, Just H, Hasenfuss G (1995) Alterations of sarcoplasmic reticulum proteins in failing human dilated cardiomyopathy. Circulation 92: 778–784
34. Michalak M, Milner RE, Burns K, Opas M (1992) Calreticulin. Biochem J 285: 681–692
35. Movsesian MA, Karimi M, Green K, Jones LR (1994) Ca^{2+}-transporting ATPase, phospholamban, and calsequestrin levels in nonfailing and failing human myocardium. Circulation 90: 653–657
36. Nagai R, Zarain-Herzberg A, Brandl CJ, Fujii J, Tada M, MacLennan DH, Alpert NR, Periasamy M (1989) Regulation of myocardial Ca^{2+}-ATPase and phospholamban mRNA expression in response to pressure overload and thyroid hormone. Proc Natl Acad Sci USA 86: 2966–2970
37. Niggli E, Adunyha ES, Penniston JT, Carafoli E (1981) Purified $(Ca^{2+}\text{-}Mg^{2+})$-ATPase of the erythrocyte membrane. J Biol Chem 256: 395–401
38. Nimer LR, Needleman DH, Hamilton SL, Krall J, Movsesian MA (1995) Effect of ryanodine on sarcoplasmic reticulum Ca^{2+} accumulation in nonfailing and failing human myocardium. Circulation 92: 2504–2510
39. Otsu K, Willard HF, Khanna VK, Zorzato F, Green NM, MacLennan DH (1990) Molecular cloning of cDNA encoding the Ca^{2+} release channel (ryanodine receptor) of rabbit cardiac muscle sarcoplasmic reticulum. J Biol Chem 265: 13472–13483
40. Philipson KD (1990) The cardiac $Na^{+}\text{-}Ca^{2+}$-exchanger. In: Langer GA (ed.) Calcium and the Heart. Raven Press, New York, pp 85–108
41. Pieske B, Kretschmann B, Meyer M, Holubarsch C, Weirich J, Posival H, Minami K, Just H, Hasenfuss G (1995) Alterations in intracellular calcium handling associated with the inverse force-frequency relation in human dilated cardiomyopathy. Circulation 92: 1169–1178
42. Pieske B, Sütterlin M, Schmidt-Schweda S, Minami K, Meyer M, Olschewski M, Holubarsch C, Just H, Hasenfuss G (1996) Diminished post-rest potentiation of contractile force in human dilated cardiomyopathy. J Clin Invest 98: 764–776
43. Piot C, Lemaire S, Albat B, Seguin J, Nargeot J, Richard S (1996) High frequency-induced upregulation of human cardiac calcium currents. Circulation 93: 120–128
44. Rasmussen RP, Minobe W, Bristow MR (1990) Calcium antagonist binding sites in failing and nonfailing human ventricular myocardium. Biochem Pharmacol 39: 691–696
45. Schillinger W, Meyer M, Kuwajima G, Mikoshiba K, Just H, Hasenfuss G (1996) Unaltered ryanodine receptor protein levels in ischemic cardiomyopathy. Mol Cell Biochem 160/161: 297–302
46. Schwinger RH, Böhm M, Schmidt U, Karczewski P, Bavendiek U, Flesch M, Krause EG, Erdmann E (1995) Unchanged protein levels of SERCA II and phospholamban but reduced Ca^{2+} uptake and Ca^{2+}-ATPase activity of cardiac sarcoplasmic reticulum from dilated cardiomyopathy patients compared with patients with nonfailing hearts. Circulation 92: 3220–3228
47. Studer R, Reinecke H, Bilger J, Eschenhagen T, Böhm M, Hasenfuss G, Just H, Holtz J, Drexler H (1994) Gene expression of the cardiac $Na^{+}\text{-}Ca^{2+}$-exchanger in end-stage human heart failure. Circ Res 75: 443–453
48. Swynghedauw B (1986) Developmental and functional adaptation of contractile proteins in cardiac and skeletal muscles. Physiol Rev 66: 710–771
49. Takahashi T, Allen PD, Lacro RV, Marks AR, Dennis AR, Schoen FJ, Grossman W, Marsh JD, Izumo S (1992) Expression of dihydropyridine receptor (Ca^{2+} cannel) and calsequestrin genes in the myocardium of patients with end-stage heart failure. J Clin Invest 90: 927–935
50. Wagenknecht T, Grassucci R, Frank J, Saito A, Inui M, Fleischer S (1989) Three dimensional architecture of the calcium channel/foot structure of sarcoplasmic reticulum. Nature 338: 167–170

Authors' address:
G. Hasenfuss, MD
Medizinische Klinik III
Universität Freiburg
Hugstetter Str. 55
79106 Freiburg, Germany

Role of cAMP in modulating relaxation kinetics and the force-frequency relation in mitral regurgitation heart failure

L. A. Mulieri, B. J. Leavitt[1], R. K. Wright[2], N. R. Alpert

Dept. Molec. Physiol. & Biophys., Given Building, University of Vermont, Burlington, USA
[1] Dept. Surgery, Given Building, University of Vermont, Burlington, USA
[2] Dept. Mathematics, University of Vermont, Burlington, USA

Abstract

The report is a discussion of previously published and newly analyzed results concerning the association between heart diseases and alterations in the force-frequency relation (FFR). The optimum stimulation frequency of the FFR is measured and compared in isolated left ventricular myocardium from non-failing hearts with atrial septal defect, coronary artery disease (without and with insulin dependent diabetes mellitus) and from failing hearts with mitral regurgitation, or idiopathic dilated cardiomyopathy. Specfically, we examine the role of altered *control* of the excitation-contraction coupling system in blunting the force-frequency relation. We use the percent slope of the FFR as a measure of changes in the frequency sensitivity of this *control*. Our finding of a linear, direct relation between optimum stimulation frequency and % slope across all disease types suggests both parameters are coupled to the same underlying mechanism. To investigate the possible role of altered *control* of the calcium pump in this mechanism, we analyzed the detailed relation between isometric twitch relaxation kinetics and stimulation frequency in mitral regurgitation myocardium (MR). In the presence of 0.5 μM forskolin the depressed slope and optimum frequency of the FFR and the prolonged half-time of twitch relaxation were all restored to values found in non-failing myocardium. We use the kinetics of isometric twitch relaxation as an index of changes in pumping rate that occur in response to changes in stimulation frequency or in intracellular cyclic adenosine monophosphate concentration. A mathematical model based on the Hill relations for calcium pump uptake rate and for isometric tension as a function of intracellular pCa is developed to simulate isometric twitch relaxation in MR and non-failing myocardium. The success of this model in simulating non-failing and failing twitch relaxation supports a proposed mechanism for the prolonged relaxation time and depressed FFR in MR involving depressed protein kinase-A activity (due to lowered cAMP or to a defect in the Ser^{16} site of phospholamban) as a mechanism of altered *control* of the calcium pump in MR heart disease.

Key words Frequency treppe – atrial septal defect – coronary artery disease – insulin dependent diabetes mellitus – idiopathic dilated cardiomyopathy – excitation-contraction coupling – calcium pump – SERCA2A – forskolin – protein kinase-A – cAMP – CaM-K

Introduction

In mitral regurgitation heart (MR) failure left ventricular circumferential fiber shortening velocity is depressed 40 % in the presence of normal was stress (7, 10, 11). Some of this depression is attributable to alterations in cross-bridge function since there is a 50 % depression of myofibrillar ATPase activity (29, 30) and an 85 % increase in cross-bridge force-time integral suggesting an increased duration of cross-bridge attachment time (16). Excitation-contraction coupling (ECC) alterations also occur. There is a blunting of the slope of the force-frequency relation ("positive frequency treppe") and a shifting of its optimum frequency (f_o) or beginning of the descending limb (negative treppe) to subnormal (15 – 120 BPM) contraction frequencies (5, 21, 22, 24). Similar abnormalities occur in end-stage failure in idiopathic dilated cardiomyopathy (IDCM) (9, 25, 31, 36). Figure 1 summarizes shifts in the peak of the force-frequency relation observed in various disease types. The rightmost three curves, atrial septal defect (ASD), coronary artery disease (CAD), and CAD with insulin dependent diabetes mellitus (CAD + IDDM) are from-non-failing (NF) hearts with normal left ventricular (LV) wall motion and normal ejection fractions

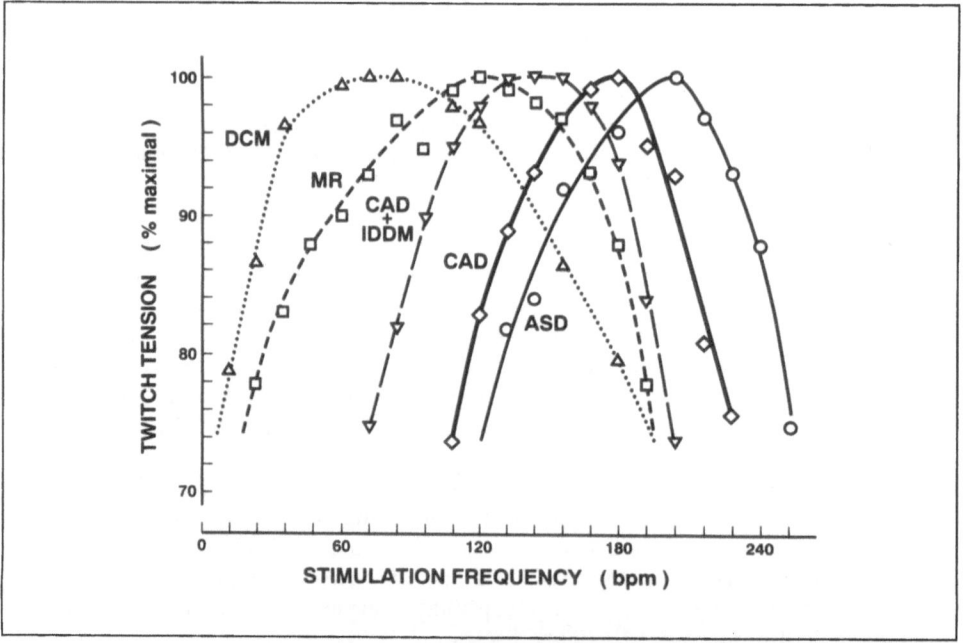

Fig. 1. Normalized force-frequency relations in human left ventricular myocardial strip preparations from diseased hearts. Isometric twitch tension at the peak of the tension-length relation divided by maximal twitch tension achieved at optimal stimulation frequency (f_o). Disease type, f_o (bpm), number of hearts, respectively are: Atrial Septal Defect (ASD), 204 ± 7, 1; Coronary Artery Disease (CAD with normal LV function), 177 ± 4, 6; Coronary artery disease + Insulin Dependent Diabetes Mellitus (CAD+IDDM with normal LV function), 142 ± 11, 6; Mitral Regurgitation (MR in NYHA class II-III heart failure), 123 ± 14, 6; Idiopathic Dilated Cardiomyopathy (DCM in NYHA class IV heart failure), 81 ± 22, 6. Krebs-Ringer solution, $[Ca^{2+}]$ = 2.5 mM, 37 ° C.

(50 % – 60 %). The two curves with peaks below 120 bpm are from patients with mitral regurgitation (MR) heart failure (NYHA II-III) or idiopathic dilated cardio-myopathy (IDCM) heart failure (NYHA IV). There is a progressive lowering of the optimum stimulation frequency as the severity of heart disease increases. Note also that the 20 % reduction in optimum frequency in the non-failing, diabetic hearts (142 vs 177) suggests a possible myocardial basis for a functional deficit in "diabetic cardiomyopathy".

Our previous studies suggest that the *quantity* of calcium cycled in a twitch response is reduced by 50 % in MR (16) and by 69 % in IDCM (17). In the latter this reduction is accompanied by a depressed amplitude of the intracellular calcium trans-ient ($[Ca^{2+}]_{Sistolic} - [Ca^{2+}]_{Diastolic}$) during the twitch (2, 13, 32) and by a blunting of the stimulus frequency dependence of its amplitude (32). One possible mechanism for this alteration in ECC is a reduced number of calcium pumps ("SERCA2" which is composed mainly of SERCA2A with only a small percentage of SERCA2B) per sarcomere as suggested by the observation (18) of a significant inverse correlation between the optimal stimulation frequency and the concentration of the sarcoplas-mic reticulum calcium pump protein in different failing hearts as well as in non-failing hearts (Fig. 1 of Hasenfuss et al., this monograph). These studies show in addition that the *slope* of the tension-frequency relation correlates directly with concentration of the calcium pump (Fig. 2 of Hasenfuss et al., this monograph). This proportionality can be explained if the quantity of calcium released per action potential becomes limited by the quantity returned to the sarcoplasmic reticulum during diastole. If pump content is reduced incomplete reuptake occurs and this is exaggerated with

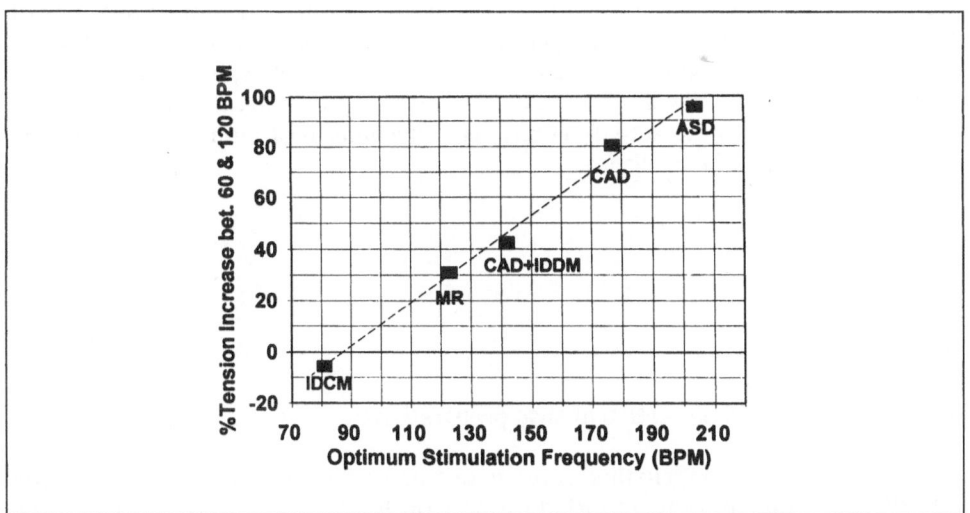

Fig. 2. Myocardial reserve vs optimum stimulation frequency in human left ventricular myocardial strip preparations from diseased hearts. Reserve is calculated as the % increase in peak twitch tension when contraction frequency is increased from 60 to 120 bpm. The following symbols are used: Atrial Septal Defect (ASD), Coronary Artery Disease with normal LV function (CAD), Coronary artery disease + Insulin Dependent Diabetes Mellitus with normal LV function (CAD+IDDM), Mitral Regurgitation with NYHA class II-III heart failure (MR), Idiopathic Dilated Cardiomyopathy with NYHA class IV heart failure (IDCM). Same preparations and conditions as in Fig. 1.

decreasing diastolic periods because the calcium pump uptake rate is insufficient to recover all of the calcium released in the previous systole. While it is recognized that changes in the sarcoplasmic reticulum ryanodine receptor or in the sodium/calcium exchanger may also contribute to alterations in the force-frequency relation (FFR), we simplify the present discussion by considering only the effects of SERCA2 on the FFR. Thus the slope of the ascending limb of the frequency treppe is considered an index of SERCA2 pumping rate reserve and is here considered as a quantitative measure of myocardial contractile reserve.

While these SERCA2 data suggest reduced calcium pumping *capacity* may contribute to the depressed myocardial contractile reserve, there is also evidence suggesting that an abnormality in *control* of the ECC system can be involved. Elevation of intracellular cAMP with forskolin can restore the positive slope of the myocardial force-frequency relation in mitral regurgitation heart failure (26, 27) and in IDCM (9, 33). In end-stage IDCM, a positive slope was also reestablished by pharmacological elevation of intracellular Na+ (37) and by anesthetics (34). In Fig. 2 the slopes of the force-frequency relations shown in Fig. 1 have been plotted as the percent increase in peak twitch tension occurring between 60 and 120 bpm (% slope). This normalization emphasizes the effects of changes in *control* of the calcium pump accompanying these myopathies and reduces the effects of changes in pump concentration on the slope of the curves. Thus the marked, progressive decline in % slope in Fig. 2 suggests that some aspects of *control* of the excitation-contraction coupling system is progressively depressed across this spectrum of diseases, independent of any depression in [SERCA2] that may also be present. Furthermore the parallel, progressive decline in optimal contraction frequency that accompanies the % slope decline suggests a common factor may contribute to both parameters.

The present discussion examines the role of altered *control* of the excitation-contraction coupling system in depressing the force-frequency relation in mitral regurgitation heart failure. We use the kinetics of isometric twitch relaxation as an index of changes in SERCA2 pumping rate (1) that occur in response to changes in stimulation frequency or in intracellular cyclic adenosine monophosphate ([cAMP]). A mathematical model is developed and used to test the possibility that altered cAMP-dependent protein kinase activity (PKA) is a mechanism of altered *control* of the calcium pump in MR heart disease.

Methods

Myocardial biopsy and dissection of strip preparations

All relaxation kinetics data in this report were obtained by further analysis of records from the same preparations reported on previously (25). Subepicardial tissue was obtained from four mitral regurgitation patients (NYHA Class II-III failure, mean LV ejection fraction = 0.64 ± 0.05) and from four coronary artery bypass patients who had normal left ventricular wall motion and normal ventricular function. Surgical biopsies from the anterior segment of the left ventricular wall were obtained shortly after cardioplegic arrest (25). Patients gave informed, written consent before participating in the study which was approved by the Committee on Human Research of The University of Vermont. There were no complications resulting from the biopsy procedure in any patient. The excised tissue was immediately submerged in room temperature, pre-oxygenated BDM-protective solution (22). After a 60-min recovery from surgical trauma the tissue was dissected into thin strips approximately 0.2 mm in diameter (22, 23). Experiments were performed on two strip preparations from each of the eight hearts biopsied.

Apparatus and measurements

Isometric twitch tension was measured at the peak of the tension-length relation (L_{max}) in each of the two muscle strip preparations simultaneously using the same apparatus, methods, and protocols as described previously (23).

The steady-state force-frequency relation of each strip was obtained at 37 °C with 5 min of stimulation at each frequency starting at 0.2 Hz (12 BPM) and increasing in 0.2 Hz increments. Repeat measurements at 1 Hz and at f_o were made to confirm stability of the FFR. Peak twitch tension and half relaxation time parameters of the steady-state myograms were measured by digital readout and averaged at each frequency across all strips in each group (23, 25). The relaxation phase of the twitch myograms were digitized at 50 ms intervals and displayed on semi-log axes. The relaxation time constants (τ_R) were evaluated from a straight line fit to each log-plot. A 30-min equilibration was allowed between Forskolin addition and subsequent redetermination of the entire force-frequency relation. The length at L_{max} (4.84 ± 0.24 mm, Mean ± SEM) and the blotted weight (0.86 ± 0.13 mg) of the active portion of each muscle strip was measured and the quotient was used to calculate its cross-sectional area.

Results and discussion

Tension-frequency relation in failing and non-failing myocardium

The average tension-frequency curves obtained from non-failing and MR-failing myocardial strips are shown in Fig. 3. Tension at the peak of the MR curve is depressed by 62 % compared with the NF (CAD) peak value (dotted curve in Fig. 3). Frequency treppe between 60 and 120 bpm recruits only 3 mN/mm² in the MR preparations compared with 12 mN/mm² in the NF preparations. Addition of 0.5 μM Forskolin restores the MR tension-frequency curve to NF values, suggesting that frequency-dependent *control* of the calcium pump has been enhanced.

Twitch relaxation kinetics in failing and non-failing myocardium

Depressed calcium pump function in MR is suggested by the longer time to half-relaxation of the isometric twitch as shown in Fig. 4. The absence of a change in slope of the relaxation time vs stimulation frequency curve suggests the *frequency sensitivity*

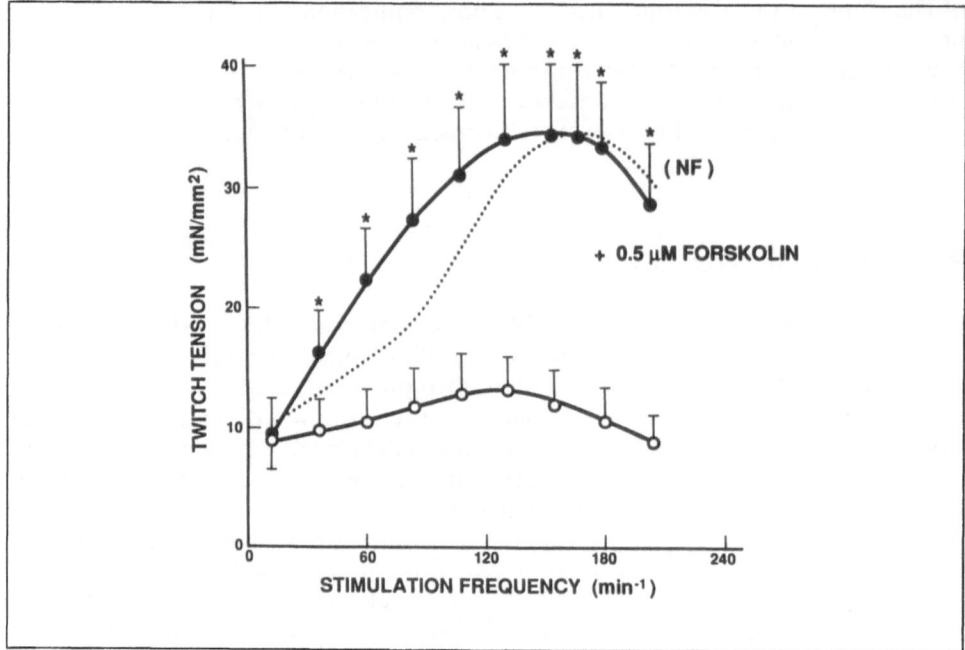

Fig. 3. Average tension-frequency curves from non-failing and failing Left Ventricular myocardial strip preparations. Dotted line: non-failing (NF) preparations (n = 8, Standard errors not shown) adapted from Mulieri et al. (27); Solid lines: mitral regurgitation (MR) preparations (n = 9) in the absence (lower curve) and presence (upper curve) of 0.5 μM Forskolin. Temperature 37 °C.

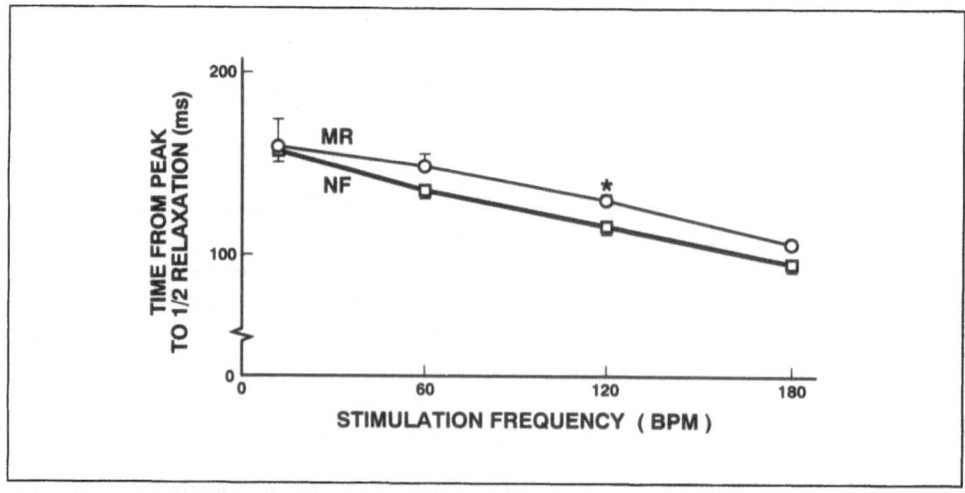

Fig. 4. Average half-relaxation time of isometric twitches vs stimulation frequency. Time from peak of twitch to 50 % relaxation of tension in non-failing (squares) and MR-failing (circles) left ventricular myocardial strip preparations. Same preparations as in Fig. 3 with * = p ≤ 0.05 for MR vs NF.

of the calcium pump control system is not impaired in MR. The *frequency sensitivity* also remains constant in the presence of Forskolin as shown by the parallel downward shift of the MR curve in Fig. 5. Forskolin reduces the half-relaxation times in MR by 50 ms compared with the values from the NF preparations (Fig. 4) in the absence of forskolin.

At physiological temperatures the decay of isometric twitch tension is more strongly controlled by calcium uptake kinetics than by cross-bridge off-rate (Bers, this monograph; and unpublished observations of cross-bridge force decay rates in NF and MR by D. W. Maughan and L. A. Mulieri, 1995). Since isometric twitch relaxation kinetics in early relaxation are controlled by the negative-velocity portion of the force-velocity relation as well as by $[Ca^{2+}]_i$, quantitation of calcium pump activity is better assessed late in the relaxation phase of the twitch after most of the series elastic stretch has been dissipated. Figure 6 shows the average relaxation myograms for MR and NF preparations at 120 bpm in the absence and presence of Forskolin. Straight lines were fitted to semi-log plots (see inset) starting 150 ms after the peak of the twitch to evaluate the time constant of relaxation (τ_R) for each preparation. Figure 7 shows the average τ_R values for both MR and NF at 120 bpm. The relaxation time constant is 57.3 ± 3.9 ms in NF and it is increased by 30 % to 74.6 ± 4.9 (p < 0.03) in the MR preparations. This 30 % increase suggests the calcium pump is running 30 % slower in MR than in NF preparations. Addition of Forskolin reduces τ_R to 29 ms in both preparations. Since τ_R in MR and NF are equal in the presence of Forskolin the 30 % longer value in the absence of Forskolin in MR compared with NF is not likely caused by the increased cross-bridge force-time integral in MR (16).

Theoretical analysis and possible mechanism of c-AMP effects

Figure 8 shows a proposed mechanisms of *control* of SERCA2 which allows independent control of twitch relaxation kinetics and of the *frequency sensitivity* of this con-

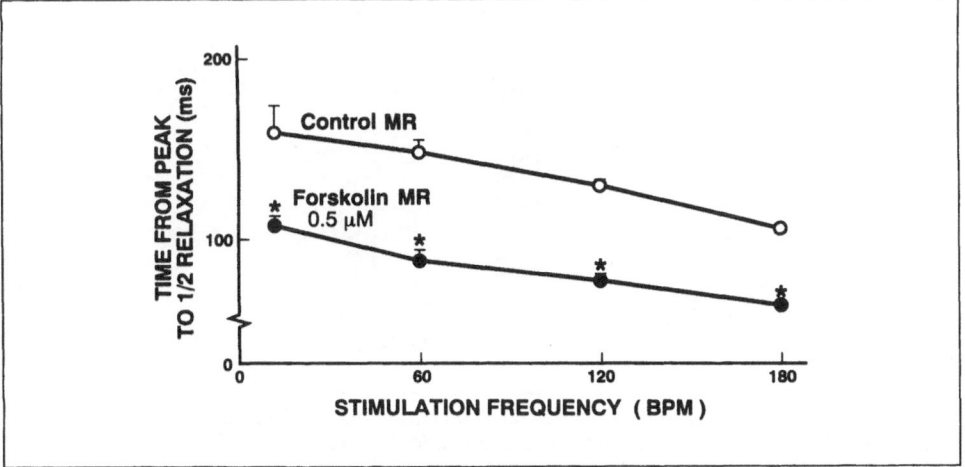

Fig. 5. Effect of Forskolin on average half-relaxation time of isometric twitches in mitral regurgitation preparations. Same MR preparations as in Fig. 4 with * = p ≤ 0.05 for Forskolin MR vs Control MR.

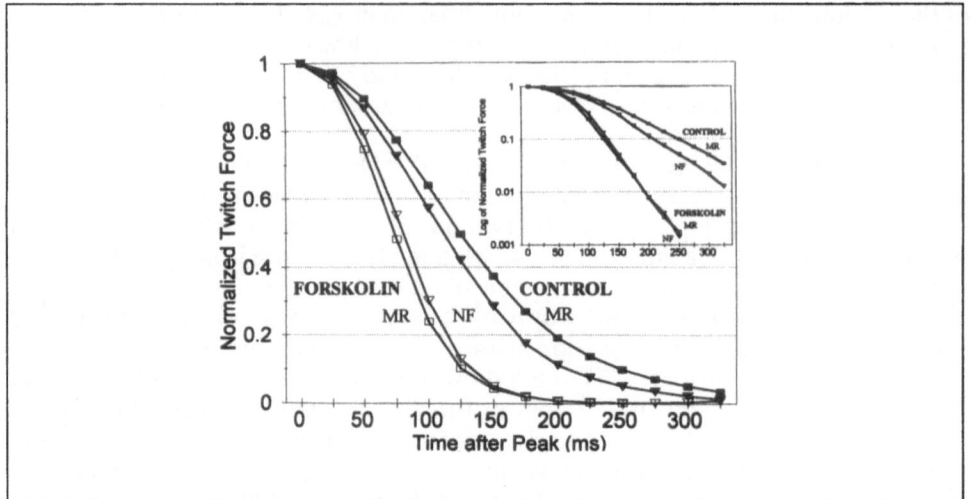

Fig. 6. Average normalized relaxation myograms in non-failing and failing myocardial strip preparations at 120 bpm. Isometric force divided by peak isometric twitch force in non-failing (NF, triangles, n = 5) and mitral regurgitation-failing (MR, rectangles, n = 5) preparations without (CONTROL, filled symbols), and with 0.5 μM forskolin (FORSKOLIN, unfilled symbols). *Inset:* Same data plotted semi-logarithmically.

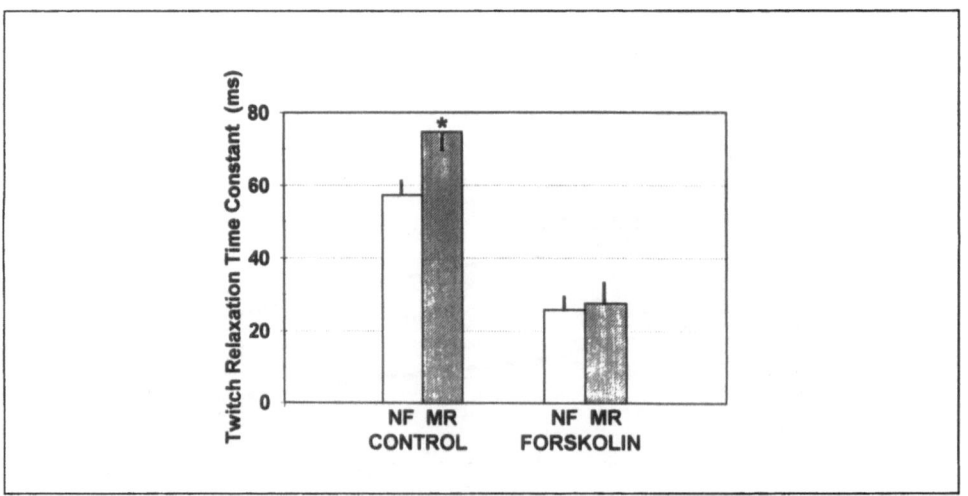

Fig. 7. Mean time constants of isometric twitch relaxation in non-failing and failing myocardial strip preparations. The following symbols and abbreviations are used: hatched bars for mitral regurgitation (MR) preparations, unfilled bars for non-failing (NF) preparations. Experiments carried out in the absence (CONTROL) and presence (FORSKOLIN) of 0.5 μM forskolin. Same preparations as in Fig. 6, 37 °C, 120 bpm.

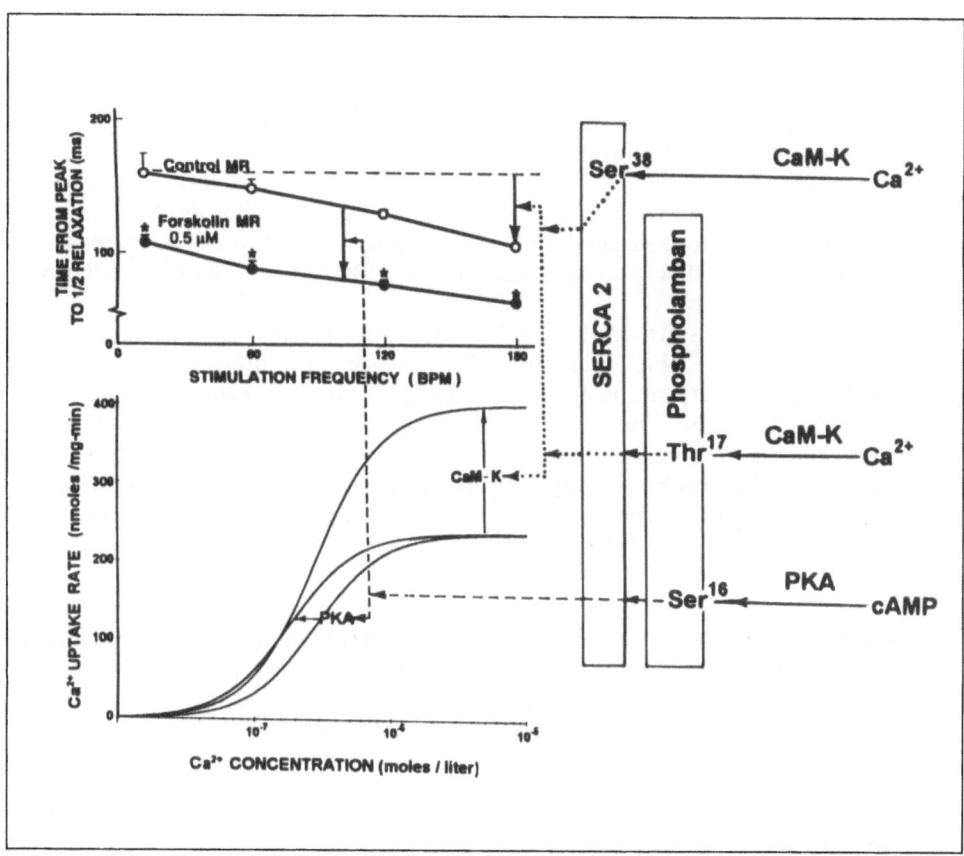

Fig. 8. Frequency-dependent and frequency-independent control of twitch relaxation kinetics. Solid, horizontal arrows: myoplasmic activating agents (Ca^{2+}, cAMP); Dashed or dotted, horizontal arrows: molecular or cellular functions controlled by site-specific phosphorylation (see below); Dashed or dotted, vertical arrows: cell function correlates of molecular functions controlled by PKA or CaM-K.

Top left panel. Frequency-dependence of half-relaxation time in mitral regurgitation (MR) heart failure in normal Krebs-Ringer (Control MR) and with 0.5 μM forskolin added (Forskolin MR), 37 °C. Data from Fig. 5.

Right panel. Mechanisms of *Control* of SR-Calcium pump (SERCA2) by *selective* phosphorylation of serine and threonine sites on SERCA2 (Ser[38]) and phospholamban (Ser[16] and Thr[17]) (19, 38, 40). PKA = cAMP-dependent protein kinase A, CaM-K = calcium-calmodulin dependent protein kinase.

Lower left panel. SERCA2 pumping rate *vs* [Ca^{2+}] calculated from the Hill relation (see Eq. (2)) with the following values for V_{max} (nmoles/mg-min), K_{50} (nM), and m, respectively: **Rightmost, lower curve** for dephosphorylated Ser[16] and Thr[17]: 238, 178 × 1.57 = 280, 1.75 (Values from Toyofuku et al. (39) with K_{50} multiplied by 1.57 according to the effect of PKA blocking shown by Bassani et al. (1) (Fig. 8A); **Left-shifted, lower curve** showing the effect of Ser[16] phosphorylation: 238, 178, 1.75; **Elevated, CaM-K curve** showing the effect of Thr[17] phosphorylation: 402, 178, 1.75 (39).

trol. As originally suggested by Schouten (35) and recently substantiated by Bassani et al. (1) calcium-calmodulin dependent protein kinase (CaM-K), by virtue of its Ca^{2+} retaining property (Ca^{2+} release rate < binding rate, see below), can confer the necessary *frequency sensitive* control of SERCA2 to account for frequency treppe.

With increasing stimulation frequency CaM-K (lower right in Fig. 8) accumulates Ca^{2+} and thereby increases the phosphorylation level of phospholamban (1, 20, 28). This accumulation occurs because Ca^{2+} is supplied to CaM-K at increasingly greater rates than its slow Ca^{2+} release rate (41) can accommodate. The resulting increase in CaM-K mediated phosphorylation of the threonine site (Thr^{17}) on phospholamban selectively (39) increases V_{max} of SERCA2 (top Hill curve at the lower left of Fig. 8) and causes the progressive decrease in the half-relaxation time of the twitch (downward slope of the Control MR curve in Fig. 8, top left). V_{max} may also be increased by direct CaM-K action (19, 41) on the serine site (Ser^{38}) of SERCA2 independently of phospholamban.

The parallel upward shifting of the relaxation time vs stimulation frequency relation that occurs with MR (Fig. 4) and the parallel downward shift caused by Forskolin (Fig. 5 or Fig. 8, top left) can be attributed to a leftward shift of the SERCA2 pumping rate vs [Ca^{2+}] relation. This shift results from c-AMP dependent protein kinase A (PKA) phosphorylation of the serine site (Ser^{16}) on phospholamban (Fig. 8, lower right). We tested the feasibility of attributing the MR-induced changes in relaxation kinetics (and in the FFR) to changes in the dissociation constant of the Hill equation relating SERCA2 pumping rate to [Ca^{2+}] by developing the following simplified model for relaxation of the isometric twitch. We restricted the analysis to only the latter portion of relaxation when series elastic stretch is largely discharged and tension decline is mainly controlled by the decline in number of attached crossbridges (see above). This assumption allows the steady-state isometric tension-pCa relation to be used to approximate instantaneous twitch tension during relaxation of the isometric twitch. The Hill equation for this relation is:

$$\text{Force production} = \frac{F}{F_{max}} = \frac{[Ca]^n}{Ca_{50}{}^n + [Ca]^n}, \tag{1}$$

where F and F_{max} represent the isometric force generated at subsaturating and saturating levels of calcium concentrations ([Ca]), respectively. Ca_{50} is the calcium concentration with produces a force equal to 50 % of F_{max} and n is a constant related to the stoichiometry of the Ca^{2+}-Troponin C-Troponin I complex. The calculated time-course of tension relaxation was obtained by substituting a time-varying expression ([Ca](t)) for [Ca] in Eq. (1). To obtain [Ca](t) we assumed the decline in [Ca] during relaxation was entirely controlled by SERCA2 pumping and that this pumping rate (V) is given by the following Hill relation:

$$\text{Calcium pump rate} = V = -\frac{d[Ca]}{dt} = \frac{V_{max}[Ca]^m}{K_{50}{}^m + [Ca]^m}, \tag{2}$$

where V and V_{max} represent calcium pumping rates at subsaturating and saturating levels of myoplasmic calcium concentrations ([Ca]), respectively, -d[Ca]/dt is the rate of disappearance of Ca^{2+} from the myoplasm, K_{50} is the [Ca] at which the pumping rate is 50 % of its maximum value, and m is a constant related Ca^{2+} binding and transport by SERCA2. Equation (2) was used to generate the pump rate curves in the lower left of Fig. 8.

Since Eq. (2) cannot be solved explicitly for [Ca](t) the alternative solution for t as a function of [Ca] was obtained by straightforward integration of (2) in inverted form to give:

$$t = \frac{[Ca]}{V_{max}} - \frac{[Ca]_{t=0}}{V_{max}} \cdot \frac{K_{50}{}^m([Ca]^{(1-m)} - [Ca]_{t=0}{}^{(1-m)}}{V_{max}{}^{(1-m)}} , \tag{3}$$

where $[Ca]_{t=0}$ is the myoplasmic calcium concentration at the start of the simulated relaxation. Equation (3) was solved numerically by Newton's method. Instabilities (i.e. negative predicted values of [Ca] that can occur in regions where the slope of the solution curve changes rapidly) were avoided by successively halving the size of the Newton steps until a positive-valued prediction was produced. The calculated numerical values of [Ca] and t were substituted into Eq. (1) to generate the time-course of isometric tension relaxation shown in Fig. 9. All calculations were implemented by a PC-based mathematical computation program (Maple V, Release 3, Waterloo Maple Software, Waterloo, Ontario).

In the absence of Ser[16] phosphorylation ($K_{50} = 280$) the relaxation time constant of the simulated twitch evaluated from the linear portion of the semi-log plot in Fig. 9 is 76 ms. This is 30 % longer than it is when this site on phospholamban is phosphorylated ($K_{50} = 178$). This simulated result corresponds well with the 30 % difference between τ_R in MR and NF and NF myocardium shown in Figs. 6 and 7.

Conclusion. The depressed % slope of the FFR in MR myocardium, in combination with the increased τ_R of twitch relaxation, are interpreted here to be caused by reduced SERCA2-Ca^{2+}ATPase activity. The restoration of the slope of the FFR in MR myocardium to its NF value by Forskolin demonstrates the role of changes in *control* of the calcium pump on the FFR and on the twitch relaxation time constant. This model-based analysis shows that phosphorylation-dependent changes in the K_{50} of the calcium pump-Hill relation alone can account for the increased τ_R of twitch relaxation in MR myocardium and presumably, for the depressed % slope of the FFR.

This analysis suggests that decreased myoplasmic [cAMP] may account for the slowed relaxation in MR. Involvement of cAMP in depressed calcium cycling in IDCM heart failure was originally suggested by Morgan et al. who demonstrated that forskolin could improve calcium cycling and increase the slope of the FFR (8, 9). Although levels of cAMP in soluble fractions prepared from non-beating, explanted IDCM hearts were not depressed (4), under more physiological conditions (37C and 30 bpm) a 63 % depression in cAMP levels has been observed (6). A similar depression may also be present in MR myocardium. It is also possible that myoplasmic [cAMP] is normal but that less in available for the phospholamban molecules that are interacting with SERCA2 molecules. Reduced availability of cAMP could be caused by competition from phospholamban molecules that are not associated with SERCA2 molecules, a condition suggested by recent observations in IDCM myocardium that SERCA2 levels are depressed in the presence of nearly normal levels of phospholamban (4, 15). Alternatively, in the presence of normal cAMP-PKA activity there could be a defect in the Ser[16] site on phospholamban or in its ability to modulate the interaction between phospholamban and SERCA2.

The present analysis also suggests the FFR improvements with forskolin in MR myocardium may be compensatory rather than curative. Restoration of NF slope values in MR myocardium (i.e., what we have termed: "reversal of the defect in the force-frequency relation" (27)) by 0.5 uM Forskolin is accompanied by a decrease in

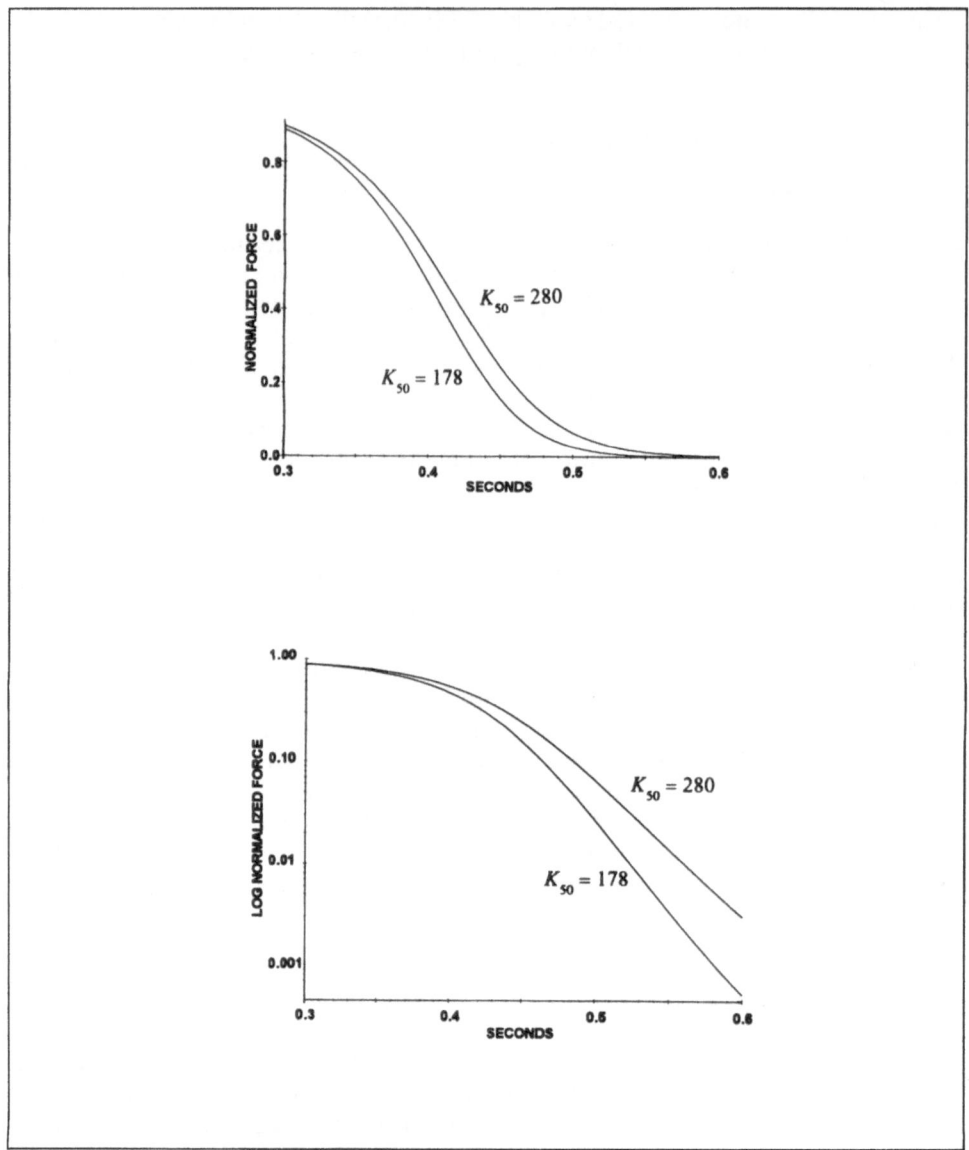

Fig. 9. Simulated twitch elaxation myograms at 120 bpm with and without phospholamban-Ser[16] phosphorylation. *Left panel.* Last 300 ms of simulated twitch relaxations with ($K_{50} = 178$) and without ($K_{50} = 280$) Ser[16] phosphorylation. *Right panel.* Same as left panel except for semi-log plotting to allow τ_R evaluation from slope of linear regions. The initial 300 ms of the simulated outputs were not used because the present, simplified model does not include the strong effect of cross-bridge cycling kinetics under negative velocity conditions on τ_R early after the peak of the twitch. Simulations were performed with the following constants.

For evaluation of the time-course of [Ca] (see Eq. (3)): $K_{50} = 175$, and 280 nM with, and without Ser[16] phosphorylation (see Fig. 8 legend for source); $m = 1.75$ (with no effect from posphorylation, Toyofuku et al. (39); $V_{max} = 400$ nM/sec (Average of values calculated from human myocardium data of Beuckelmann et al. (2) Fig. 3 (using Eq. (2) with $m = 1.75$ and $K_{50} = 178$ nM and correcting for the lower stimulation frequency) and the data of Hasenfuss et al. (17), Fig. 5 (with correction for non-SERCA2 contribution to tension independent heat according to Blanchard et al. (3)); $[Ca]_{t=0} = 200$ nM from Beuckelmann et al. (2).

For evaluation of time-course of force decay (Eq. 1): $F_{max} = 1$; [Ca] values from Eq. (3); n and $Ca_{50} = 4$ and 500 nM, respectively (average of values from Gwathmey and Hajjar (12) and Hajjar et al. (14).

τ_R to values that are 50 % shorter than in NF in absence of Forskolin. Because this abnormally short relaxation time constant accompanies restoration of the FFR in MR, we conclude that this restoration may include a compensation for an additional defect in calcium pumping that is not related to PKA *control* of SERCA2. In this case, if a lower forskolin concentration – adjusted to just achieve restoration of τ_R – were used, the defect in slope of the FFR would not be completely reversed. This result would be expected if an additional defect, possibly a reduced SERCA2 protein concentration, were also present in MR myocardium.

Acknowledgements   We thank Richard Lachapelle for apparatus maintenance and technical support and Julie Lovelette and Debra Pratt for typing and secretarial support. Supported in part by: USPHS P01HL2800-13.

REFERENCES

1. Bassani RA, Mattiazzi A, Bers DM (1995) CaMKII is responsible for activity-dependent acceleration of relaxation in rat ventricular myocytes. Am J Physiol 268: H703–12
2. Beuckelmann DJ, Nabauer M, Erdmann E (1992) Intracellular calcium handling in isolated ventricular myocytes from patients with terminal heart failure [see comments]. Circulation 85: 1046–1055
3. Blanchard EM, Mulieri LA, Alpert NR (1990) Dynamic calcium requirements for activation of rabbit papillary muscle calculated from tension-independent heat. Am J Cardiol 65: 8G–11G
4. Bohm M, Reiger B, Schwinger RH, Erdmann E (1994) cAMP concentrations, cAMP dependent protein kinase activity, and phospholamban in non-failing and failing myocardium. Cardiovasc Res 28: 1713–1719
5. Buckley NM, Penefsky ZJ, Litwak RS (1972) Comparative force-frequency relationships in human and other mammalian ventricular myocardium. Pflugers Arch 332: 259–270
6. Danielsen W, v. der Leyen H, Meyer W, Neumann J, Schmitz W, Scholz H, Starbatty J, Stein B, Doring V, Kalmar P (1989) Basal and isoprenaline-stimulated cAMP content in failing versus nonfailing human cardiac preparations. J Cardiovasc Pharmacol 14: 171–173
7. Eckberg DL, Gault JH, Bouchard RL, Karliner JS, Ross J Jr (1973) Mechanics of left ventricular contraction in chronic severe mitral regurgitation. Circulation 47: 1252–1259
8. Feldman MD, Copelas L, Gwathmey JK, Philips P, Warren SE, Schoen FJ, Grossman W, Morgan JP (1987) Deficient production of cyclic AMP: pharmacologic evidence of an important cause of contractile dysfunction in patients with end-stage heart failure. Circulation 75: 331–339
9. Feldman MD, Gwathmey JK, Philips P, Schoen F, Morgan JP (1988) Reversal of the force-frequency relationship in working myocardium from patients with end-stage heart failure. J Applied Cardiology 3: 273–283
10. Goldfine HL, Aurigemma GP, Gaasch WH (1992) Mechanism of reduction in ejection fraction following mitral valve replacement for mitral regurgitation. Circulation 86: I-660
11. Goldman ME, Mora F, Guarino T, Fuster V, Mindich BP (1987) Mitral valvuloplasty is superior to valve replacement for preservation of left ventricular function: an intraoperative two-dimensional echocardiographic study. J Am Coll Cardiol 10: 568–575
12. Gwathmey JK, Hajjar RJ (1990) Relation between steady-state force and intracellular $[Ca^{2+}]$ in intact human myocardium. Index of myofibrillar responsiveness to Ca^{2+}. Circulation 82: 1266–1278
13. Gwathmey JK, Slawsky MT, Hajjar RJ, Briggs GM, Morgan JP (1990) Role of intracellular calcium handling in force-interval relationships of human ventricular myocardium. J Clin Invest 85: 1599–1613
14. Hajjar RJ, Gwathmey JK, Briggs GM, Morgan JP (1988) Differential effect of DPI 201–106 on the sensitivity of the myofilaments to Ca^{2+} in intact and skinned trabeculae from control and myopathic human hearts. J Clin Invest 82: 1578–1584
15. Hasenfuss G, Meyer M, Schillinger W, Pieske B, Scheffler A, Holubarsch C, Reinecke H (1994) Expression of sarcoplasmic reticulum proteins in failing and non-failing human myocardium. Circulation 90: I-216
16. Hasenfuss G, Mulieri LA, Blanchard EM, Holubarsch C, Leavitt BJ, Ittleman F, Alpert NR (1991) Energetics of isometric force development in control and volume-overload human myocardium. Comparison with animal species. Circ Res 68: 836–846

17. Hasenfuss G, Mulieri LA, Leavitt BJ, Allen PD, Haeberle JR, Alpert NR (1992) Alteration of contractile function and excitation-contraction coupling in dilated cardiomyopathy. Circ Res 70: 1225–1232
18. Hasenfuss G, Mulieri LA, Leavitt BJ, Alpert NR (1994) Influence of isoproterenol on contractile protein function, excitation-contraction coupling, and energy turnover of isolated nonfailing human myocardium. J Mol Cell Cardiol 26: 1461–1469
19. Hawkins C, Xu A, Narayanan N (1994) Sarcoplasmic reticulum calcium pump in cardiac and slow twitch skeletal muscle but not fast twitch skeletal muscle undergoes phosphorylation by endogenous and exogenous Ca^{2+}/calmodulin-dependent protein kinase. Characterization of optimal conditions for calcium pump phosphorylation. J Biol Chem 269: 31198–31206
20. Mattiazzi A, Hove-Madsen L, Bers DM (1994) Protein kinase inhibitors reduce SR Ca transport in permeabilized cardiac myocytes. Am J Physiol 267: H812–20
21. Mulieri LA, Hasenfuss G, Ittleman F, Allen PD, Blanchard EM, Alpert NR (1989) Alterations in the force-frequency relation in stage III-IV failing human myocardium. Circulation 80: II-75
22. Mulieri LA, Hasenfuss G, Ittleman F, Blanchard EM, Alpert NR (1989) Protection of human left ventricular myocardium from cutting injury with 2,3-butanedione monoxime. Circ Res 65: 1441–1449
23. Mulieri LA, Hasenfuss G, Leavitt B, Allen PD, Alpert NR (1992) Altered myocardial force-frequency relation in human heart failure [see comments]. Circulation 85: 1743–1750
24. Mulieri LA, Ittleman FP, Leavitt BJ, Alpert NR (1992) Altered tension-frequency relation of human myocardium in volume overload heart failure. J Mol Cell Cardiol 24 (III): S44
25. Mulieri LA, Leavitt BJ, Hasenfuss G, Allen PD, Alpert NR (1992) Contraction frequency dependence of twitch and diastolic tension in human dilated cardiomyopathy (tension-frequency relation in cardiomyopathy). Basic Res Cardiol 87 Suppl 1: 199–212
26. Mulieri LA, Leavitt BJ, Ittleman FP, Martin BJ, Haeberle JR, Alpert NR (1992) Depressed myocardial force-frequency curve in mitral regurgitation heart failure is partially reversed by forskolin. Circulation 86: I-861
27. Mulieri LA, Leavitt BJ, Martin BJ, Haeberle JR, Alpert NR (1993) Myocardial force-frequency defect in mitral regurgitation heart failure is reversed by forskolin. Circulation 88: 2700–2704
28. Napolitano R, Vittone L, Mundina C, Chiappe de Cingolani G, Mattiazzi A (1992) Phosphorylation of phospholamban in the intact heart. A study on the physiological role of the Ca^{2+}-calmodulin-dependent protein kinase system. J Mol Cell Cardiol 24: 387–396
29. Pagani ED, Alousi AA, Grant AM, Older TM, Dziuban SW Jr, Allen PD (1988) Changes in myofibrillar content and Mg-ATPase activity in ventricular tissues from patients with heart failure caused by coronary artery disease, cardiomyopathy, or mitral valve insufficiency. Circ Res 63: 380–385
30. Peters TJ, Wells G, Oakley CM, Brooksby IA, Jenkins BS, Webb-Peploe MM, Coltart DJ (1977) Enzymic analysis of endomyocardial biopsy specimens from patients with cardiomyopathies. Br Heart J 39: 1333–1339
31. Pieske B, Hasenfuss G, Holubarsch C, Schwinger R, Bohm M, Just H (1992) Alterations of the force-frequency relationship in the failing human heart depend on the underlying cardiac disease. Basic Res Cardiol 87 Suppl 1: 213–221
32. Pieske B, Kretschmann B, Schmidt-Schweda S, Minami K, Posival H, Just H, Hasenfuss G (1993) Alterations in intracellular calcium handling are a major cause for the inverse force-frequency relationship in the failing human myocardium. Circulation 88: I-373
33. Pieske B, Trost S, Sutterlin M, Posival H, Minami K, Hasenfuss G (1994) Influence of forskolin on the force-frequency relationship in human nonfailing and end-stage failing myocardium. Circulation 90: I-211
34. Schmidt U, Schwinger RH, Bohm M (1995) Halothane restores the altered force-frequency relationship in failing human myocardium. Anesthesiology 82: 1456–1462
35. Schouten VJ (1990) Interval dependence of force and twitch duration in rat heart explained by Ca^{2+} pump inactivation in sarcoplasmic reticulum. J Physiol (Lond) 431: 427–444
36. Schwinger RH, Bohm M, Erdmann E (1992) Inotropic and lusitropic dysfunction in myocardium from patients with dilated cardiomyopathy. Am Heart J 123: 116–128
37. Schwinger RH, Bohm M, Muller-Ehmsen J, Uhlmann R, Schmidt U, Stablein A, Uberfuhr P, Kreuzer E, Reichart B, Eissner HJ (1993) Effect of inotropic stimulation on the negative force-frequency relationship in the failing human heart. Circulation 88: 2267–2276
38. Talosi L, Edes I, Kranias EG (1993) Intracellular mechanisms mediating reversal of beta-adrenergic stimulation in intact beating hearts. Am J Physiol 264: H791–7
39. Toyofuku T, Curotto Kurzydlowski K, Narayanan N, MacLennan DH (1994) Identification of Ser[38] as the site in cardiac sarcoplasmic reticulum Ca^{2+}-ATPase that is phosphorylated by Ca^{2+}/calmodulin-dependent protein kinase. J Biol Chem 269: 26492–26496

40. Voss J, Jones LR, Thomas DD (1994) The physical mechanism of calcium pump regulation in the heart [see comments]. Biophys J 67: 190–196
41. Xu A, Hawkins C, Narayanan N (1993) Phosphorylation and activation of the Ca^{2+}-pumping ATPase of cardiac sarcoplasmic reticulum by Ca^{2+}/calmodulin-dependent protein kinase. J Biol Chem 268: 8394–8397

Authors' address:
Louis A. Mulieri, PhD
Dept. Molec. Physiol. & Biophys.
Given Building, University of Vermont
Burlington, VT 05405, USA

Contributions of Ca^{2+}-influx via the L-type Ca^{2+}-current and Ca^{2+}-release from the sarcoplasmic reticulum to $[Ca^{2+}]_i$-transients in human myocytes

D. J. Beuckelmann

Department of Medicine III, University of Cologne, Cologne, Germany

Abstract

Experiments were performed to determine the relative contributions of direct Ca^{2+}-entry through the L-type Ca^{2+}-current and of Ca^{2+}-release from the sarcoplasmic reticulum (s.r.) to the intracellular $[Ca^{2+}]_i$-transient in isolated human atrial and ventricular myocytes from patients with severe heart failure and from non-failing controls. Cells were isolated from explanted hearts of patients undergoing transplantation because of severe heart failure due to dilated or ischemic cardiomyopathy or from donor hearts which could not be transplanted for technical reasons. Ca^{2+}-current densities were -2.1 ± 0.6 pA/pF in atrial cells, -4.8 ± 0.5 pA/pF in cells from patients with heart failure and -3.2 ± 0.5 pA/pF in non-failing controls. $[Ca^{2+}]_i$-transients were significantly smaller in heart failure (370 ± 33 nM) compared to ventricular cells from non-failing hearts (760 ± 69 nM, $p < 0.05$). Atrial myocytes had average $[Ca^{2+}]_i$-transients of 505 ± 38 nM. After incubation in ryanodine the average $[Ca^{2+}]_i$-transients were not significantly different between different cell types.

The results indicate that the relative contribution of Ca^{2+} released from the sarcoplasmic reticulum to the $[Ca^{2+}]_i$-transient is significantly smaller in heart failure. The absolute contribution of the L-type Ca^{2+}-current to the transient seemed to be comparable in all cell types investigated. As the $[Ca^{2+}]_i$-transient in the presence of ryanodine was comparable in size in all cells, changes of the intracellular $[Ca^{2+}]_i$-transient in heart failure are mainly due to alterations of s.r. function in these cells.

Key words Human myocytes – sarcoplasmatic reticulum – Ca^{2+}-release – L-type Ca^{2+}-current, Ca^{2+}-entry

Introduction

The mechanism of release of Ca^{2+} from the sarcoplasmic reticulum (s.r.) has been demonstrated to be due to Ca^{2+}-induced Ca^{2+}-release (1, 12). The key element of this mechanism is that Ca^{2+}-release from the s.r. is "triggered" by Ca^{2+} provided by the "fast component" of the sarcolemmal Ca^{2+}-current. The major part of the systolic

[Ca^{2+}]$_i$-transient is therefore due to Ca^{2+}-release from the s.r. into the cytoplasm. However, a part of the [Ca^{2+}]$_i$-transient is due to direct influx through the voltage-gated Ca^{2+}-channel. This part of the [Ca^{2+}]$_i$-transient that is due to direct influx as the Ca^{2+}-current varies between species. It is small in rats where the major component of Ca^{2+} entering the cytoplasm is released from the s.r. but the current provides the predominant part of Ca^{2+} in frog myocytes.

Intracellular [Ca^{2+}]$_i$-handling has been shown to be significantly altered in patients with terminal heart failure (6). In single ventricular myocytes isolated from hearts of these patients whose disease was due to dilated or ischemic cardiomyopathy systolic [Ca^{2+}]$_i$-transients were reduced, diastolic [Ca^{2+}]$_i$-levels were increased and the rate of diastolic decay of [Ca^{2+}]$_i$ was significantly slowed (2). However, the density of the triggering Ca^{2+}-current has been demonstrated to be unchanged in heart failure (2, 10). Therefore, the relative contribution of direct entry of Ca^{2+} via the Ca^{2+}-current to [Ca^{2+}]$_i$-transient has to be different in patients with heart failure.

The purpose of the present study was to determine the relative contributions of the L-type Ca^{2+}-current and of Ca^{2+} released from the sarcoplasmic reticulum to the intracellular [Ca^{2+}]$_i$-transient in human atrial and ventricular myocytes and their possible changes in severe heart failure.

Methods

Patients

Ventricular cells were prepared from six hearts of patients with end-stage heart failure due to dilated cardiomyopathy (DCM, n = 3) or ischemic cardiomyopathy (ICM, n = 3) undergoing transplantation. Patients' age was 54 ± 3 years, ♂ : ♀ was 5:1, cardiac index was 2.3 ± 0.2 l/min/m^2, ejection fraction was 30 ± 4 %. All patients received digoxin and diuretics and were under vasodilator therapy. No catecholamines or β-adrenoceptor blocking drugs were given during 48 hours before the operation. Results were compared with ventricular cells isolated from three normal human hearts without cardiac disease that could not be transplanted for technical reasons. Atrial myocytes were isolated from eight right atrial appendages from patients undergoing bypass surgery for coronary artery disease without any signs of heart failure. Informed consent was obtained from all patients prior to the operation.

Cell isolation

The isolation procedure has been described in detail before (2). A part of the left ventricular wall was excised together with its artery branch. The wall segment was then perfused via this artery branch: 30 min with a nominally Ca^{2+}-free modified Tyrode's solution (138 mM NaCl; 4 mM KCl; 1 mM MgCl$_2$; 10 mM Glucose; 0.33 mM NaH$_2$PO$_4$; 10 mM Hepes; pH 7.3 with addition of NaOH, 37 °C), followed by 40 min with the same solution with added collagenase (type II, 56 mg/50 ml, Worthington) and protease, (type XIV, 6 mg/50 ml, Sigma Chemicals). Finally, the enzyme was washed out for 15 min with modified Tyrode's solution that contained 200 μM Ca^{2+}. As tissue digestion was maximal within the ventricular wall with the endocardial and epicardial layers almost undigested, cells were prepared from areas within the central one third of the myocardial width. Ventricular cells were disaggregated by mechanical agitation, and, after filtering through a nylon mesh, stores in Tyrode's solution containing 2.0 mM Ca^{2+} at room temperature.

Atrial myocytes were isolated using a modification of the method described by Bustamante et al. (3).

The living cell yield was approximately 5 – 8 %. Only cells with clear cross striation without significant granulation or spontaneous contraction were selected for experiments. They did contract upon field stimulation as judged by visual control.

Solutions and loading of cells with fura-2

After establishing whole cell recording the electrode solution was allowed to exchange with the cytoplasm. It was composed of 0.050 mM fura-2 (Molecular Probes); 120 mM Cs-glutamate; 10 mM CsCl; 1 mM $MgCl_2$; 5 mM NaCl; 10 mM Hepes (cesium salt); and 2 mM Mg-ATP; pH was 7.2 with addition of KOH. Positive pressure to the electrode was never applied to avoid potential disintegration of intracellular structures during such procedure.

Cells were superfused, at 35 °C, with a modified Tyrode's solution containing 2.0 mM $CaCl_2$; 140 mM NaCl; 10 mM CsCl; 1 mM $MgCl_2$; 10 mM Glucose; 10 mM Hepes (Na^+-salt); pH was 7.3 with addition of NaOH. Cs^+ was added to the solutions to block K^+-currents that might interfere with the measurements of Ca^{2+}-currents.

Functional inhibition of the sarcoplasmic reticulum

The sarcoplasmic reticulum was functionally inhibited by incubation of the cells in modified Tyrode's solution to which ryanodine had been added: 2.0 mM $CaCl_2$; 140 mM NaCl; 10 mM CsCl; 1 mM $MgCl_2$; 10 mM Glucose; 10 mM Hepes (Na^+-salt); 1 μM ryanodine; pH 7.3. Cells were incubated for at least 10 min in ryanodine to assure a complete block of s.r. Ca^{2+}-release.

Measurements of $[Ca^{2+}]_i$-transients and Ca^{2+}-currents

Experiments were carried out using standard whole-cell recording techniques employing a patch-clamp amplifier model EPC-7 (LIST Instruments) with a 100 mOhm feedback resistor. The method of measuring $[Ca^{2+}]_i$ has been described in detail before (2). Briefly, for fluorescence recordings UV light, emitted from a 75 watt Xenon arc lamp passed through 10 nm interference filters (340 nm or 380 nm wavelengths) and was reflected by a dichronic mirror centered at 405 nm into the objective for excitation of the Ca^{2+}-indicator in the cell. Fluorescence emitted from the cell passed through the objective and a 510 – 540 nm bandpass filter and was directed into a photomultiplier tube (PMT). Fluorescence and current recordings were digitized (1 kHz) and stored for off-line analysis according to the method described by Grynkiewicz et al. (5).

The average pipette resistance in ventricular cells was 2 – 2.5 MOhms, for current measurements in atrial cells the pipette electrodes had resistances of 3 – 4 MOhms. Series resistance was compensated for as much as possible (30 – 60 %).

Statistical analysis

Mean values ± standard deviations are shown. Mann-Whitney non-parametric analysis was used for statistical evaluation of the data and p-values < 0.05 were considered significant.

Results

[Ca^{2+}]$_i$-handling in atrial myocytes

The dependence of Ca^{2+}-currents and [Ca^{2+}]$_i$-transients on clamp-pulse potential is shown in Fig. 1. The cell membrane was clamped from a holding potential of -80 mV after a 100 ms prepulse to -45 mV to inactivate the Na$^+$-current for 300 ms to $+10$ and $+70$ mV. When the membrane was depolarized to $+10$ mV there was a fast rise of [Ca^{2+}]$_i$ to a maximum of 700 nM. Upon repolarization from $+70$ mV to -45 mV a repolarization transient was elicited. After the cell was incubated in 1 μM ryanodine the [Ca^{2+}]$_i$-transient in this myocyte was reduced by approximately 75 % and the repolarization transient was abolished. [Ca^{2+}]$_i$-currents were largely unchanged.

[Ca^{2+}]$_i$-handling in ventricular myocytes of non-failing hearts

In Fig. 2 the same protocol as in Fig. 1 was used in a ventricular myocyte isolated from a non-failing heart. Upon depolarization for 300 ms to $+10$ mV [Ca^{2+}]$_i$ increased to 800 nM and upon repolarization from $+70$ mV a repolarization transient was elicited. The Ca^{2+}-current was larger than in atrial myocytes as ventricular cells had a larger cell surface. After incubation in 1 μM ryanodine the [Ca^{2+}]$_i$-transient in this myocyte was reduced by 75 % and the [Ca^{2+}]$_i$-transient upon repolarization was abolished.

[Ca^{2+}]$_i$-handling in ventricular myocytes from terminally failing hearts

In Fig. 3 the same protocol was used as in Fig. 1 and 2 in a ventricular myocyte isolated from a heart of a patient with terminal heart failure due to dilated cardiomyo-

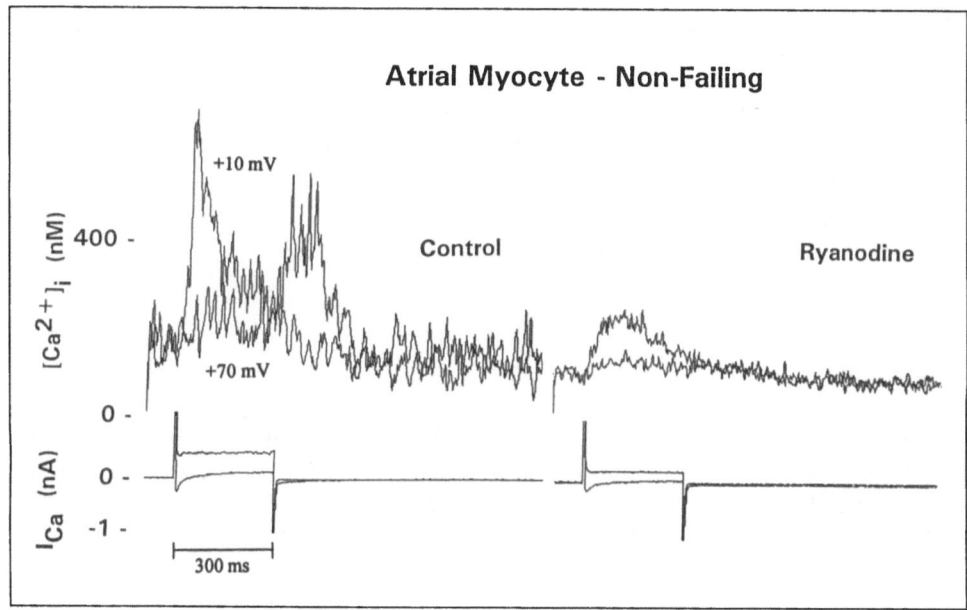

Fig. 1. Atrial myocyte. Ca^{2+}-current and $[Ca^{2+}]_i$-transient upon depolarization from -45 mV to $+10$ mV and $+70$ mV in the absence and in the presence of ryanodine (1 μM). Upon depolarization to $+10$ mV $[Ca^{2+}]_i$ increased from 160 nM to 700 nM, after addition of ryanodine the $[Ca^{2+}]_i$-transient was reduced to 200 nM. The $[Ca^{2+}]_i$-transient upon repolarization from -70 mV to -45 mV was abolished by ryanodine.

pathy. Upon depolarization of the cell membrane to $+10$ mV $[Ca^{2+}]_i$-increased to 400 nM and upon repolarization from $+70$ mV a small repolarization transient was elicited. Incubation of the cell in ryanodine reduced the $[Ca^{2+}]_i$-transient in this myocyte by 30 % and abolished the repolarization-transient. The Ca^{2+}-current was not significantly altered after incubation in ryanodine.

$[Ca^{2+}]_i$-transients and Ca^{2+}-current densities in human myocytes

Average Ca^{2+}-current densities and $[Ca^{2+}]_i$-transients upon depolarization to $+10$ mV are shown in Fig. 4. There was a significant reduction of $[Ca^{2+}]_i$-transients in ventricular myocytes from patients with heart failure (370 ± 33 nM compared to ventricular cells from control hearts (760 ± 69 nM, $p < 0.05$). Atrial myocytes had an average $[Ca^{2+}]_i$-transient of 505 ± 38 nM. Although there was a trend towards a higher Ca^{2+}-current density in cells from patients with heart failure (-4.8 ± 0.5 pA/pF) compared to controls (-3.2 ± 0.5 pA/pF) this difference did not reach statistical significance. However, there was a significant difference between Ca^{2+}-current densities in atrial cells (-2.1 ± 0.6 pA/pF) and ventricular cells from patients with heart failure ($p < 0.05$).

[Ca^{2+}]$_i$-transients in human myocytes after incubation in ryanodine

Average Ca^{2+}-current densities and [Ca^{2+}]$_i$-transients upon depolarization to $+10$ mV after incubation in 1 μM ryanodine are summarized in Table 1. No significant differences of [Ca^{2+}]$_i$-transients could be found between the three groups after incubation in ryanodine.

Discussion

The purpose of this study was to investigate whether the relative contribution of the L-type Ca^{2+}-current to the intracellular [Ca^{2+}]$_i$-transient may differ in isolated human myocytes from right atrium and ventricular myocardium of patients with severe heart failure or without any sign of heart failure. It was found that the [Ca^{2+}]$_i$-transient upon depolarization to $+10$ mV was significantly reduced in myocytes iso-

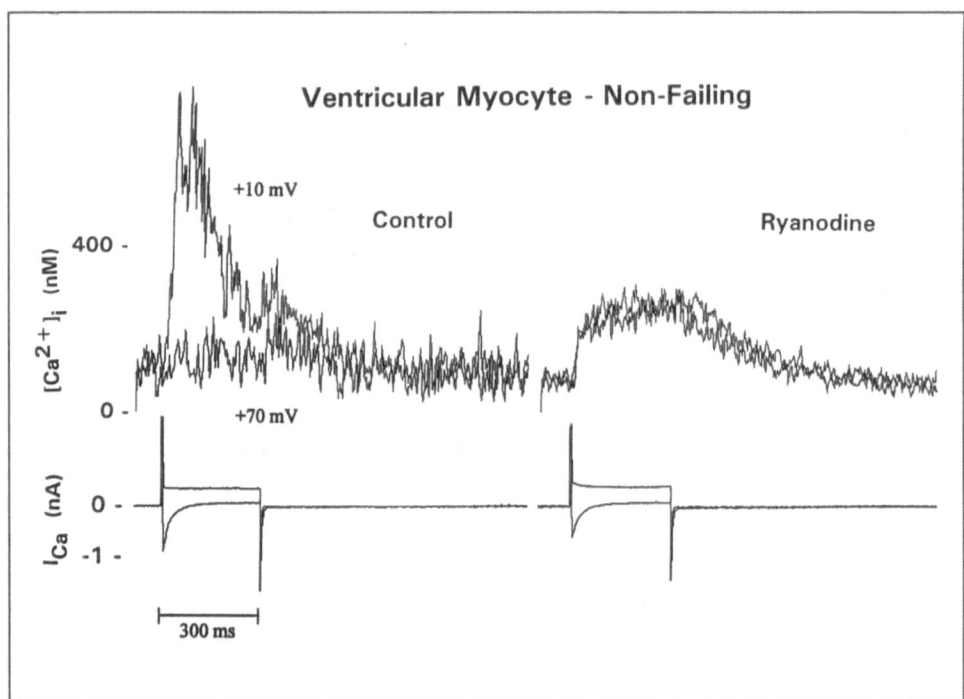

Fig. 2. Ventricular myocyte (non-failing). Ca^{2+}-current and [Ca^{2+}]$_i$-transient upon depolarization from -45 mV to $+10$ mV and $+70$ mV in the absence and in the presence of ryanodine (1 μM). Upon depolarization to $+10$ mV [Ca^{2+}]$_i$ increased from 100 nM to 700 nM, after addition of ryanodine the [Ca^{2+}]$_i$-transient was reduced to 250 nM. The [Ca^{2+}]$_i$-transient upon repolarization from -70 mV to -45 mV was abolished by ryanodine.

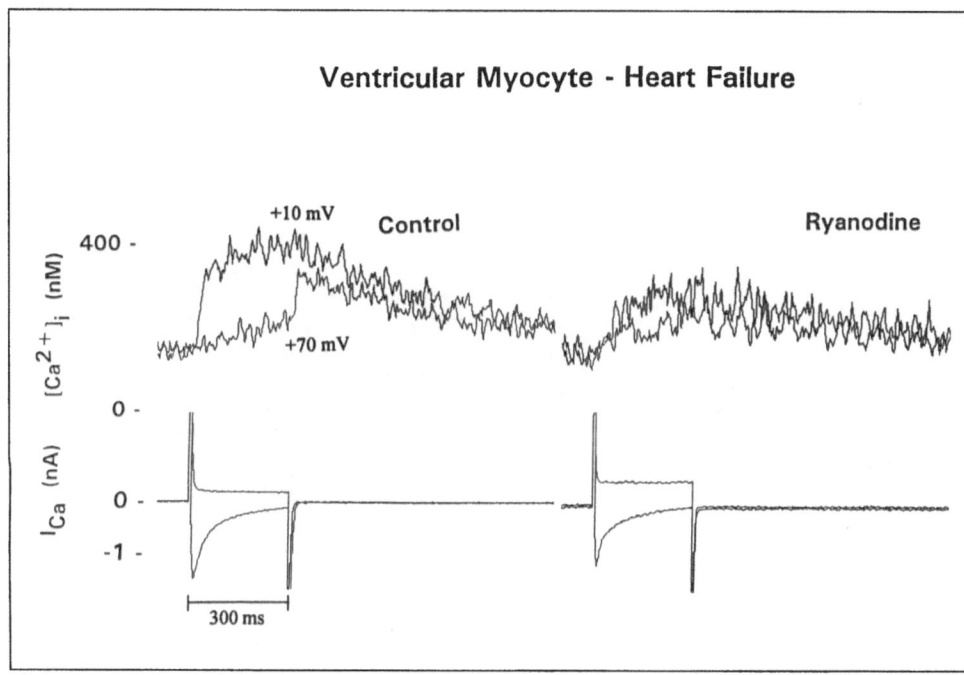

Fig. 3. Ventricular myocyte (heart failure). Ca^{2+}-current and $[Ca^{2+}]_i$-transient upon depolarization from -45 mV to $+10$ mV and $+70$ mV in the absence and in the presence of ryanodine (1 μM). Upon depolarization to $+10$ mV $[Ca^{2+}]_i$ increased from 180 nM to 400 nM, after addition of ryanodine the $[Ca^{2+}]_i$-transient was reduced to 350 nM. The small $[Ca^{2+}]_i$-transient upon repolarization from -70 mV to -45 mV was abolished by ryanodine.

lated from patients with severe heart failure as has been shown before in these cells (2). Although in this study there was a trend towards an increase in Ca^{2+}-current density in cells from patients with heart failure this difference did not reach statistical significance due to large variations of the Ca^{2+}-current size, hence the Ca^{2+}-current density was unchanged. An unchanged Ca^{2+}-current density has been confirmed by other groups (10). However, in animal models of heart failure a decrease of Ca^{2+}-current density has been demonstrated in most cases (7, 8, 11). In our experiments current densities in atrial myocytes seemed to be smaller than in ventricular cells, although a statistical difference could only be found between atrial cells and ventricular cells from patients with heart failure. Current densities were comparable to those found by other authors (10). Therefore, alteration of intracellular $[Ca^{2+}]_i$-handling in heart failure cannot be explained by alterations of L-type Ca^{2+}-currents in these cells.

Ryanodine is an alkaloid that locks the Ca^{2+}-release channel of the sarcoplasmic reticulum in a half open state (14). Although Ca^{2+}-uptake into the sarcoplasmic reticulum is not directly inhibited the opening of the s.r. release channel effectively inhibits s.r. function (13). Although there was a trend towards smaller currents in the ryanodine groups, there were no significant alterations of the Ca^{2+}-currents by incubation in ryanodine as has been shown in other species (9, 16). The trend towards a smaller Ca^{2+}-current after incubation in ryanodine was probably caused by an insignificant run-down of the Ca^{2+}-current.

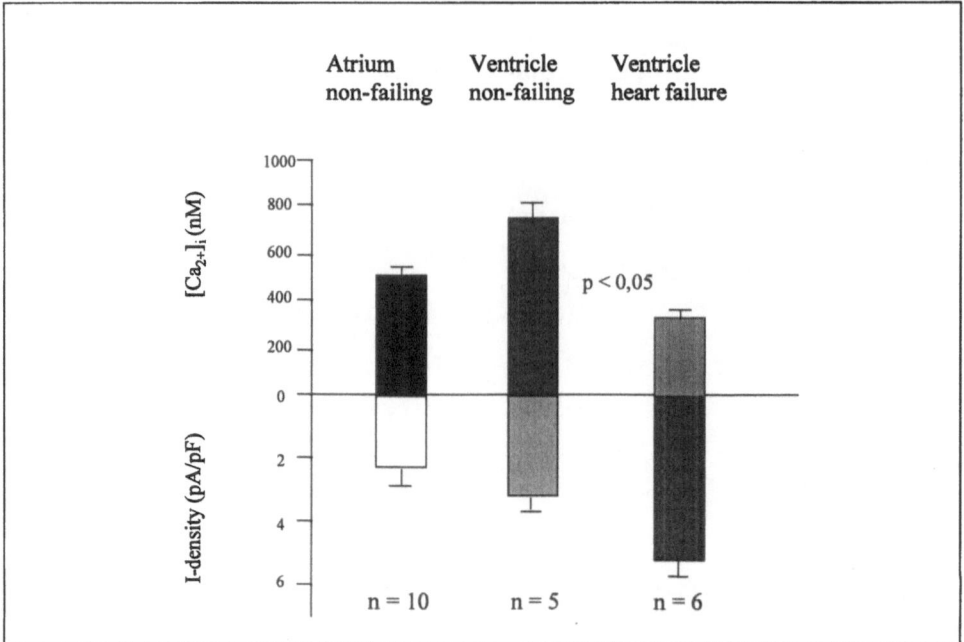

Fig. 4. $[Ca^{2+}]_i$-transients and Ca^{2+}-current densities in atrial and ventricular myocytes from patients with and without severe heart failure.

Table 1. Ca^{2+}-current densities and $[Ca^{2+}]_i$-transients after incubation in 1 μM ryanodine

	Ca²⁺-current density (pA/pF)	[Ca²⁺]ᵢ-transient (nM)
Atrial myocyte non-failing n = 10	2.0 ± 0.7	282 ± 25
Ventricular myocyte non-failing n = 5	3.0 ± 0.5	305 ± 14
Ventricular myocyte failing n = 6	4.4 ± 0.5	296 ± 10

Ca^{2+}-current densities and $[Ca^{2+}]_i$-transients were measured during depolarization to $+10$ mV. Cells were incubated in 1 μM ryanodine for at least 10 min. n indicates the number of cells investigated.

Our experiments show that the $[Ca^{2+}]_i$-transients in human atrial and ventricular myocytes were significantly altered by incubation with ryanodine. The size of the $[Ca^{2+}]_i$-transient was markedly reduced and the transient upon repolarization from positive potentials was abolished. This $[Ca^{2+}]_i$-transient upon repolarization has been postulated to be a marker of an intact s.r. Ca^{2+}-release function (1). Thus, incubation of human myocytes in 1 μM ryanodine effectively inhibited the s.r. Ca^{2+}-release function. Between groups there were significant differences. In atrial myocytes and in ventricular myocytes from patients without heart failure the systolic $[Ca^{2+}]_i$-transient was decreased by 44 %. The effect of ryanodine on the $[Ca^{2+}]_i$-transients in cells of patients with heart failure was significantly less pronounced. $[Ca^{2+}]_i$-transients were reduced by only 20 %. Therefore, the relative contribution of Ca^{2+} released from the sarcoplasmic reticulum is significantly smaller in heart failure. Figure 3 clearly shows that a major part of the $[Ca^{2+}]_i$-transient in myocytes from patients with heart failure was due to direct influx of Ca^{2+} through the Ca^{2+}-current. Furthermore, the $[Ca^{2+}]_i$-transient in the presence of ryanodine was comparable in size in all cells (Fig. 1 – 3), indicating that changes of the intracellular $[Ca^{2+}]_i$-transient in heart failure are mainly due to alterations of s.r. function in these cells. The absolute contribution of the L-type Ca^{2+}-current seemed to be comparable in all cell types investigated.

Although an alteration of other Ca^{2+}-transport mechanisms cannot be excluded from these experiments, no obvious difference in the kinetics of the $[Ca^{2+}]_i$-transients in heart failure compared to controls could be found in the presence of ryanodine. It has been shown that the protein expression and mRNA-levels of the Na^+/Ca^{2+}-exchanger are increased in heart failure (4, 15). However, the present results indicate that alterations of the Na^+/Ca^{2+}-exchanger or of the sarcolemmal Ca^{2+}-ATPase seem to have only minor influences on intracellular $[Ca^{2+}]_i$-handling under conditions of an uncoupling of the sarcoplasmic reticulum. This does not exclude the possibility that there may be a significant impact of alterations of the Na^+/Ca^{2+}-exchanger on $[Ca^{2+}]_i$-handling when the s.r. function is intact.

Acknowledgements Supported by the Deutsche Forschungsgemeinschaft (Be 1113/2–3) and the Zentrum für Molekulare Medizin Köln # 4 (BMWFT 01 KS 9502).

REFERENCES

1. Beuckelmann DJ, Wier WG (1988) Mechanism of release of calcium from sarcoplasmic reticulum of guinea-pig cardiac cells. The Journal of Physiology (London) 405: 233–255
2. Beuckelmann DJ, Näbauer M, Erdmann E (1992) Intracellular calcium handling in ventricular myocytes from patients with terminal heart failure. Circulation 85: 1046–1055
3. Bustamante JO, Watanabe T, Murphy DA, McDonald TF (1982) Isolation of single atrial and ventricular cells from the human heart. Canadian Medical Association 126: 791–793
4. Flesch M, Putz F, Schwinger RHG, Böhm M (1996) Functional relevance of an enhanced Na^+-Ca^{2+}-exchanger in the failing human heart. Annals of the NY Academy of Science 779: 539–542
5. Grynkiewicz G, Poenie M, Tsien RY (1985) A new generation of Ca^{2+}-indicators with greatly improved fluorescence properties. The Journal of Biological Chemistry 260: 3440–3450
6. Gwathmey JK, Copelas L, MacKinnon R et al. (1987) Abnormal intracellular calcium handling in myocardium from patients with end-stage heart failure. Circulation Research 61: 70–76
7. Krüger C, Erdmann E, Näbauer M, Beuckelmann DJ (1994) Intracellular calcium handling in ventricular myocytes from cardiomyopathic hamsters (strain BIO 14.6) with congestive heart failure. Cell Calcium 16: 500–508
8. Li GR, Ferrier GR, Howlett SE (1995) Calcium currents in ventricular myocytes of prehypertrophic cardiomyopathic hamsters. American Journal of Physiology 268: H999–H1005
9. Marban E, Wier WG (1985) Ryanodine as a tool to determine the contributions of calcium entry and calcium release to the calcium transient and contraction of cardiac purkinje fibers. Circulation Research 56: 133–138
10. Mewes T, Ravens U (1994) L-type calcium current of human myocytes from ventricle of non-failing and failing hearts and from atrium. Journal of Molecular and Cellular Cardiology 26: 1307–1320
11. Ming Z, Nordin C, Siri F, Aronson RS (1994) Reduced calcium current density in single myocytes isolated from hypertrophied failing guinea-pig hearts. Journal of Molecular and Cellular Cardiology 26: 1133–1143

12. Näbauer M, Calewaert G, Cleemann L, Morad M (1989) The mechanism of Ca^{2+}-release in mammalian cardiac myocytes requires Ca^{2+} influx through the Ca^{2+}-channel. Science 244: 800–803
13. Nagasaki K, Fleischer S (1988) Ryanodine sensitivity of the calcium release channel of sarcoplasmic reticulum. Cell Calcium 9: 1–7
14. Rousseau E, Smith JS, Meissner G (1987) Ryanodine modifies the gating behavior of single Ca^{2+}-release channels. American Journal of Physiology 253: C364–C368
15. Studer R, Reinecke H, Bilger J, Eschenhagen T, Böhm M, Hasenfuss G, Just H, Hotz J, Drexler H (1994) Gene expression of the cardiac Na^{+}-Ca^{2+}-exchanger in endstage heart failure. Circulation Research 75: 443–453
16. Wier WG, Yue DT, Marban E (1985) Effects of ryanodine on intracellular $[Ca^{2+}]_i$-transients in mammalian cardiac muscle. Federation Proceedings 44: 2989–2993

Authors' address:
Dirk J. Beuckelmann MD
Department of Medicine III
University of Cologne
Joseph-Stelzmann-Straße 9
50935 Cologne, Germany

Molecular and cellular aspects of re-entrant arrhythmias

A. G. Kleber, V. Fast

Department of Physiology, University of Bern, Bern, Switzerland

Abstract

In recent years it has become evident that myocardial tissue undergoes remodeling in diseased states such as myocardial infarction and hypertrophy which affects membrane channels, cell-to-cell coupling as well as the connective tissue matrix. Although the detailed mechanisms of ventricular arrhythmias in ventricular hypertrophy are not known, studies carried out by computer simulations or high resolution mapping of electrical activity have suggested a complex interaction between changing ionic currents at the level of the cell membranes, altered cell-to-cell coupling and altered macroscopic structure. The present report summarises these recent developments and their potential relevance for arrhythmogenesis.

Key words Anisotropic conduction – cell cultures – microscopical conduction – current-to-load mismatch

Introduction

Cardiac arrhythmias associated with a variety of pathophysiologic states are traditionally divided into disturbances of impulse formation and impulse conduction. In normal cardiac function, impulse formation is confined to a limited number of pacemaker regions, the sino-artrial node, the atrio-ventricular junction and the His-Purkinje system. In pathological states, rapid impulse formation is either generated by circulating excitation with re-entry, which may involve relatively large regions of the atria and/or the ventricles (macro-reentry) (1, 2) or by so-called focal activity. Repetitive rapid electrical activity emerging from a focus, i.e. a small circumscribed region of excitable tissue, can be caused by a variety of mechanisms: Automatic or triggered activity, brought about by electrically unstable cells which produce repetitive membrane oscillations at different levels of membrane potential (early and delayed afterdepolarizations (e.g. (3, 4) or reentry confined to a small mass of tissue (5, 6). Such relatively small re-entrant circuits have been shown or postulated to underlie, for example, AV-nodal tachycardia (7) or ventricular premature beats (8).

Several investigators have emphasized the relationship between normal or remodeled cellular or tissue architecture and cardiac arrhythmias. Both remodeling at the level of membrane channels or connexons and remodeling at the level of connective tissue may increase the likelihood of occurrence of arrhythmias. The recent developments of sophisticated computer models (4, 9, 10) and of high-resolution mapping techniques of electrical activity (11, 12) have provided the tools which may help to understand the relation between the changes observed at the molecular and cellular level, the propagation disturbances and the resulting arrhythmias. It this context, it is important to realize that cardiac arrhythmias, per definition, always involve a complex system which is composed of a large mass of tissue in which different compartments (intracellular space, interstitial space, vascular space) interact. The present report summarizes recent developments made in research on cardiac impulse propagation at a cellular level. Some of the findings are likely to stimulate further research in defined pathophysiological settings, such as chronic myocardial infarction and hypertrophy. However, it seems too early to provide conclusive evidence about the dominance of a certain arrhythmogenic mechanism in cardiac hypertrophy and failure, although it is well known that this particular state of disease is associated with a high incidence of sudden cardiac death and that electrical disturbances and failure of mechanical function are closely interrelated.

Discontinuous conduction and arrhythmogenesis

The basic mechanism for circus movement re-entry arrhythmias is illustrated schematically in Fig. 1. The effect of an obstacle present in a wavefront of propagation is to deviate the otherwise homogenous wavefront into a rotating vortex, which becomes self-sustaining if it encounters non-refractory tissue at a site which had been previously excited. The basic principle of such circus movement was already

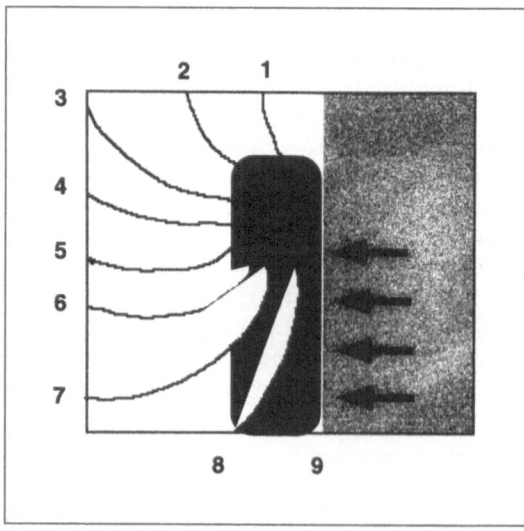

Fig. 1. Schematic explanation of circus movement with re-entry in a quadrangular area of excitable tissue. The right (grey part) of the tissue is excited homogenously from right to left. An obstacle (black area) leads to deviation of the wavefront, which circulates around the obstacle. The unidirectional block is illustrated by the dark arrows. The relative instants of excitation are represented by the isochrone lines from 1–9. At time 6 the excitation enters the previous zone of block from the rear and re-excites the originally excited area at time 9. The electrophysiological conditions for the occurrence of unidirectional block and for re-entry are multiple and listed in the text.

described early in this century (13), it was then modified to explain several types of cardiac arrhythmias. All these various types of circus movement have certain basic features in common: The wavefront must encounter a zone of tissue where local electrical inhomogeneity is present. This inhomogeneity may concern 1) the ionic properties of the cell membranes giving rise to different types of action potentials (inhomogeneity in electrical driving force), or requiring various amounts of local input current to generate a regenerative response (inhomogeneity in electrical excitability), 2) local gradients in the resistive properties of the diffusive medium (cellular coupling, resistive properties of the extracellular space), or 3) combinations of the above conditions. Also, such changes may be permanent (e.g., in remodeling after myocardial or ventricular hypertrophy (14), or they may be purely functional (e.g., inhomogeneity of refractoriness in acutely ischemic tissue (1). It is important to note that some of the above-mentioned changes are only needed to set the initial condition for the deviation of the impulse, the so-called "unidirectional conduction block". Once the disturbance is initiated, an arrhythmia can take place in a perfectly homogenous electrical medium (15).

In discussing the mechanism responsible for initiation, it is therefore important to ask the question of whether some of the physiological properties of myocardial tissue may already represent an arrhythmogenic substrate, which will become manifest in the case some additional condition in a certain disease state is fulfilled, for instance a local decrease in the action potential amplitude or a change in action potential duration. The crucial importance of myocardial architecture for the generation of arrhythmias was shown in several studies: Spach et al. (see e.g. 16) showed that in normal atrial tissue, a ventricular premature beat can be conducted in direction transversal to the main axis of the muscle fibers whereas it may get blocked in longitudinal direction. As a result, deviation of the impulse with re-entry occurred. Dillon et al. (17) showed that in tissue surviving from myocardial infarction, circus movement with re-entry occurred in strict topological relation to fiber architecture, the re-entrant circuits exhibiting an elliptic shape with a central zone of block corresponding to a zone separating longitudinally oriented fiber bundles. De Bakker et al. (18, 19) demonstrated that apparently slow macroscopic conduction in tissue surviving from infarction corresponded at a microscopical level to fast conduction taking a very long and complex "zig-zag"pathway across the scar tissue. This again confirmed a close relationship between tissue architecture and propagation.

Discontinuities induced by individual cell borders

Cell cultures grown in a predetermined pattern offer the possibility to assess the effect of gap junctions on the inhomogeneity in conduction in dense cellular networks. In such dense cellular networks, propagation can be studied as a function of cell-to-cell coupling alone, i.e., without interference from larger resistive barriers formed by connective tissue sheets or blood vessels. A technique to produce such cultures from dissociated neonatal rat myocytes has recently been described by our laboratory (20). Figure 2 illustrates two different types of growth patterns, 1) a chain of single cells growing in series (Fig. 2A) and a "street" of cells, consisting of 5–6 cells in width (Fig. 2B). As shown in Figs. 3 and 4, the conduction pattern in these two structures is distinctly different, and the difference allows to assess the role of gap junctions to induce discontinuities in conduction at a microscopical level. Since cells in single cell chains only exhibit end-to-end but no side-to-side connections, the conduction time along a cell chain is solely determined by action potential propagation within the cytoplasm and through the connexons located at the cell poles. The conduction patterns obtained in these strands are shown in Fig. 3B for a single experiment (12). The conduction time along 30 μm within a single cell is relatively short whereas the conduction time along the same distance is significantly longer if an end-to-end cell connection is interposed. The difference between the two conduction times corresponds to the transfer time at the connexons between the two cells and

a

b

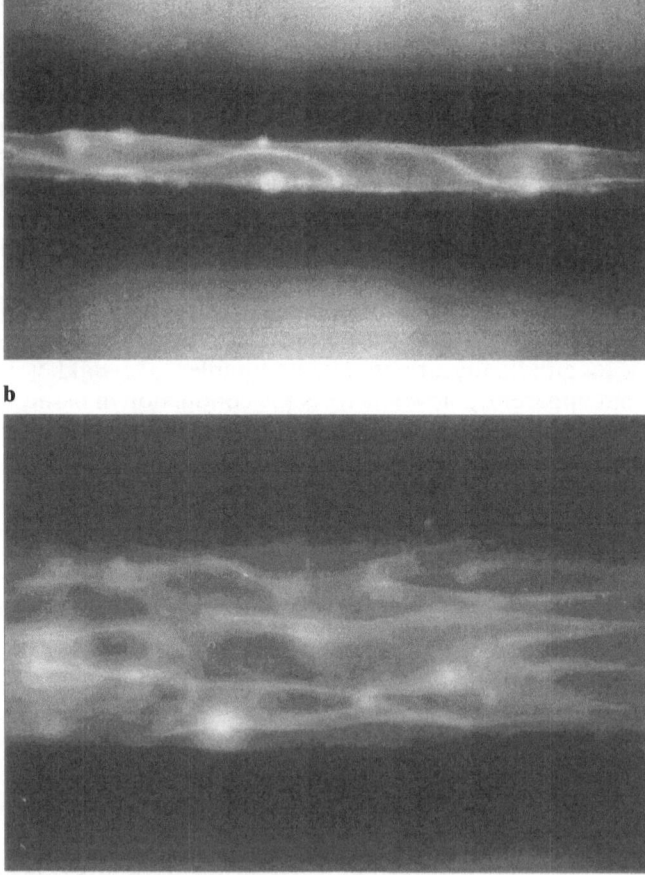

Fig. 2. Panel A: Fluorescent image of a one-dimensional synthetic strand of neonatal rat myocytes growing in a 2-μm-wide channel. Cells are stained with the voltage-sensitive dye RH-237. **Panel B:** Fluorescent image of a two-dimensional synthetic strand of neonatal rat myocytes growing in a 80-μm-wide channel. These channels contained four – six cells in cross-section. Reproduced from ref. (12) with permission.

amounts to 80 μs in this experiment. The average intracellular (cytoplasmic) conduction (Fig. 3C) along a distance of 30 μm is 38 $\pm$ 25 μs (n = 37). The average conduction time from one cell to the follower cell amounts to 118 $\pm$ 40 μs (n = 27), yielding a mean transfer time through an end-to-end cell connection of 80 μs. The analogous experiment carried out in a cell strand consisting in average of 5–6 cells in width, is illustrated in Fig. 4B, the collected data are shown in Fig. 4C. In the wider strands, the average cytoplasmic conduction time is longer than in the single cell chains, and the average cell-to-cell conduction time is shorter, the mean transfer time across an end-to-end cell connection amounting to 32 μs (versus 80 μs in the single cell chain). It is important to note that the macroscopic conduction velocities in both the single

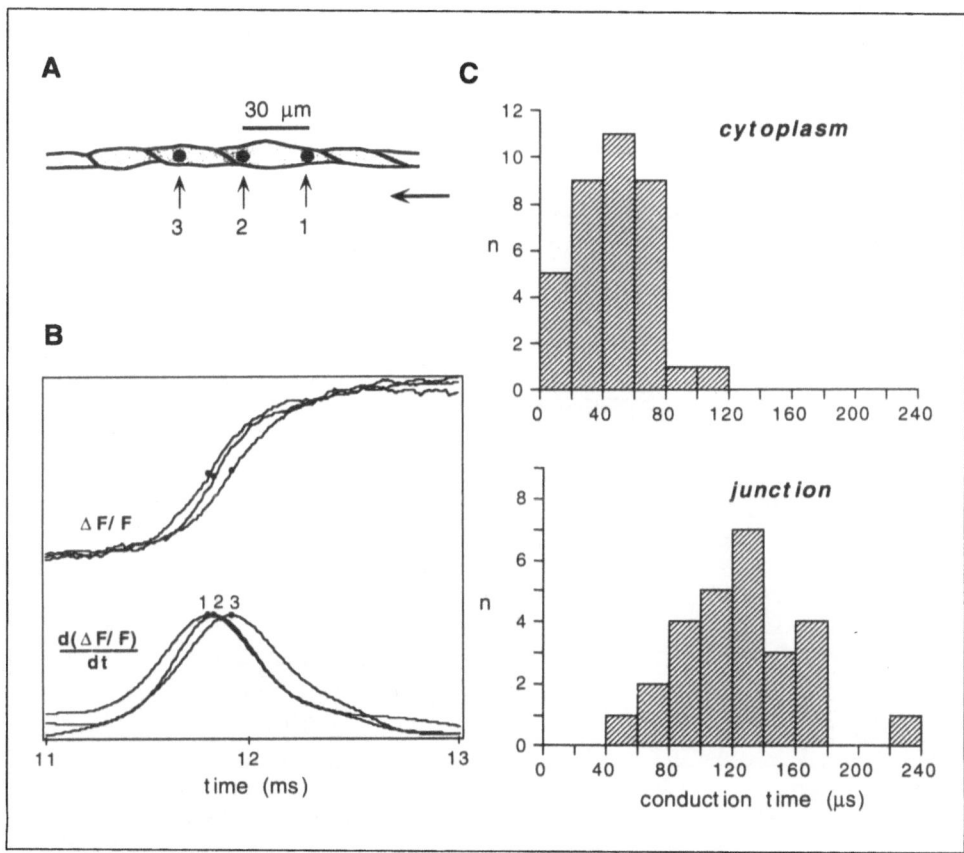

Fig. 3. Impulse propagation in one-dimensional cell chains. **Panel A:** Picture of a portion of a cell chain, reproduced from the bright-field illumination photograph. Position and size of membrane areas sensed by the three diodes are indicated by filled circles. Arrow indicates direction of propagation. **Panel B:** Potential-dependent fluorescence change $\Delta F/F$ recorded by the diodes given on Panel A and their superimposed derivatives d($\Delta F/F$)/dt. Activation times are depicted by points. Cytoplasmic conduction time = 30 μs, junctional conduction time = 110 μs. **Panel C:** Histograms of conduction times from all experiments. The average cytoplasmic conduction time (t = 38 $\pm$ 25 μs, n = 37) was markedly shorter than the average junctional conduction time (t = 118 $\pm$ 40 μs, n = 27, p < 0.0001). The mean difference, attributed to the conduction delay induced by the gap junctions, amounted to 80 μs which is 51 % of overall conduction time. Reproduced from ref. 12 with permission.

cell chains and the wide streets are the same. Comparison between the conduction times between these two structures therefore demonstrates that the lateral apposition of single cell chains to a cell strand decreases the degree of inhomogeneity induced by the end-to-end cell connections. This so-called "averaging effect" can best be explained by looking at the magnitude and direction of electrotonic current flowing between neighboring cells at the instant a given site reaches threshold for rapid Na$^+$ inward current, as explained in Fig. 5. This figure is taken from a computer model simulating propagation in cellular networks, which has been adopted to the electrical parameters characterizing the cultured chains and streets (12). It depicts the currents flowing into or from a given measuring site: If the wavefront of propaga-

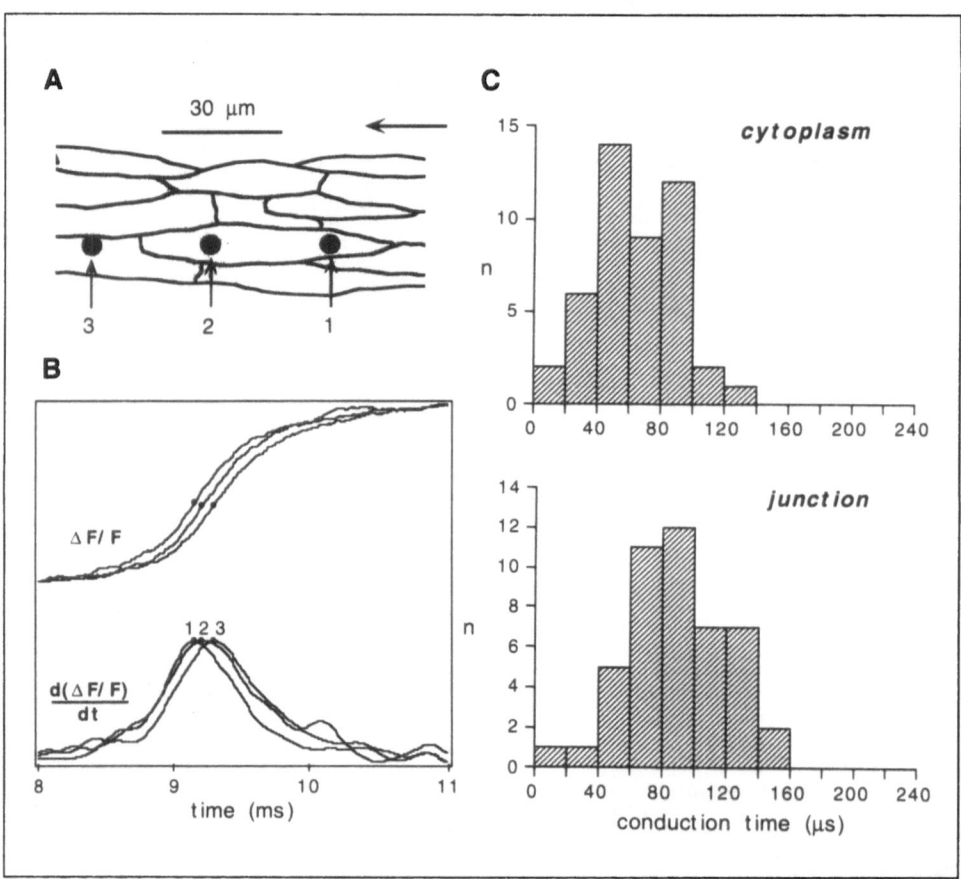

Fig. 4. Impulse conduction in two-dimensional cell strands. **Panel A:** Picture of a wide cell strand (4–6 cells in width) reproduced from a bright-field illumination photograph. Position and size of membrane areas sensed by the three diodes are indicated by filled circles. Arrow indicates direction of propagation. **Panel B:** Fluorescence changes $\Delta F/F$ and their superimposed derivatives $d(\Delta F/F)/dt$ recorded by diodes given on Panel A. Cytoplasmic conduction time = 60 μs, junctional conduction time = 80 μs. **Panel C:** Histograms of conduction times from all experiments. The average cytoplasmic conduction time was 57 ± 26 μs (n = 46) and the junctional conduction time was 89 ± 39 μs (n = 48, p < 0.001). The gap junctional conduction delay amounted to 32 μs which is 22 % of overall conduction time. Reproduced from ref. (12) with permission.

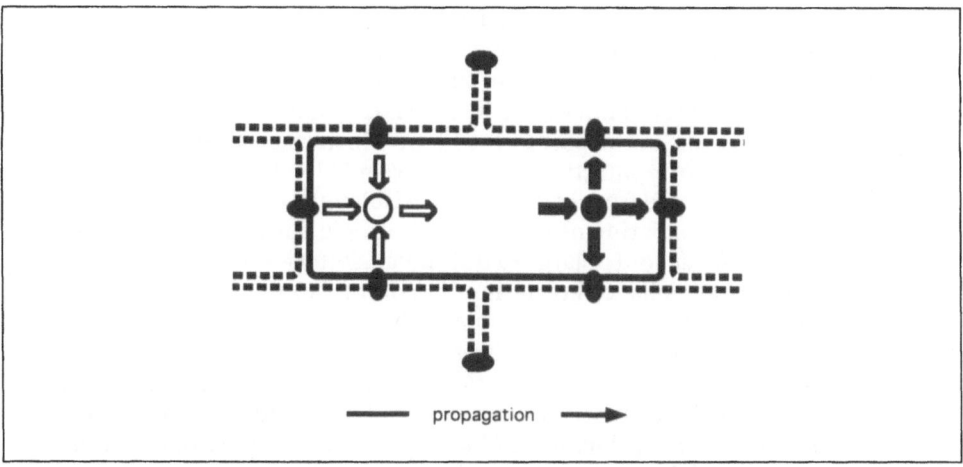

Fig. 5. Schematic diagram showing local current flow in a cell of a two-dimensional strand coupled to six neighboring cells. Gap junctions are symbolized by filled oval dots. The electrotonic currents flowing in the wavefront of propagation (horizontal arrows) and between laterally apposed cells (vertical arrows) are depicted at the instants of local activation for a point distal to the end-to-end cell connection (open symbols) and a point proximal to the end-to-end connection (filled symbols). The direction of these currents is given by the computed potential distribution at the two instants of activation. At the distal point lateral convergence of local current accelerates activation; at the proximal point lateral divergence delays activation. Both divergence and convergence of local currents through lateral connections are responsible for the reduced inhomogeneity of propagation in two-dimensional strands. Reproduced from ref. (12) with permission.

tion reaches, in a given cell, a point immediately beyond an end-to-end connection (point 1), the wavefront will lag slightly behind the front in the two neighboring cells, because these two cells do not encounter a resistive barrier at that site. Consequently, this point will receive local electrotonic current from both neighboring rows in addition to the normal electrotonic current flowing in the direction of the wave front. Sites immediately beyond an end-to-end connection will therefore depolarize earlier in presence of lateral coupling and, consequently, the transition time across the longitudinal cell-to-cell connection will become shorter and the cytoplasmic conduction time will become longer. The opposite process takes place at the cell end (point 2), where local current from this site is fed to the two neighboring cells. This divergence of local electrotonic current results in shortening of the transition time across the longitudinal cell-to-cell connection and prolongation of the cytoplasmic conduction time. As an overall result, conduction becomes more homogenous by lateral apposition and coupling of cells. Both the comparison of average conduction times as well as the type of computer model chosen provide knowledge about the average behavior of the cellular network. A variability of both cytoplasmic and cell-to-cell conduction times is suggested from the histograms in Figs. 3 and 4, and expected from the variability in cell shape, the variability in lateral apposition of individual cells, as well as from the variability in connexin distribution. This variability has been simulated recently in a computer model taking into account the stochastic architecture of adult myocytes (9).

Most experiments performed in isolated ventricular and atrial tissue have shown that the maximal upstroke velocity of the transmembrane action potential, dV/dt_{max}, is higher during transverse than during longitudinal propagation (21–24). This difference was taken to indicate a different mechanism for propagation in longitudinal versus transverse direction and related to the intrinsic arrhythmogenic substrate of anisotropic tissue. Whether or not this difference is explained by the specific arrangement of the gap junctions in the part of the tissue which consists of densely coupled cells or by the presence of connective tissue sheets and blood vessels separating fiber bundles cannot be answered from experiments in isolated tissue because of methodological limitations. An experiment showing anisotropic conduction in a dense network of cultured cells, (devoid of large extracellular clefts) is illustrated in Fig. 6 (25). Such type of experiments have shown that, in contrast to the in vivo experiments, average dV/dt_{max} in transverse and longitudinal directions are not different. Although the interpretation of such results is not unequivocal, they indicate that at a moderate degree of anisotropy (e.g. ventricular tissue) the discrete arrangement of gap junctions at the cell borders is not directly responsible for the direction-dependent differences in dV/dt_{max}. Similar findings have been recently obtained in computer simulations (26). They indirectly attribute a crucial importance to the resistive barriers larger than the gap junctions for explaining direction-dependent differences in dV/dt_{max} and arrhythmogenicity. Modification of gap junctional coupling will nevertheless modulate the effects of large resistive barriers, as discussed below.

Discontinuities induced by macroscopic changes in tissue geometry

Discontinuities in myocardial architecture exist at several levels. In addition to discontinuities imposed by cell borders (as described in the paragraph above), connective tissue sheets and microvessels may act as resistive barriers (27). A propagating impulse is expected to 1) collide with such a barrier and 2) to travel around resistive barriers wherever it encounters excitable tissue. The sites, where these deviations from homogenous and linear spread occur, are known to be susceptible for conduction block, because of so-called "impedance-to-load mismatch".

A basic model to investigate the effect of impedance-to-load mismatch and obtained by using the technique of patterned growth of cultured cells (described above) is shown in Fig. 7A (28). In this model, the impulse traveling along the small "street" has to excite the large tissue mass beyond the expansion, and therefore, to furnish local excitatory current to a large surface of excitable membranes downstream. As a consequence local slowing of conduction is to be expected, and eventually, conduction block occurs if the width of the street reaches a critical diameter, h_c. Although, at first glance, this simple macroscopical geometry bears no resemblance to the longitudinally oriented resistive barriers encountered in intact tissue, the biophysical principle governing impulse transmission at such sites is very similar. Thus, current-to-load mismatch has been described at a single ended obstacle or so-called pivoting point (Fig. 7B) forcing the wavefront to a curved shape or at a narrow "isthmus" or "gate" of excitable tissue interposed between connective tissue sheets (Fig. 7C) (29). An experiment measuring impulse transmission at a tissue expansion is shown in Fig. 8. This figure depicts optically measured action potential upstrokes

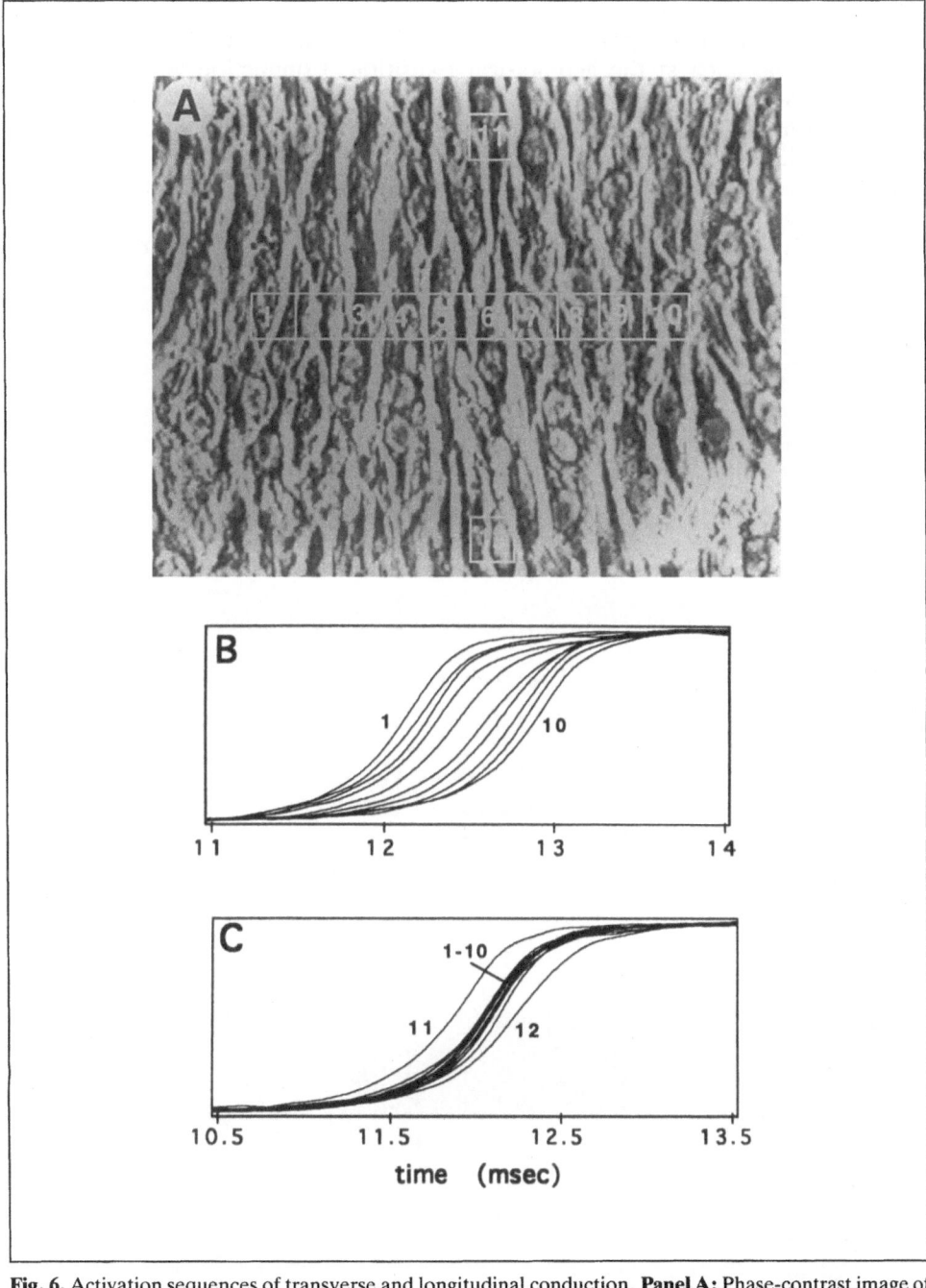

Fig. 6. Activation sequences of transverse and longitudinal conduction. **Panel A:** Phase-contrast image of the cell culture and photodiodes. Numbers within rectangles indicate photodiode numbers. **Panel B:** Normalized optical upstrokes recorded by the photodiodes shown on Panel A during *transverse conduction*. **Panel C:** Normalized optical upstrokes recorded from the same localization during *logitudinal conduction*. Both action potential upstrokes during longitudinal and transverse conduction show a variability in the maximal upstroke velocity indicating local variability in current flowing into membrane capacitance. However, no significant difference between mean values in tranverse versus longitudinal direction can be detected. Reproduced from ref. (25) with permission.

during conduction from a small street across the expansion into a large excitable area. Typically, the action potentials exhibit a biphasic upstroke which is due to the impedance mismatch at the geometrical transition. Conduction velocity at such expansions gets smaller with decreasing street width until it occasionally blocks if the streets are only 1–2 cells in width. Due to the asymmetry of the tissue, conduction in the inverse direction accelerates with decreasing street width.

The question relevant to anisotropic conduction is whether such resistive obstacles take part in impulse deviation and discontinuous conduction in vivo, and whether they contribute to anisotropy, i.e. whether their effects depend on the direction of the

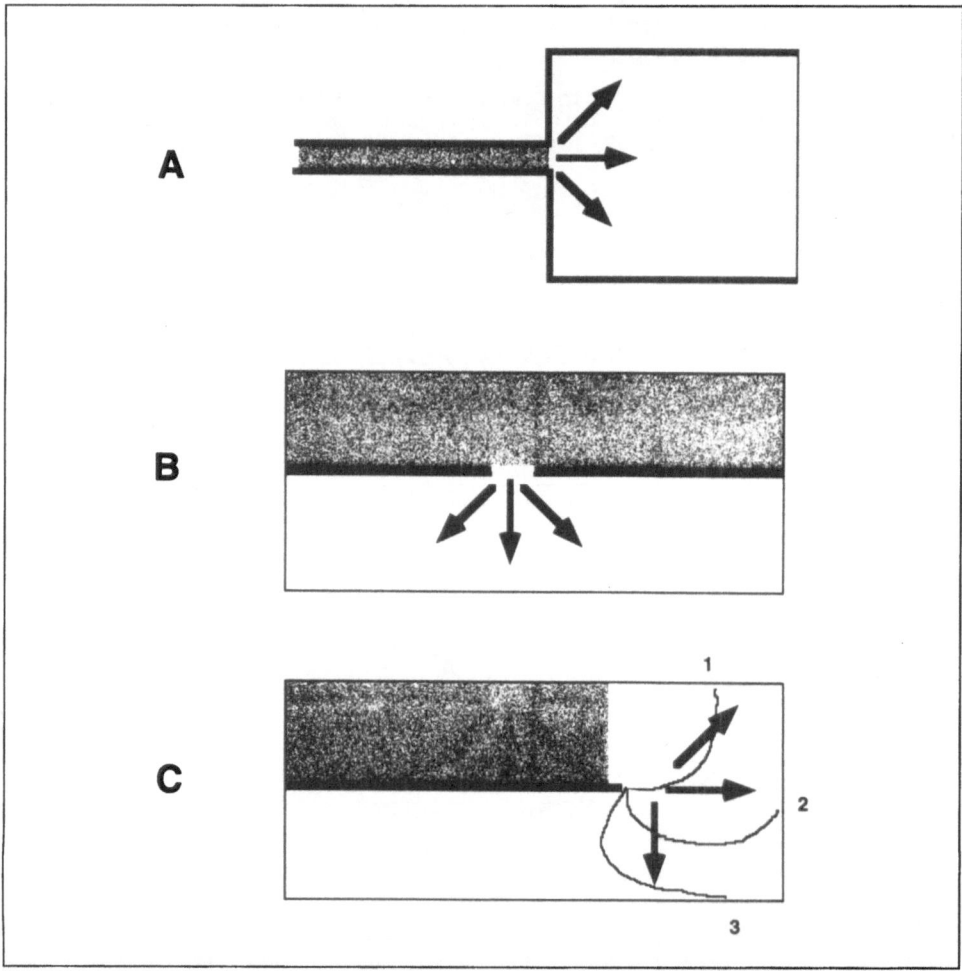

Fig. 7. Different types of "current-to-load mismatch" in cardiac tissue. In each scheme, the excited area is symbolized by the dark shading. The black lines indicate the tissue boundaries or the resistive obstacles, the arrows symbolize divergence of the electrotonic current which is produced by the ionic membrane channels in the excited area upstream. **A)** Abrupt tissue expansion, as discussed in Figs. 8–10. **B)** Connective tissue sheet separating two excitable areas with gate or isthmis. **C)** Connective tissue sheet, producing partial separation of two excitable areas, with excitation turning around the end of the obstacle ("pivoting point"). Curved isochrones at relative times 1 to 3 illustrate circus movement.

wavefront spread. An important role for connective tissue sheets separating bundles of excitable myocytes, which are longitudinally oriented and thus anisotropic, has been given by Spach et al., see (16) who observed both discontinuities in action potential upstrokes and extracellular electrograms during transverse but not during

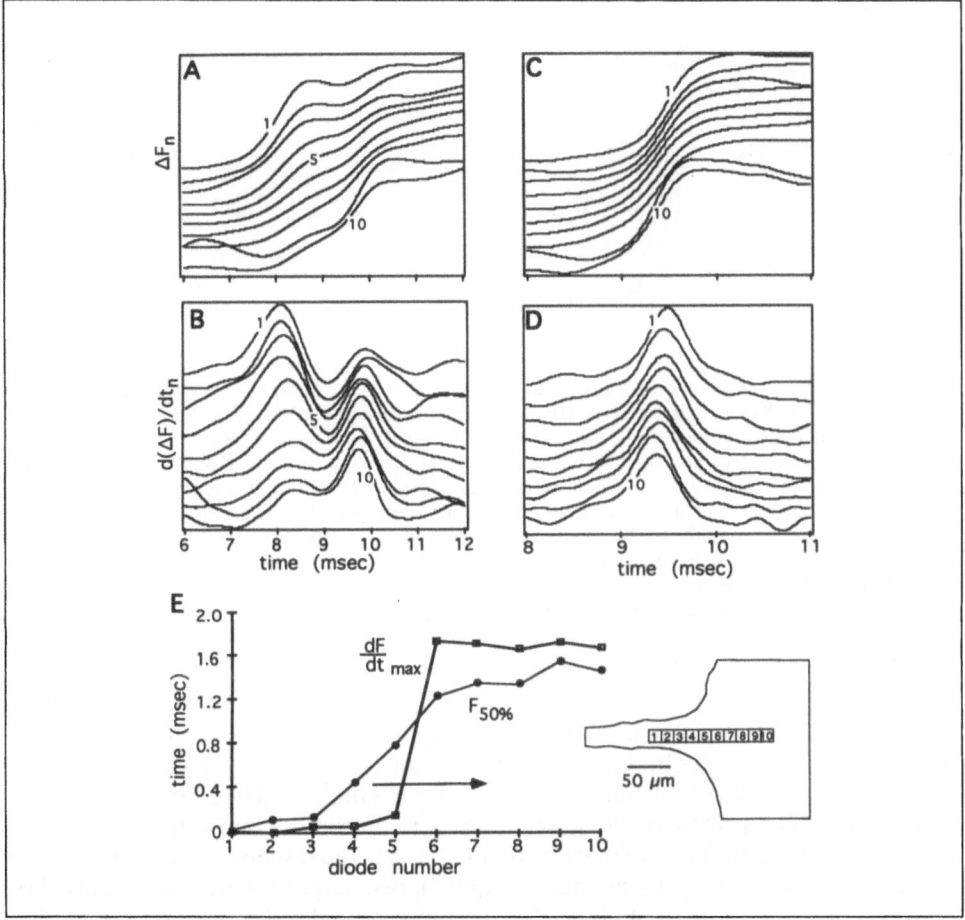

Fig. 8. Anterograde and retrograde impulse conduction at the region of abrupt expansion in a cell culture. **Bottom right.** Schematic presentation of an abrupt tissue expansion. The width of the small cell strand emerging into the large area (corresponding to the geometry shown in Fig. 7 A) amounts to 22 μm. The grid shows the localization of photodiodes with numbers. An individual diode covers a cell membrane area of 14 $\times$ 14 μm^2. The spacing between borders of individual diodes is 1 μm. **Panels A and C:** Normalized optical upstrokes (ΔF_n) of transmembrane action potentials recorded during anterograde conduction (A) from the strand into the large area and during retrograde conduction (C). Numbers on traces indicate corresponding photodiode numbers. Time was measured from the beginning of the recording interval. Stimulation pulse was delivered at t = 5 ms. **Panel B and D:** Normalized first time derivatives of corresponding optical signals, dF/dt$_n$. Two rising phases can be seen on optical upstrokes ΔF_n corresponding to the two maxima on derivative traces dF/dt$_n$. **Panel E:** Time sequences of dF/dt$_{max}$ (quadrangles) and F$_{50\%}$ (circles) calculated from the recordings on Panels A and B. Data are plotted relative to the moment of dF/dt$_{max}$ at the site number 10 which was considered to be zero. Note that the geometrical expansion induces a conduction delay during anterograde spread (Panel A) while propagation is fast during spread from the large area into the strand (Panel C). Reproduced from ref. (28) with permission.

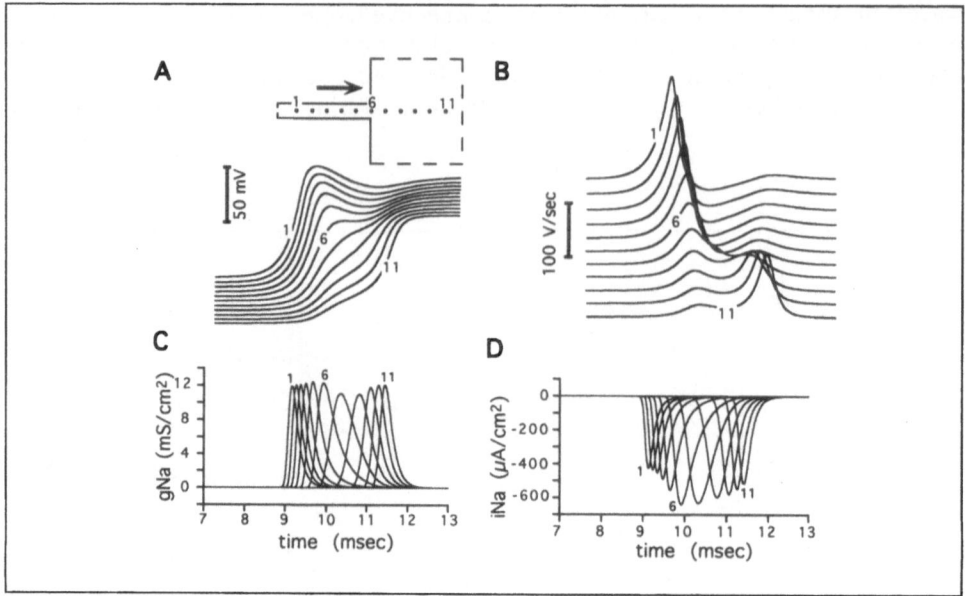

Fig. 9. Computer simulation of impulse conduction in a structure with abrupt expansion. Transmembrane action potentials V (Panel A), first time derivative of action potential dV/dt (Panel B), sodium conductance gNa (Panel C), and sodium current iNa (Panel D) calculated during impulse propagation from a narrow strand into a large area are shown. Time was measured from the onset of stimulus. The geometrical structure is indicated on the inset of Panel A (analogue geometry to Figs. 7A and 8). The 11 recording points were 30 μm apart. The arrow indicates the direction of propagation. The strand width was 120 μm. The strand length was 3 mm (only a short strand portion is shown). The length and the width of the large area were 3 mm and 2 mm correspondingly. Note that there is an increase in the maximum sodium current at the tissue expansion, demonstrating a feedback effect of tissue geometry on activation of local ionic currents. Reproduced from ref. (28) with permission.

longitudinal direction in such tissue. Especially, it was emphasized that such structural remodeling appears in human hearts with age (30). Comparing discontinuities at a relatively large level (obstacles introduced by connective tissue separating whole cell bundles or carrying blood vessels) with the discontinuities due to the discrete gap junction distribution, one might argue that the larger the discontinuity the larger the susceptibility of occurrence of conduction block in a stage of depressed excitability. However, the situation is likely to be far more complex because of interaction between the macroscopic tissue geometry, gap junctional coupling and activation of ionic membrane currents.

Interaction between macroscopic and cellular alterations

Experimental data and computer simulations suggest mutual and complex interactions between the discontinuities at smaller (cellular) and larger (connective tissue, vasculature) scales. An example of the effect of an abrupt tissue expansion on the activation of membrane currents is shown in Fig. 9. This figure depicts the simulated time-course of the fast Na^+ inward current, I_{Na}^+, at consecutive locations along an abrupt tissue expansion (28). As can be seen, there is a significant increase of I_{Na}^+ at the sites where the conduction delay is maximal. The increase in depolarizing current contributes to maintenance of conduction at the expansion and to prevention of conduction block. It is explained by the slower rate of depolarization at the expansion with respect to steady-state conduction which allows the Na^+ channels enough time to fully activate. Inversely, partial inhibition of the fast Na^+ inward current (e.g., by pharmacological blockade) is expected to increase the probability for the occurrence of conduction block at a tissue expansion. Therefore not only primary changes in ionic current flow at the level of the cell membranes will determine conduction or block at a site of a change in macroscopical tissue architecture, but the macroscopical tissue architecture itself will have a feedback interaction on the activation of ionic membrane channels.

In addition to interaction between macroscopical tissue architecture and activation of ionic membrane channels, similar interactions can be postulated with gap junctional coupling. In Fig. 10, a simulated geometrical expansion contains a network of excitable elements in which both the resistive interconnections and the membrane ionic currents can be modified. These modifications do affect the minimal width of the street, h_c, at which conduction block occurs. If the values of the resistors between

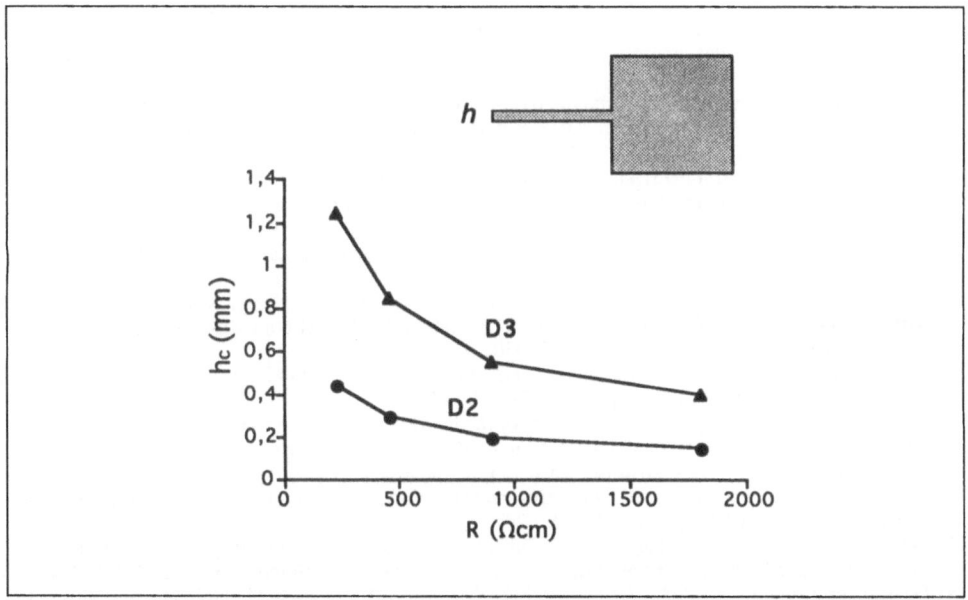

Fig. 10. Dependence of critical strand width, h_c, on intracellular resistivity R. **Inset:** Schematic illustration of an abrupt tissue expansion. A small strand of width h emerges into a large area. If h decreases unidirectional conduction block occurs at the critical width h_c. **Graph:** The critical width, h_c, is plotted as a function of the intracellular resistivity R given in Ωcm for a two-dimensional expansion (D2) and a three-dimensional expansion (D3). This simulation demonstrates that an event at a molecular level (cellular uncoupling) can modulate the effect of macroscopical tissue geometry to produce conduction block at the critical width h_c. Reproduced from ref. (31) with permission.

the excitable elements (simulating a decrease in cell-to-cell coupling) are increased (within a certain range) the minimal width h_c decrease, i.e. propagation across the site of impedance-to-load mismatch gets safer and the probability for occurrence of conduction block lower (31). The safer propagation is explained by the higher resistances decreasing the amount of electrotonic current loss downstream of the abrupt geometrical tissue transition. It contrasts to steady-state propagation in tissue without a change in geometry where a decrease in cell-to-cell coupling is always associated with a decrease in velocity.

REFERENCES

1. Janse M, Wit A (1989) Electrophysiological mechanisms of ventricular arrrhythmias resulting from ischemia and infarction. Physiological Reviews 69: 1049–1169
2. Allessie MA, Bonke FIM, Schopman FJC (1977) Circus movement in rabbit atrial muscle as a mechanism of tachycardia. III. The "leading circle" concept: a new model of circus movement in cardiac tissue without the involvement of an anatomical obstacle. Circ Res 41: 9–18
3. January CT, Riddle JM (1989) Early afterdepolarizations: mechanism of induction and block. A role for L-type Ca2+ current. Circ Res 64: 977–990
4. Luo CH, Rudy Y (1994) A dynamic model of the cardiac ventricular action potential. II. afterdepolarizations, triggered activity, and potentiation. Circ Res 74: 1097–1113
5. Jalife J, Moe GK (1981) Excitation, conduction, and reflection of impulses in isolated bovine and canine cardiac Purkinje fibers. Circ Res 49: 233–247
6. Wit AL, Cranefield PF, Hoffman BF (1972) Slow conduction and reentry in the ventricular conducting system. II. Single and sustained circus movement in networks of canine and bovine Purkinje fibers. Circ Res 30: 11–22
7. Janse MJ, Van Capelle FJL, Freud GE, Durrer D (1971) Circus movement within the AV node as a basis for supraventricular tachycardia as shown by multiple microelectrode recording in the isolated rabbit heart. Circ Res 28: 403–414
8. Antzelevitch C, Bernstein MJ, Feldman HN, Moe GK (1983) Parsystole, reentry, and tachycardia: a canine preparation of cardiac arrhythmias occurring across inexcitable segments of tissue. Circulation 68: 1101–1115
9. Spach MS, Heidlage JF (1995) The stochastic nature of cardiac propagation at a microscopic level-electrical description of myocardial architecture and its application to conduction. Circ Res 76: 366–380
10. Leon LJ, Roberge FA (1991) Directional characteristics of action potential propagation in cardiac muscle. A model study. Circ Res 69: 378–395
11. Rohr S, Salzberg BM (1994) Multiple site optical recording of transmembrane voltage (MSORTV) in patterned growth heart cell cultures: assessing electrical behavior, with microsecond resolution, on a cellular and subcellular scale. Biophys J 67: 1301–1315
12. Fast VG, Kléber AG (1993) Microscopic conduction in cultured strands of neonatal rat heart cells measured with voltage-sensitive dyes. Circ Res 73: 914–925
13. Mines G (1913) On the dynamic equilibrium of the heart. J Physiol (London) 46: 349–383
14. Boyden P, Jeck C (1995) Ion channel function in disease. Cardiovasc Res 29: 312–318
15. Fast VG, Pertsov AM (1990) Drift of a vortex in the myocardium. Biophysics 35: 489–494
16. Spach MS, Josephson ME (1994) Initiating reentry: The role of nonuniform anisotropy in small circuits. J Cardiovasc Electrophysiol 5: 182–209
17. Dillon SM, Allessie MA, Ursell PC, Wit AL (1988) Influences of anisotropic tissue structure on reentrant circuits in the epicardial border zone of subacute canine infarcts. Circ Res 63: 182–206
18. De Bakker JMT, Van Capelle FJL, Janse MJ, Tasseron S, Vermeulen JT, Dejonge N, Lahpor JR (1993) Slow conduction in the infarcted human heart – zigzag course of activation. Circulation 88: 915–926
19. De Bakker JMT, Van Capelle FJL, Janse MJ, Vanhemel NM, Hauer RNW, Defauw JJAM, Vermeulen FEE, Dewekker PFAB (1991) Macroreentry in the infarcted human heart – the mechanism of ventricular tachycardias with a focal activation pattern. J Am Coll Cardiol 18: 1005–1014
20. Rohr S, Schölly DM, Kleber AG (1991) Patterned growth of neonatal rat heart cells in culture. Morphological and electrophysiological characterization. Circ Res 68: 114–130

21. Delmar M, Michaels DC, Johnson T, Jalife J (1987) Effects of increasing intercellular resistance on transverse and longitudinal propagation in sheep epicardial muscle. Circ Res 60: 780–785
22. Kadish AH, Spear JF, Levine JH, Moore EN (1986) The effects of procainamide on conduction in anisotropic canine ventricular myocardium. Circulation 74: 616–625
23. Tsuboi N, Kodama I, Tayama J, Yamada K (1985) Anisotropic conduction properties of canine ventricular muscles. Jpn Circ J 49: 487–498
24. Spach MS, Miller WTI, Gezelowitz DB, Barr RC, Kootsey JM, Johnson EA (1981) The discontinuous nature of propagation in normal canine cardiac muscle. Evidence for recurrent discontinuities of intracellular resistance that affect the membrane currents. Circ Res 48: 39–54
25. Fast VG, Kleber AG (1994) Anisotropic conduction in monolayers of neonatal rat heart cells cultured on collagen substrate. Circ Res 75: 591–595
26. Fast VG, Kleber AG (1994) Conduction velocity and shape of action potential upstroke in a computer model of an anisotropic heart cell monolayer. Circulation 90: I-40
27. Sommer JR, Scherer B (1985) Geometry of cell and bundle appositions in cardiac muscle: light microscopy. Am J Physiol 248: H792–H803
28. Fast VG, Kleber AG (1995) Cardiac tissue geometry as a determinant of unidirectional conduction block: assessment of microscopic excitation spread by optical mapping in patterned cell cultures and in a computer model. Cardiovasc Res 29: 697–707
29. Cabo C, Pertsov AM, Baxter WT, Davidenko JM, Gray RA, Jalife J (1994) Wave-front curvature as a cause of slow conduction and block in isolated cardiac muscle. Circ Res 75: 1014–1028
30. Spach MS, Dolber PC (1986) Relating extracellular potentials and their derivatives to anisotropic propagation at a microscopic level in human cardiac muscle. Evidence for electrical uncoupling of side-to-side fiber connections with increasing age. Circ Res 58: 356–371
31. Fast VG, Kleber AG (1995) Block of impulse propagation at an abrupt tissue expansion: evaluation of the critical strand diameter in 2- and 3-dimensional computer models. Cardiovasc Res 30: 449–459

Authors' address:
Prof. Dr. André G. Kleber
Department of Physiology
University of Bern
Bühlplatz 5
3012 Bern, Switzerland

Subject Index

α-adrenoceptor 124
α-adrenoceptor stimulation 125, 131
α-CaM kinase II 49
α-tropomyosin (a-Tm) 105, 110, 114
acidic phospholipids 87
actin activated ATPase activity 110
actin filament sliding 110
actin-activated myosin ATPase 115
actin-cross-bridge reaction 106
action potentials 7
aequorin 123, 124, 126, 127, 128, 136
affinity of Troponin C for Ca²⁺ 124
alternative splicing 89, 90
angiotensin 124
angiotensin II 92, 98, 101
anisotropic conduction 186
ANP 101
antisense oligonucleotides 29, 68
arrhythmogenic potential 77
arrhythmogenic substrate 186
atrial myocytes 168, 172
atrial septal defect 152
autoradiogram 29

β-adrenergic stimulation 26, 56
β-adrenoceptor 124
β-adrenoceptor stimulation 123, 125, 131, 136, 137
β-MHC molecule 110
β-MHC gene 105
β-myosin heavy chain (β-MHC) 105, 108
β-Tm 115
binding state 108
butanedione-monoxime 125

c-AMP dependent protein kinase A (PKA)
  phosphorylation 162
Ca²⁺ affinity 46
Ca²⁺ ATPase 17, 18, 19, 20, 22, 23, 25, 26, 27, 28,
  31, 34, 35, 36, 39, 40, 41, 44, 46, 48, 49, 50, 56,
  116, 156, 159, 161, 163
Ca²⁺ ATPase isoforms 42
Ca²⁺ channel 49, 50
Ca²⁺ concentration 163
Ca²⁺ current 12, 171, 175
Ca²⁺ current density 142, 173, 175
Ca²⁺ entry 169
Ca²⁺ extrusion 11
Ca²⁺ handling 141
Ca²⁺ handling proteins 141
Ca²⁺ induced calcium release 143
Ca²⁺ influx 12
Ca²⁺ overload 77
Ca²⁺ pump 17, 152

Ca²⁺ pump rate 162
Ca²⁺ release 50, 168, 169
Ca²⁺ release channel 40, 48, 56
Ca²⁺ release channel (ryanodine receptor) 39
Ca²⁺ removal 4
Ca²⁺ sensitivity of the myofilaments 135
Ca²⁺ storage proteins (calsequestrin and calreticulin)
  141, 145
Ca²⁺ transients 123
Ca²⁺ transport 1
Ca²⁺ transport systems 9
Ca²⁺ uptake 19, 35, 46, 50, 146
Ca²⁺ uptake into the sarcoplasmic reticulum 175
Ca²⁺/calmodulin-dependent 63
Ca²⁺/calmodulin-dependent phosphorylation 43
Ca²⁺/calmodulin-dependent protein kinase (CaMK)
  39, 40, 41, 43, 44, 46, 48, 49, 50, 55, 56, 63, 152,
  161
Ca²⁺ᵢ handling 175
Ca²⁺ᵢ transients 5, 6, 7, 11, 12, 168, 171, 173, 174,
  176
caffeine 3, 4
caffeine contractures 4
calmidazolium 55, 61
calmodulin 40, 44, 48, 58, 85, 87, 88, 89
calmodulin binding domain 87
calpain 85, 87
calreticulin 145, 148
calsequestrin 145, 146, 148
CaMKII 58, 61
cAMP 56, 58, 61, 152, 163
cAMP-dependent protein kinase 40, 55, 56
carboxyeosin 9
cardiac arrhythmias 179
cardiac hypertrophy 1, 12
cardiac hypertrophy and failure 77
cardiac myocyte 1
cardiac sarcoplasmic reticulum 55, 57
cardiac troponin T (cTnT) 105, 110
cardiomyocytes 92
cardiomyopathy 105
caveolae 101
cell connection 183
cell culture 92
cell isolation 170
cell shortening 3
cell-to-cell conduction time 183
cell-to-cell connection 185
cell-to-cell coupling 179
cGMP-dependent protein kinase 55, 102
chimeras 20
chimeric constructs 88
clamp-pulse potential 172
coexpression system 20

computer simulations 179
conduction time 183
contractility 25, 35, 124
cooperative activation 106, 108
coronary artery disease 152
COS-1 cells 19
cross-bridge off-rate 159
cross-bridge reaction 116
cross-bridge states 108
cultured cells 186
current-to-load mismatch 186
cytoplasmic conduction 183

deletion mutants of TnT 111
developmental differences in cardiac Ca^{2+}
  handling 79
diacylglycerol 136
diastole 25
dihydropyridine 142
dihydropyridine binding 142
dilated or ischemic cardiomyopathy 80, 141, 152,
  168, 170
Drosophila melanogaster 114

electron density mapping 114
electrostatic interactions 18
embryonic development 79
endogenous peptides 124
endothelin 123, 124, 125, 131
endothelin-receptor 123
eosin (tetrabromofluorescein) 9
ET-receptor stimulation 136
exchanger isoforms 67
excitation-contraction coupling 123, 124, 152, 156

familial hypertrophic cardiomyopathy (FHC) 105,
  113, 114, 115, 116
ferret 1, 7, 8
ferret myocytes 9
fluorescein analogues 9
fluorescence 1
focal activity 179
force-frequency relation (FFR) 124, 125, 128, 134,
  137, 152, 156, 157, 163
forskolin 152, 156, 159, 163, 165
Frank-Starling law of the heart 124
Frank-Starling mechanism 123, 125, 127, 134,
  135, 136
fura-2 171

guinea-pig 3

heart failure 12, 80, 123, 141, 177
heart-rate inotropism 124
high-resolution mapping 179, 180
human myocytes 169
hypertrophy 98

impedance-to-load mismatch 186
in situ hybridization 27, 28
indo-1 3
inheritance 105
inotropic 123
inotropic mechanisms 133
insulin dependent diabetes mellitus 152
intra-cellular Ca^{2+} concentration 123
inwardly directed current 78
ionic currents 179
isometric force 128, 157
isoproterenol 33, 35, 56, 92, 98, 131, 133

KN-62 49

L-type Ca^{2+} channels 2, 68, 142
L-type Ca^{2+} current 168, 169, 175
length-dependent activation 135, 136
length-tension curves 28
lusitropic effects 123

macro-reentry 179
missense mutations 105
mitochondrial Ca^{2+} transport 5
mitochondrial Ca^{2+} uniporter 1, 2, 4, 7
mitochondrial Ca^{2+} uptake 3, 4, 8
mitral regurgitation 152
muscle strip preparations 123
mutagenesis system 20
myf5 92
myf6 92
myocardial contractility 124, 134
myocardial contraction 26
myocardial growth 89
myocytes 5, 7, 9, 11, 168, 172
myoD 92
myofibrillar ATPase activity 154
myofilament activation 105, 106, 114, 115
myogenic cells 97
myogenic differentiation 89, 90, 94, 97, 101
myogenin 92

Na^+ channels 68
Na^+-dependent Ca^{2+} uptake 78
Na^+/Ca^{2+} exchange 1, 2, 3, 4, 5, 7, 8, 9, 11, 12, 67,
  68, 156
Na^+/Ca^{2+} exchange current 12, 72
Na^+/Ca^{2+} exchange proteins 67, 71
Na^+/Ca^{2+} exchanger 12, 77, 78, 89, 137, 141, 148,
  177
Na^+/Ca^{2+} exchanger activity 77, 78
Na^+/Ca^{2+} exchanger expression 81
Na^+/Ca^{2+} exchanger isoforms 69
Na^+/H^+ exchanger 136
Na^+/K^+-ATPase 101
NCX1 67, 69, 70
NCX2 70
NCX3 70

neonatal rat cardiomyocytes 98
neonatal rat ventricular myocytes 12
newborn rats 77

optimum stimulation frequency 152
overload-induced hypertrophy 80
oxalate-supported Ca²⁺ uptake 78

patch-clamp 171
peptide PLB-24 62
pharmacological interventions 123
phenylephrine 92, 98, 131
phorbol esters 12
phospholamban (PLN) 17, 18, 19, 20, 22, 23, 25,
    26, 27, 28, 29, 30, 31, 33, 34, 35, 36, 39, 40, 41,
    43, 44, 48, 49, 50, 55, 56, 62, 116, 141, 145, 146,
    162
phospholamban knock-out 25, 28, 33, 35
phospholamban knock-out mice 26
phospholamban over-expression 35
phosphoprotein 25
phosphorylation 17, 26, 40, 44, 48, 49, 50, 55, 57,
    62, 63
PKG 63
plasma membrane Ca-pump (PMCA) 85
PLB-24 55, 56, 57, 58
PMCA 90, 99, 100, 101, 102
PMCA splicing variants 94
poison peptides 114
polymerase chain reaction 27
post-rest behavior 124, 125, 128
post-rest modulation 134
potocytosis 101
pressure overload-induced hypertrophy 77
propranolol 131
protein kinase A (PKA) 17, 50, 58, 63, 87, 152
protein kinase C 12, 87, 136
protein phosphatase 49

rabbit 1, 4, 5, 7, 8, 9, 11
rabbit myocytes 68
rapid cooling contractures 3
rat 1, 5, 11
rat cardiac myocytes 68
rat myocytes 4
re-entry arrhythmias 179, 180
relaxation 1, 2, 3, 4, 8, 9, 11,12, 25, 26, 32, 39, 46,
    50, 152
relaxation phase 157
relaxation time constant 163
remodeling 179
responsiveness of the myofilaments for Ca²⁺ 133
rest decay 128
rest intervals 123
reverse Na-Ca exchange 70
ryanodine 168, 174
ryanodine 175
ryanodine receptor 51, 144, 148, 156

S1 region 108
sarcolemmal Ca²⁺ ATPase 1, 2, 3, 4, 5, 7, 9, 68, 89,
    91, 148, 177
sarcomere formation 108
sarcoplasmic reticulum 1, 2, 17, 56, 62, 168, 169,
    171
sarcoplasmic reticulum calcium pump and
    phospholamban 145
sarcoplasmic reticulum calcium release channel
    (ryanodine receptor) 141
SERCA 90
SERCA 1 19, 39, 42, 44, 49
SERCA2a 19, 152, 155
SERCA2b 19
SERCA3 19
shortening 1
SHR 89, 98
slowing of the cross-bridge cycle 116
SR Ca²⁺ content 12
SR Ca²⁺ release 69
SR Ca²⁺ uptake 5, 8, 56
SR Ca²⁺ ATPase 1, 2, 9, 12, 39, 43, 44, 48, 78, 80,
    137, 141, 145, 146, 148
SR Ca²⁺ ATPase expression 12
SR Ca²⁺-ATPase mRNA 12
SR Ca²⁺ pump 3, 6, 7
SR Ca²⁺ release channel (ryanodine receptor) 143
SR membranes 44
synthetic peptide (PLB-24) 56

tension-length relation 157
thapsigargin 5, 7
thick filament 108
thin filament protein mutations 110
TnC binding 113
TnT1 110
TnT2 110, 113
total cytoplasmic Ca²⁺ 9
transgenic mice 115
triggered activity 179
1,4,5-trisphosphate-receptor 101
tropomyosin 105, 106
troponin 45, 106
troponin C (TnC) 106, 114, 124
troponin I (TnI) 106, 113
troponin T (TnT) 105, 106, 110, 111, 112, 114
truncation 115

unidirectional conduction block 181

ventricular arrhythmias 179
ventricular hypertrophy 179
verapamil 12
voltage clamp 11

whole cell voltage clamp 3
whole cell recording techniques 171

XIP 68